Genetics and
Mental Retardation
Syndromes

D0965409

Genetics and Mental Retardation Syndromes

A New Look at Behavior and Interventions

by

Elisabeth M. Dykens, Ph.D.
University of California, Los Angeles

Robert M. Hodapp, Ph.D.
University of California, Los Angeles

and

Brenda M. Finucane, M.S.
Elwyn Training and Research Institute
Elwyn, Pennsylvania

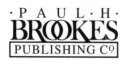

·P·A·U·L·H·
BROOKES
PUBLISHING C?

Baltimore · London · Toronto · Sydney

Paul H. Brookes Publishing Co.
Post Office Box 10624
Baltimore, Maryland 21285-0624

www.brookespublishing.com

Typeset by Integrated Publishing Solutions, Grand Rapids, Michigan.
Manufactured in the United States of America by
Versa Press, East Peoria, Illinois.

Any information about medical treatment contained herein is in no way
meant to substitute for a physician's advice or expert opinion; readers should
consult a medical practitioner if they are interested in more information.

Photographs courtesy of the authors and Elwyn Training and Research
Institute.

Library of Congress Cataloging-in-Publication Data

Dykens, Elisabeth M.
  Genetics and mental retardation syndromes : a new look at behavior and
interventions / by Elisabeth M. Dykens, Robert M. Hodapp, Brenda M.
Finucane.
     p.   cm.
  Includes bibliographical references and index.
  ISBN 1-55766-471-4
  1. Mental retardation—Genetic aspects.   2. Behavior genetics.   I. Hodapp,
Robert M.   II. Finucane, Brenda M.   III. Title.

RC570.2 .D95 2000
616.85'88042—dc21   00-040389

British Library Cataloging in Publication data are available from the British
Library.

Contents

About the Authors

Elisabeth M. Dykens, Ph.D., Associate Professor in Residence, Department of Psychiatry, Child and Adolescent Division, University of California, Los Angeles, California 90024

Dr. Dykens is a child clinical psychologist who has worked with individuals with many different disorders, both clinically and in research. She is particularly interested in the interconnections among genes, brain, and behavior—more specifically, in maladaptive behavior–psychopathology in individuals who have Prader-Willi syndrome, Williams syndrome, or other disorders. Co-author of *Behavior and Development in Fragile X Syndrome* (Sage Publications, 1994), Dr. Dykens has also published numerous studies on the behavior of people with mental retardation. She is a member of the scientific advisory boards of several national syndrome organizations, the steering committee of the National Institute of Child Health and Human Development, the Gatlinburg Society for Research and Theory in Mental Retardation, and the research and evaluation committee for Special Olympics International.

Robert M. Hodapp, Ph.D., Associate Professor, Graduate School of Education and Information Studies, University of California, Los Angeles, California 90095

Dr. Hodapp is a developmental psychologist who has examined how children with different mental retardation syndromes develop and interact with their families. A leading proponent of developmental approaches to children with disabilities, Dr. Hodapp's interests relate to the so-called "indirect effects" of genetic mental retardation disorders on others, intellectual strengths and weaknesses in Down syndrome, and the possibilities of etiology-based educational interventions. He is the author of *Development and Disabilities: Intellectual, Sensory, and Motor Impairments* (Cambridge University Press, 1998), and co-editor of the *Handbook of Mental Retardation and Development* (Cambridge University Press, 1998). Dr. Hodapp is also a member of the editorial boards of the *American Journal on Mental Retardation* and *Mental Retardation*.

Brenda M. Finucane, M.S., Director, Genetic Services, Elwyn Training and Research Institute, Elwyn, Pennsylvania 19063

Ms. Finucane is a genetics counselor who serves as Director of Genetic Services at Elwyn Training and Research Institute, one of the United

States' oldest multiservice agencies for people with mental retardation. She is the recipient of the 1994 Jane Engelberg Memorial Fellowship from the National Society of Genetics Counselors for her work with women with mental retardation; this work also resulted in her book, *Working with Women with Mental Retardation* (Elwyn Training and Research Institute, 1998). Ms. Finucane is also the author of *What's So Special about Genetics? A Guide for Special Educators* (Elwyn Training and Research Institute, 1996), and *Fragile X Syndrome: A Handbook for Families and Professionals* (National Fragile X Foundation, 1993) and the editor of several parent support group newsletters. She has thus led the way in promulgating etiology-based interventions to parents and educators.

Preface

Depending on one's perspective, this book appears too late, too early, or right on time. Those subscribing to the "too late" position would argue that the idea that specific genetic disorders differ in behavioral outcomes is several decades old. William Nyhan coined the term *behavioral phenotype* back in 1972, and the British-based Society for the Study of Behavioural Phenotypes is now more than a decade old. One could also argue that we have long known about the behavioral effects of several genetic disorders. The best example concerns Down syndrome. Since its identification in the 1860s, small groups in Britain and the United States have intensively studied many different aspects of cognition in Down syndrome, as well as language, adaptive and maladaptive behavior, and even family functioning and etiology-based interventions. Similarly, in recent years unresolved issues involving either behavior or genetics have spurred many behavioral studies on disorders such as fragile X syndrome, Prader-Willi syndrome, and Williams syndrome.

In contrast, others would argue that we simply do not yet know enough to devote an entire book to behavioral phenotypes—that our book comes too early in this field's history. "Too-early-ists" also marshall some interesting arguments. They note, for example, that studies of Down syndrome constitute almost half of the behavioral studies on all genetic mental retardation disorders combined, while most of the remaining 750 different genetic mental retardation syndromes do not feature even a single behavioral study. Even with a recent increase in etiology-based studies, little agreement exists about basic issues. Questions such as "What constitutes a behavioral phenotype?" and "What is the best way (or ways) to perform etiology-based research?" are either inadequately addressed or debated among those interested in etiology-based approaches. Even less well considered are questions of possible indirect effects and of etiology-based therapeutic, educational, or other interventions. Thus, some believe it is simply too early to summarize a field that seems so ill-defined.

Weighing both of these perspectives, our response is that this book is, indeed, well timed—occurring neither too early nor too late in the history of this field. To us, these conflicting facts imply only that the field is uneven and lacks coherence.

Acknowledging the field's variability, this book looks both backward and forward. Given this book's Janus-like sensibility, we made several decisions about content and structure as we were writing. In terms of content, we have chosen not to review the current behavioral knowledge of a large number of genetic syndromes. Udwin and Dennis (1995) have already done an excellent job with this difficult task; for most syndromes, we could add little to their efforts. Instead, we felt it better to spend most of our energies reviewing behavioral information about only those syndromes on which more specific, detailed behavioral studies already exist. Although our decision highlights problems in the field itself, we feel strongly that it is best to provide selective, rather than comprehensive, coverage.

We have also considered both the type and level of this book's content. Our sense in recent years has been that many social scientists and parents are attempting to understand the behavioral effects of genetic mental retardation syndromes. Our presentations are therefore aimed at nongenetically trained workers: those behavioral scientists, practitioners, and family members who desire to learn more about etiology-based behavioral findings and issues. To this aim, we have tried to keep material on the "new genetics" in Chapter 2 user-friendly and to provide relatively nontechnical explanations of various genetic etiologies throughout the book.

In summing up what is currently known, then, we provide up-to-date information on genetic and behavioral implications of four well-researched disorders: Down syndrome, Williams syndrome, fragile X syndrome, and Prader-Willi syndrome. For each syndrome, we first provide basic information about cause, prevalence, and physical and medical characteristics. More detailed information is then provided about cognitive, linguistic, adaptive and maladaptive behaviors, families, education, and interventions. We devote a single chapter apiece to each of these four disorders (Chapters 3–6). In another chapter (Chapter 7) we cover several other intriguing mental retardation syndromes on which less is known at present, though they will inevitably receive increased research attention in future years.

In addition to summarizing, however, we also envision this book as moving the field forward. In the book's first two chapters, we therefore discuss the basics of genetic mental retardation syndromes' direct and indirect effects (Chapter 1), as well as provide a nontechnical primer on the new genetics (Chapter 2). At the book's end (Chapter 8), we discuss a variety of research issues that we hope will lead to a more coherent and expanded body of knowledge on mental retardation syndromes and, subsequently, advances in interventions and services. Our hope is that this book will spur more and more behavioral workers to embark on etiology-based research.

Acknowledgments

In writing this book, we acknowledge the efforts of many people. We particularly thank Beth Rosner and Tran Ly for their help in pointing out infelicities of writing, collecting and checking references, and providing unfailingly cheerful assistance (usually with little or no notice). At Paul H. Brookes Publishing Company we thank Jessica Allan and January Layman-Wood as well as Leslie Eckard for her able copyediting. Much of our research and this book was supported, in part, by Grants #R0135684 and #P0103008 from the National Institute of Child Health and Human Development.

Many of our etiology-based ideas were sharpened by the wit and wisdom of our mentors, James Leckman, Ed Zigler, and Donald Cohen, and we owe them many thanks. We have also been blessed to work with many collaborators and students over the years: Suzanne Cassidy, Bryan King, Bhavik Shah, Joan Overhauser, Ann Smith, B.J. Goff, Kevin Walsh, Connie Kasari, Stephanny Freeman, Deborah Fidler, Cindy Wijma, Tran Ly, Beth Rosner, and Linda Masino. We also thank Elwyn Training and Research Institute for its unwavering support, especially Elliott Simon and Marv Rosen for their inspiration and encouragement.

A special thank you goes to the individuals and their families whose photographs are sprinkled throughout the book; each of these photos is indeed worth a thousand words. Many thanks as well to Stuart Williams for the use of his outstanding artwork, and to Special Olympics International for their photographs of athletes with Down and Williams syndromes. We are grateful as well to other organizations for their enthusiastic support of our research: the Prader-Willi Association (USA); the Prader-Willi California Foundation; the Prader-Willi Syndrome and Down Syndrome Clinics at the University of California, Los Angeles; the Prader-Willi Clinic at the University of Connecticut; the National Williams Syndrome Association; the Down Syndrome Association of Los Angeles; the 5p- Society; and PRISMS (Parents and Researchers Interested in Smith-Magenis Syndrome).

Finally, we remain very grateful to all of the families who have helped us in our research over the years. As two of us are new parents ourselves (and the third has been a parent for several years), we have a new appreciation for that special mixture of joys and trials that parenting brings. We appreciate, too, that different sense of time—where does it go?—that makes parents' participation in our studies even more special. We hope that, in some small measure, this book is worth all of their efforts.

To our children:
Daniel, Amy, & Alexander James Arthur

I

AN INTRODUCTION TO BEHAVIORAL AND GENETIC ISSUES

1

Toward Etiology-Based Work

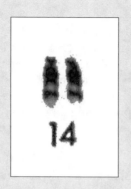

14

This book goes beyond mere description to advance a larger argument. Simply put, we argue that genetic disorders affect various aspects of behavior, from cognition and language to adaptive and maladaptive behaviors.

Over the past few decades, advances in human genetics have brought revolutionary changes to the mental retardation field. With new genetic causes of mental retardation discovered each year, more than 750 genetic mental retardation etiologies have now been identified (Opitz, 1996). And, given the success of the Human Genome Project, these rapid advances show no signs of slowing. Indeed, in the late 1990s geneticists estimated that the chemical structure of each of the 100,000 human genes would be known by the year 2003 (Goodman, 1998), leading to a better understanding of the connections between particular genes and specific human behaviors (i.e., "gene–behavior correlations"). These advances mark a new era in our understanding of and interventions for people who have mental retardation.

Looking back, it is startling to see how far we have come in so short a time. Until Watson and Crick's discoveries were reported in 1953, the world did not even know the basic structure of the human chromosome, how many chromosomes human beings posessed, or how genes operated. In 1959, Lejeune, Gautier, and Turpin discovered that most cases of Down syndrome are caused by an extra—or third—chromosome 21 (i.e., trisomy 21). A decade later Lubs (1969) first observed the pinched, "fragile" site of fragile X syndrome, and, over the past two decades, discoveries in fragile X syndrome, as well as in Prader-Willi syndrome and Angelman syndrome, led to new models of human disease. In short, these advances are promoting a new way of looking at a variety of human disorders and permanently changing the disability field as a result.

This book describes these remarkable genetic advances as they apply to behavioral issues within specific mental retardation syndromes. To promote understanding of the behavioral characteristics of several genetic mental retardation disorders, we provide in each chapter descriptions of causes, prevalence, and basic physical characteristics for each syndrome, along with more in-depth understandings of many different behavioral characteristics.

GENETICS AND BEHAVIOR: A CRITICAL LINK

This book goes beyond mere description to advance a larger argument. Simply put, we argue that genetic disorders affect various aspects of behavior, from cognition and language to adaptive and maladaptive behaviors. More indirectly, the behaviors often exhibited by people with a particular genetic disorder also influence how others react. In the first few decades of the new millennium genetic disorders will also increasingly influence the choice of which specific psychological, educational, or other therapies are most effective for individuals with a given syndrome. To us, then, genetic disorders matter in understanding the behaviors of people with mental retardation.

The assertion that "genetic disorders matter" is obvious to some researchers, anathema to others. Indeed, to professionals in many disciplines, our argument will seem so obvious that it is hardly worth stating. To these people, the importance of genetic etiology shows itself every day. In other disciplines, however, workers cringe at the idea of etiology-based research or intervention. To these individuals, our arguments concerning the importance of genetic etiology on behavior seem obviously wrong, at odds with major philosophies in the field, and heretical to good science or practice.

The assertion that "genetic disorders matter" is obvious to some researchers, anathema to others.

How, then, can we best reconcile such diametrically opposed views on the same topic? We first offer answers to several common criticisms of etiology-based approaches.

COMMON CRITICISMS OF ETIOLOGY-BASED APPROACHES

Common criticisms of etiology-based approaches typically fall into one or more of the following general categories.

"Syndromes Rarely Occur"

Many mental retardation workers dismiss genetic syndromes as unimportant because of the low prevalence estimates of such conditions. They note that disorders such as 5p- (cri-du-chat) syndrome occur in only 1 per 50,000 births, whereas Prader-Willi syndrome and Williams syndrome occur in about 1 per 15,000–20,000 births. Even Down syndrome, the most common genetic-chromosomal cause of mental retardation, occurs in only about 1 per 700 live births.

This view is consistent with the long-held belief that only 25% of people with mental retardation have known "organic" causes for their developmental delay. These pre-, peri-, or postnatal insults are thought to occur mostly among those with severe and profound mental retardation. The remainder of people with mental retardation, up to 75% (and supposedly almost all with mild mental retardation), are thought to have "nonspecific" or "cultural-familial" causes related to their syndromes (e.g., Drash, 1992; Zigler, 1967).

Population studies, however, have revealed a gradual shift in these percentages. As of 2000, genetic disorders probably account for about one third of all occurrences of mental retardation (Matalainen, Airaksinen, Mononen, Launiala, & Kaariainen, 1995). Furthermore, individuals with Down syndrome, fragile X syndrome, Prader-Willi syndrome, Williams syndrome, and other genetic etiologies compose from 10% to 50% of individuals with mild mental retardation (Rutter, Simonoff, & Plomin, 1996). At the very least, these percentages show that not all cases of mild mental retardation are nonspecific or "cultural-familial" in nature. These prevalence rates also do not include the many people whose mental retardation is caused by fetal alcohol syndrome, premature birth, and other "organic but not genetic" causes. Altogether, approximately 50% of people with mental retardation show some form of organic etiology (Matalainen et al., 1995; Zigler & Hodapp, 1986).

Although one can only estimate the percentages of people with genetic mental retardation syndromes, several points seem clear. First, with remarkable advances in molecular genetics, additional mental retardation syndromes are being discovered every year (Moser, 1992). The number of identified genetic conditions can be expected to increase in the years to come.

Second, improved genetic techniques now more accurately diagnose individuals with many of these syndromes. Whereas currently many individuals with certain genetic disorders were only diagnosed in the later childhood or adult years, diagnoses during infancy or early childhood should occur for increasing numbers of individuals over the next few decades. And, as more and more people are diagnosed with a more complete list of genetic disorders, such disorders will account for growing percentages of people with mental retardation. Workers critical of etiology-based approaches will find it increasingly difficult to disregard genetic syndromes as too rare to bother with.

"Syndromes Provide Only Unnecessary Labels"

People with mental retardation have historically been classified according to their level of cognitive and adaptive impairment—the distinction between mild, moderate, severe, or profound mental retardation found in most behavior studies in the field. Departing from traditional nomenclature, some workers no longer label the people with mental retardation themselves, preferring instead to label their needs for environmental supports (American Association on Mental Retardation, 1992). In this spirit, some fear that genetic diagnoses further stigmatize people already identified as having mental retardation (Goodman, 1990). To some, genetic diagnoses may even be seen as highlighting an immutable difference (i.e., one's chromosomes) relative to those without mental retardation.

In contrast, we argue that the behavioral effects of genetic disorders are not unchangeable and that diagnoses can help in intervention efforts. We note, for example, the effectiveness of many environmental interventions that are based on these diagnoses, such as the long-term use of a specialized diet to alleviate the genetically based disorder phenylketonuria (PKU). Children with PKU do not metabolize the amino acid phenylalanine. By following a specific, phenylalanine-free diet from infancy, however, the severe/profound mental retardation related to PKU can be circumvented, so only subtle cognitive and attention problems exist (Waisbren, Brown, de Sonneville, & Levy, 1994).

So, too, can other interventions partially alleviate the effects of many genetic mental retardation disorders. By utilizing characteristic behavioral profiles found in each syndrome, we can develop more targeted, fine-grained, and effective interventions. These interventions can be applied in many areas, including behavioral management, education, pharmacotherapy, psychotherapy, and even the transition from child to adult services. To the extent possible, examples are provided later in this book of syndrome-specific studies that guide treatment and shed new light on how and when to intervene.

"Syndromes Don't Matter for Inclusion or Other 'Practical' Concerns"

A related criticism of etiology-based approaches distinguishes between "basic" and "applied" issues within the mental retardation field. Several professionals thus suggest that phenotypic research, though it may describe basic aspects of behavioral functioning, is meaningless for more practical, applied concerns. In essence, these individuals argue that because the outcome (mental retardation) is more or less the same for everyone, why should subtle behavioral differences from one syndrome to another matter for education, group home placement, or supported employment?

However, as we are increasingly understanding, syndromes do matter for inclusion and other aspects of life for people with mental retardation. To cite only one example, parents of children with Prader-Willi syndrome versus with Down syndrome show many differences (as well as some similarities) in the educational services that they desire for their children. In general, parents of children with Prader-Willi syndrome desire more specialized services and services related to help in specific academic areas (e.g., arithmetic), whereas parents of children with Down syndrome desire placements that are more integrated with their child's age-mates or are in their own neighborhood school (Hodapp, Freeman, & Kasari, 1998). More ominously, the hyperphagia (i.e., excessive overeating) and food-seeking behavior associated with Prader-Willi syndrome make the complications of obesity the leading cause of death for people with this syndrome (Dykens & Cassidy, 1996). Thus, for schools, group homes, and other environments that serve one or more individuals with Prader-Willi syndrome, a tension exists between people's rights to self-determination and the need to stop them from literally eating themselves to death (Dykens, Goff, et al., 1997). In short, only by attending to etiology can one address these everyday, life-determining issues in people with mental retardation.

"People with Different Syndromes All Behave the Same"

The final criticism of etiology-based approaches is rooted in a long-standing belief that people with different etiologies behave similarly. Consider the following statements, spanning three decades:

- "Rarely have behavioral differences characterized different etiological groups" (Ellis, 1969, p. 561).

- "There is now considerable skepticism as to the usefulness of classifying mental retardation by form, due primarily to our current inability to separate biological and psychological forces" (MacMillan, 1982, p. 60).

- "Most special educators do not believe that etiology is pertinent to their function" (Kahn, 1988, p. 550).

- "Classification systems based on etiology or clinical types have little value in education" (Blackhurst & Birdine, 1993, p. 425).

- "In general, the focus of educational programs varies according to the degree of the student's retardation" (Hallahan & Kauffman, 1997, p. 138).

These statements, concerning both research and intervention, highlight the most commonly mentioned argument against etiology-based work. For decades, the prevailing sentiment has been that genetic etiology simply does not matter. This view is a well-established tradition in the field—a legacy inherited from researchers and clinicians working during a time when we understood much less about genetic disorders and their effects than we do today. Spurred by genetic advances, then, there is no better time to question this legacy, to better understand how, when, and why genetic syndromes make a difference in research and intervention. Yet, most traditions die hard, in part because they become woven into the very fabric of a much larger culture.

Spurred by genetic advances, then, there is no better time to question this legacy, to better understand how, when, and why genetic syndromes make a difference in research and intervention.

MENTAL RETARDATION'S TWO CULTURES OF BEHAVIORAL RESEARCH

In determining why some people dismiss genetic etiology while others consider it the cornerstone of their research, it appears that behavioral researchers in the mental retardation field can be divided into two separate cultures (Hodapp & Dykens, 1994). We borrow this two-cultures metaphor from C.P. Snow (1959/1993), a British chemist and novelist who in the late 1950s identified what he called the two cultures of science versus the humanities. In particular, Snow noted that workers in the sciences versus those in the humanities spoke their own technical languages that were mutually unintelligible. The two groups published in different journals, held different standards for training and excellence, and socialized in different circles. With his own firsthand knowledge of both cultures, Snow saw rich potential for cross-cultural collaborations and was troubled that neither group seemed to understand or respect the other.

On a smaller scale, we find two cultures in the field of mental retardation research as well. Unlike Snow's cultures, however, mental retardation's two cultures share a common interest in the behavior of people with mental retardation. One culture consists of researchers, primarily psychologists (of various types) and special educators, who conduct studies using mixed or heterogeneous groups of subjects. In this approach, people with any number of different syndromes or with unknown etiologies are grouped together. The resulting data are used to analyze subjects by IQ level, age, gender, living status, or other variables of interest. This mixed-group approach dominates most behavioral research in mental retardation.

Strengths and Weaknesses

The research conducted by this mixed-group culture possesses both strengths and weaknesses (see Table 1.1). On the positive side, these professionals are expert in measuring a wide range of behavior. This culture has therefore led the way in measuring key features of mental retardation, such as adaptive and maladaptive behavior, social competence, speech and language, cognition, achievement, quality of life, and family functioning. Yet, these same workers fail to appreciate that individuals with different genetic disorders may vary in their behaviors.

In contrast, researchers in the second culture examine the behavior of people with specific genetic diagnoses. These workers typically have a more biomedical orientation and include clinical and medical geneticists, genetic counselors, psychiatrists, and pediatricians. As experts in the chromosomal, the medical, and the physical intricacies of genetic syndromes, these individuals have led the way in applying new genetic techniques to people with mental retardation, ultimately identifying the genetic causes of old and new syndromes. Yet, these same researchers are often quite naïve about the complexities of measuring behavior.

Specifically, although geneticists and other etiology-based workers view behavior as important, they often describe it in superficial ways.

Table 1.1.   The two cultures of behavioral research in mental retardation

Culture of behavioral reseach	Main characteristics	Professions (with some overlap)	Strengths	Weaknesses
Mixed etiology	Group by degree of disability, age, or living status Less regard for genetic etiology	Behavioral psychologists Special educators Clinical psychologists Social workers	Advances in behavioral measurement	Often less aware of advances in genetics and molecular genetics Often less appreciation for impact of genetic etiology on research or intervention
Etiology	Group by etiology De-emphasize degree of disability	Geneticists Genetic counselors Child psychiatrists Pediatricians Psychiatrists	Advances in molecular genetics	Often less sophisticated in behavioral measurement Often less application of findings to pertinent issues in larger mental retardation field

To researchers in this culture, behavior is often cast as part of the "clinical features" or "natural history" of a particular syndrome, described along with the syndrome's salient physical, medical, and genetic characteristics. For example, behavior is typically summarized in terms of the percentage of subjects whom the examiner judges to be "overactive" or whose speech is characterized as "sing-songy." Researchers might also describe a participant's personality as "friendly" or his or her ataxic movements as "puppet-like." Such vague (even pejorative) behavioral descriptions persist despite the careful, well-established behavioral assessments developed by clinical psychologists, psycholinguists, personality psychologists, and physical therapists.

In several surveys, we have found that approximately 90% of empirical journal articles in the "mixed" culture—such as the *American Journal on Mental Retardation, Mental Retardation, Research in Developmental Disabilities,* and the *Journal of Intellectual Deficiency Research*—feature heterogeneous research groups. Conversely, more than 90% of behavioral mental retardation articles appearing in medically oriented journals such as the *American Journal of Medical Genetics, Journal of Child*

Psychology and Psychiatry, and *Journal of the American Academy of Child and Adolescent Psychiatry and Allied Disciplines,* are considered etiology based (Dykens, 1996a; Hodapp & Dykens, 1994).

Granted, several exceptions also exist to this general pattern. The *Journal of Intellectual Disability Research,* for example, features a higher percentage of etiology-based articles (about 30%; Hodapp & Dykens, 1994). Furthermore, there is a rich research tradition in the study of Down syndrome, with almost as many empirical articles having been published about Down syndrome as there have been for all of the other 750 genetic etiologies of mental retardation combined (Hodapp, 1996a).

Overall, though, the pattern still holds: Sophisticated behavioral research is generally performed by psychologists when they use mixed etiological groups, whereas biomedically oriented personnel perform etiology-based research that is generally less sophisticated behaviorally. Our point is not to assert that different disciplines publish in different journals but instead that professionals from the two different cultures need to join their respective strengths.

Yet, some joining of mental retardation research's two cultures may be underway. For example, in November 1995, more than 375 special educators attended the first-ever conference called "Genetics in the Classroom," sponsored by Elwyn Training and Research Institute; and the 1996 Gatlinburg conference sponsored by the National Institute of Child Health and Human Development (NICHD) was devoted to genetics and behavior. Similarly, NICHD's conference called "Cross-Disciplinary Collaboration" (1995) was partly focused on behavior in different genetic disorders. In addition, the British-based Scientific Society for the Study of Behavioural Phenotypes is now more than a decade old, and at least one book (O'Brien & Yule, 1995) and one special journal issue (Dykens, in press) have been devoted to behavioral issues in different genetic syndromes. We consider this book, *Genetics and Mental Retardation Syndromes: A New Look at Behavior and Interventions,* an additional effort to build bridges between the two cultures of behavioral research in mental retardation.

UNDERSTANDING BEHAVIORAL PHENOTYPES

As a first step in joining the two cultures of behavioral research, one must address these three questions:

1. How do genetic disorders operate?
2. What do we mean when we say that genetic disorders "matter" for research and intervention?

3. How, in fact, should one think about the effects of one versus another genetic disorder?

To answer these questions it is necessary to consider what are called *behavioral phenotypes*. The term, first introduced by William Nyhan (1972), is borrowed from biology and concerns the distinction between one's genetic makeup (*genotype*) and one's ultimate physical characteristics (*phenotype*). In this sense, however, the phenotypic outcome goes beyond such physical characteristics as height, facial features, or a predisposition to certain health problems (e.g., heart disease, strabismus); the phenotypic outcome also includes behavior. In short, a behavioral phenotype implies connections between one's genes and one's behavior, and that different genetic disorders might somehow influence individuals' behavior.

> *In short, a behavioral phenotype implies connections between one's genes and one's behavior, and that different genetic disorders might somehow influence individuals' behavior.*

Until this point, most etiologically oriented professionals would agree. But now the issue becomes what, exactly, is a behavioral phenotype? Two contrasting definitions have been proposed. In the first, Flynt and Yule argued that "a behavioral phenotype should consist of a distinctive behavior that occurs in almost every case of a genetic or chromosomal disorder, and rarely (if at all) in other conditions" (1994, p. 666). In contrast to this extremely strict definition, however, most etiologically oriented professionals adopt a more probabilistic view of behavioral phenotypes. That is, behavioral phenotypes involve "the heightened probability or likelihood that people with a given syndrome will exhibit certain behavioral and developmental sequelae relative to those without the syndrome" (Dykens, 1995c, p. 523). To better understand the implications of these conflicting definitions, the next section discusses in more depth the complex issues surrounding the connections between genetic disorders and behaviors.

Specificity of Behavioral Phenotypes: Three Views

At present, three views describe the connections between genetic disorders and behavior (Hodapp, 1997b).

No Specificity   The first view, traditionally held by mixed-group behavioral researchers, is that genetic disorders are nonspecific in their effects. Thus, if a child has Down syndrome, fragile X syndrome, or Prader-Willi syndrome, then that child has mental retardation, in much

Etiology   **Outcomes**

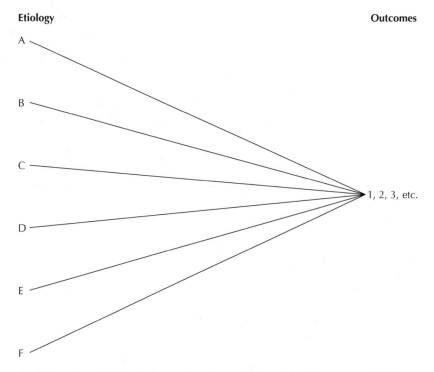

Figure 1.1.   Viewpoint 1: Syndromes produce nonspecific effects. (From Hodapp, R. M. [1997]. Direct and indirect behavioral effects of different genetic disorders of mental retardation. *American Journal on Mental Retardation, 102,* 70; reprinted by permission.)

the same way that any child has mental retardation. To quote Ellis again, "Rarely have behavioral differences characterized different etiological groups" (1969, p1. 561). According to this view, then, physical or other characteristics may differ, but behavior remains essentially the same regardless of what caused any person's mental retardation.

This *nonspecific* sense of behavioral phenotypes is shown in Figure 1.1. In this graph, different genetic disorders lead to the single outcome of mental retardation. This nonspecific view has traditionally characterized most work by psychologists, special educators, and other behavioral and social scientists in mental retardation. To this day, most of these researchers and practitioners find little value in studies or interventions based on the individual's type of mental retardation. And, at least on the most global level, a no-specificity view makes sense, for many different genetic and other causes of mental retardation all lead to lower intellectual and adaptive functioning. This "all roads lead to a single outcome" perspective also holds for all behaviors.

Total Specificity   In direct contrast to the nonspecificity perspective is the view that different genetic disorders have unique behavioral

Etiology **Outcomes**

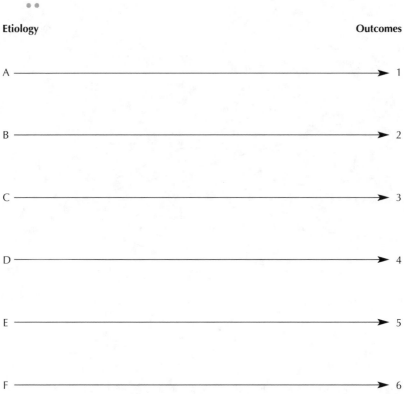

Figure 1.2.   Viewpoint 2: Syndromes produce totally specific effects. (From Hodapp, R. M. [1997]. Direct and indirect behavioral effects of different genetic disorders of mental retardation. *American Journal on Mental Retardation, 102,* 70; reprinted by permission.)

outcomes. Flynt and Yule best exemplified this view when they asserted that a behavioral phenotype "occurs . . . rarely (if at all) in other conditions" (1994, p. 666). This perspective might be described as one of *total specificity*. That is, a particular genetic disorder leads to a unique behavioral outcome. This view is illustrated in Figure 1.2, in which each genetic disorder leads to a behavior (or behaviors) not shared by other genetic disorders. In essence, one road leads to one (and only one) outcome, while another road leads to another.

One can identify several instances of total specificity. According to Nyhan's (1972) original writings, it appears that individuals with Lesch-Nyhan syndrome are unique in exhibiting extreme self-mutilation behaviors, which do not appear in any other syndrome to anywhere near this degree. Similarly, at present Prader-Willi syndrome is the only syndrome to show extreme hyperphagia and food ideation (Dykens & Cassidy, 1996), and other syndromes may also be unique in one or more of their characteristic behaviors. Although the "state of the art" in behav-

Table 1.2.   Genetic etiologies with possibly unique associated behaviors

Genetic syndrome	Behavior(s) possibly unique to a particular syndrome
Prader-Willi syndrome	Hyperhagia, food ideation
Lesch-Nyhan syndrome	Extreme self-injury
Down syndrome	Better visual versus auditory receptive abilities
Smith-Magenis syndrome	Putting objects into body orifices; bodily self-hugging
Williams syndrome	High-level language abilities in face of lower overall mental age and extremely poor visuospatial functioning
Rett syndrome	Stereotypic hand movements (described as "hand washing" or "hand wringing")
Angelman syndrome	Ataxic gait
Cri-du-chat syndrome	"Cat cry" during infancy

ioral research does not allow us to say with certainty exactly which syndrome's behaviors are or are not unique, Table 1.2 lists some possibly unique behaviors in several genetic mental retardation syndromes.

Partial Specificity   The third and final view might be called *partial specificity*. In partial specificity, a few different genetic disorders lead to a single outcome. This outcome is different from the "usual" findings in mixed samples of children who have mental retardation, but it is not unique to only one genetic disorder. Two or three genetic disorders might lead to a single outcome, even as most other types of mental retardation do not share that outcome. Figure 1.3 shows this partial specificity view graphically.

Although examples of total and partial specificity are sprinkled throughout this book, partial specificity is probably the most commonly occurring effect of genetic disorders of mental retardation (Hodapp, 1997b). Consider the pattern of intellectual strengths and weaknesses generally shown by individuals with Prader-Willi syndrome. On one IQ test, the Kaufman Assessment Battery for Children (K-ABC; Kaufman & Kaufman, 1983), intellectual abilities are divided up into *sequential processing* (involving serial, step-by-step processing), *simultaneous processing* (involving holistic, gestalt processing), and *achievement* (or knowledge of learned facts, reading, arithmetic, and so forth). Compared with their performances in simultaneous processing and in achievement, children with Prader-Willi syndrome show a pronounced weakness in sequential, or serial, processing (Dykens, Hodapp, Walsh, & Nash, 1992a). This weakness in sequential processing does not characterize

Etiology **Outcomes**

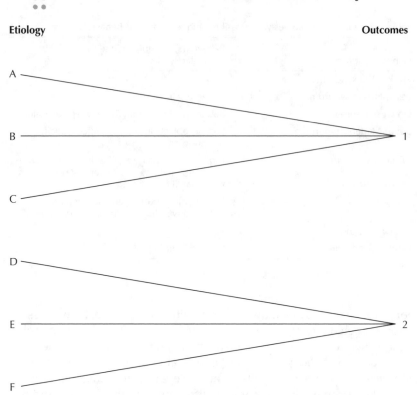

Figure 1.3. Viewpoint 3: Syndromes produce partially specific effects. (From Hodapp, R. M. [1997]. Direct and indirect behavioral effects of different genetic disorders of mental retardation. *American Journal on Mental Retardation, 102,* 70; reprinted by permission.)

other, "mixed" groups of people with mental retardation but is also found in boys with fragile X syndrome (Dykens, Hodapp, & Leckman, 1987; Kemper, Hagerman, & Altshul-Stark, 1988) and in individuals with Smith-Magenis syndrome (Dykens, Finucane, & Gayley, 1997). The sequential processing weakness is thus different from individuals with mental retardation in general, but it is not unique to only one genetic syndrome.

This discussion of behavioral phenotypes—and the differences between nonspecific, totally specific, and partially specific behavioral effects—is also more than an intellectual enterprise. As we note in subsequent chapters, instances of partial specificity might indicate that some shared pathways exist from genes to behavior, pathways that will become better understood as time goes on. Conversely, total specificity implies that, whatever the genetic anomaly, its effects seem unique. In these cases a single pathway probably exists from the genetic anomaly, to its biochemical effects, to brain structure, to behavior. Similarly, partial and total specificity also relate to shared versus unique intervention approaches, a topic that we also return to in later chapters.

Consistency

Total versus partial specificity relates to what might be called a "between-groups" question, the degree to which groups with one genetic syndrome differ behaviorally from groups with another syndrome. In contrast, other types of questions can also be asked, specifically those involving "within-group" issues. Within-group issues involve variations within a specific group from one person to another. One might examine, for instance, variations among different members of a particular social class, ethnic group, religion, place, or organization. All of these people, even though they may belong to the same group, are not identical—a fair amount of "within-group variation" occurs within any large group.

In this case, the question concerns whether everyone—or only some people—with a particular disorder shows that disorder's characteristic behavior. The question has been called one of consistency by Pennington, O'Connor, and Sudhalter (1991). As before, divergent definitions of behavioral phenotypes provide different views. Flynt and Yule thus emphasized "a distinctive behavior that occurs in almost every case of a genetic or chromosomal disorder" (1994, p. 666), whereas Dykens noted that behavioral phenotypes involve "the heightened probability or likelihood" that people with a given syndrome will exhibit certain behavior (1995c, p. 523).

Again, we favor the more probabilistic view, the idea that many—but not all—individuals with a specific genetic syndrome show that syndrome's "characteristic" behaviors. As we demonstrate in later chapters, rarely are genetic disorders totally determinative in their effects on behavior. Moreover, rarely do all group members show any one of a syndrome's characteristics—even those apart from behavior. Witness, for example, Pueschel's (1990) finding that only 57% of infants with Down syndrome display that syndrome's characteristic epicanthal folds around the eyes (although higher percentages of people who have Down syndrome may show them by later ages).

New Avenues for Research

Apart from the factual questions involving within-syndrome variability, such probabilistic views of behavioral phenotypes also open interesting avenues for research. Why, for example, does one person display behaviors characteristic of a syndrome, whereas another person with the same syndrome does not? Is there some slight genetic difference from one person to another? Has the environment in some ways prevented an existing predisposition from occurring? Whatever the ultimate explanation, the important point is that few—possibly no—genetic disorders lead to behaviors that are observed in every person with that disorder. Variability exists in even the most characteristic of a syndrome's behaviors, and *why* that variability exists is among the most interesting questions that face etiology-oriented researchers (Dykens, 1995c, 1999; Fidler & Hodapp, 1998).

Whatever the ultimate explanation, the important point is that few—possibly no—genetic disorders lead to behaviors that are observed in every person with that disorder.

OTHER ISSUES INVOLVING BEHAVIORAL PHENOTYPES

In addition to the basic definitional questions described above, other issues also arise when considering behavioral phenotypes. These questions relate to changes with age, variations across different behaviors, and indirect effects. Although these issues arise repeatedly throughout this book, we provide a brief introduction of each here.

Changes with Age

In discussing whether the behaviors associated with a particular genetic disorder are unique or shared, and whether these behaviors affect all or only some individuals, one might get the impression that behavioral phenotypes are static. That is, it might seem as though people exhibit behaviors characteristic of a particular syndrome similarly at every age.

But just as different individuals vary in the degree to which they exhibit a syndrome's characteristic behaviors, so, too, do behaviors change with age. Some behaviors become more prominent with a person's increasing chronological age, others less prominent. To take only one example, Prader-Willi syndrome has often been considered a "two-stage" disorder (Dykens & Cassidy, 1996). During the first few years of life, infants with Prader-Willi syndrome characteristically display failure to thrive: These infants have hypotonia during the early years, with decreased arousal, a weak cry, and poor reflexes, leading to a poor suck that causes feeding problems. Indeed, parents are often pleased when, around 2–4 years of age, feeding improves. Unfortunately, feeding improves too much, such that hyperphagia and food preoccupation begin. In effect, often the underweight infant and toddler who has difficulty feeding later becomes the hyperphagic and often morbidly overweight child and adult. Chronological age may matter when examining whether any etiology's behavioral characteristics are present, absent, or more versus less prominent.

Such changes in thinking are also in line with the relatively new field of developmental psychopathology (Cicchetti & Cohen, 1995). Following a developmental psychopathological approach, there is an interesting interplay between typical and atypical development. Thus, psychiatric disorders such as depression or oppositional defiant disorder may show themselves differently in children of various ages, or may have precursor behaviors that make it more likely that a child will have (or avoid) a certain condition. In mental retardation syndromes as well, characteristic behaviors change with age, may have particular precursors, and must be considered in light of the child's age and level of functioning (i.e., mental age; Hodapp & Zigler, 1995). These points, though seemingly obvious, are often overlooked.

Variations Across Different Behaviors

In examining Figures 1.1, 1.2, and 1.3, one might also get the impression that a particular genetic disorder differs on every behavior from one or all other disorders. Such does not appear to be the case. Instead, a particular genetic disorder may differ from other disorders on one specific aspect of behavior and be similar to all or some other disorders on others.

A good example again occurs in Prader-Willi syndrome. Prader-Willi syndrome seems unique in its hyperphagia and food ideation. To date, no other genetic disorder has been identified that displays these food-related behaviors. The characteristic weaknesses that these children show in sequential processing, however, seem shared with children who have Smith-Magenis syndrome and fragile X syndrome (and, possibly, some other genetic etiologies as well). Thus, Prader-Willi syndrome, a disorder that seems unique in one aspect of behavior (hyperphagia), is, at the same time, similar to some other genetic etiologies in terms of intellectual profiles.

Although we detail these issues more in later chapters, such "same and different" combinations may ultimately tell us much about gene–behavior relations and about the ways that different behavioral domains go together. For now, we note only that disorders differ in terms of some behaviors, but are similar on others.

Indirect Effects

A third complication involves indirect effects. So far, we have discussed only the direct effects of genetic disorders (Dykens, 1999). We have briefly noted how a genetic disorder predisposes individuals to specific intellectual strengths and weaknesses, particular maladaptive behaviors, and other areas that are presumably directly affected by the deletion, trisomy, or other genetic anomaly. But genetic disorders may also have indirect effects. Because people with Prader-Willi syndrome typically show hyperphagia and life-threatening obesity, or children with Down syndrome seldom show severe psychopathology, might not these behaviors influence members of the child's environment to respond in different ways?

This idea of indirect effects owes much to studies of both at-risk children and behavior genetics (Hodapp, 1999). In a 30-year study of at-risk children living on the Hawaiian island of Kauai, Werner (1993) noted that children who seemed resilient even in the face of difficult environments often showed attributes allowing them to elicit care from surrounding adults. For example, a child from a broken, abusive home might nonetheless fare well if he or she is friendly and outgoing, thereby eliciting substitute parenting from teachers, coaches, ministers, or others.

Similarly, the behavior geneticist Sandra Scarr (1993) noted that interactions between children and their environments can often be characterized as "evocative." That is, children often evoke specific responses from adults. Following Bell's (1968) model of adult–child interactions, children's different behaviors—possibly even their different physical or other characteristics—elicit specific behaviors from parents and others. To take only the most obvious examples, parents soothe crying infants and stimulate underactive ones, performing what Bell and Harper (1977) referred to as "upper- and lower-limit" controls. In essence, adults attempt to keep their children "within normal bounds" with reference to behavior, which presumably helps children themselves extract needed social and tangible resources from the environment.

Children with mental retardation may also elicit helpful environments, which may partially relate to etiologically specific characteristics. For example, children with Down syndrome demonstrate a basic interest in people, lower levels of psychopathology, and actual or perceived upbeat personalities; all may partially account for lower stress levels among their families (Hodapp, 1997b, 1999; see Chapter 3). Although the field scarcely understands genetic disorders' indirect effects, such effects seem worth considering. To appreciate fully the effects of genetic disorders on behavior, an understanding of both direct and indirect effects is important.

SOME FURTHER THOUGHTS

In presenting this brief introduction to genetic disorders and their effects, we acknowledge our own and the field's shortcomings. No one can simultaneously know everything about all aspects of behavior and about all aspects of what has been called "the new genetics." Having a fair grasp of even one culture is difficult, and for any one person to have total understanding of both cultures is probably impossible. In the same way, the field itself is limited in its understandings of the behavioral effects of most genetic disorders. Thus, although some 750 different genetic disorders have now been associated with mental retardation (Opitz, 1996), not a single behavioral study exists of the vast majority of them. Both personal and disciplinary limits to knowledge suggest caution, even humility.

HOW TO USE THIS BOOK

How, then, should one sum up behavioral effects of different genetic etiologies? We have chosen to divide this book into three sections. Section I, which is divided into two chapters, gives an overview of issues related to defining and measuring behavioral phenotypes and explains advances in the so-called "new genetics" that are relevant to syndromic diagnoses. These two chapters provide the conceptual background necessary for understanding the behavioral information provided later about each disorder.

Section II, consisting of Chapters 3 through 7, describes phenotypic data and intervention implications for the disorders themselves. But given that most disorders lack adequate behavioral information for anyone to attempt all but the most cursory of behavioral descriptions, we have chosen to focus on a small number of disorders (see Udwin & Dennis, 1995, for behavioral descriptions of other genetic disorders). We review, in one chapter apiece, those disorders on which a reasonable amount of behavioral data is available—Down syndrome, Williams syndrome, fragile X syndrome, and Prader-Willi syndrome. An additional chapter summarizes five other intriguing syndromes that have less behavioral research associated with them, but that nevertheless hold great promise for future phenotypic studies—velocardiofacial syndrome, Rubinstein-Taybi syndrome, Smith-Magenis syndrome, Angelman syndrome, and 5p- syndrome.

In reviewing behavioral research conducted on each syndrome, we follow a set structure. For each syndrome, we describe as much as is currently known about 1) basic genetics, prevalence, and physical phenotype; 2) cognitive and linguistic functioning; 3) adaptive and mal-adaptive functioning–psychopathology; and 4) implications for intervention (educational–vocational, therapeutic services, and family support). At times, the presentation of the information is uneven because more information exists in some syndromes (e.g., Down syndrome) than in others (e.g., 5p- syndrome).

Section III, consisting of a concluding chapter, points toward new directions. Here we highlight themes from across the syndromes and discuss the strengths and limits of etiology-based approaches for both research and intervention. We conclude by offering new research directions, including specific recommendations for the syndromic studies that we feel will increasingly characterize mental retardation behavioral work during the 21st century.

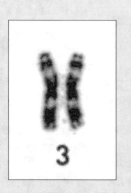

3

2

Applying the New Genetics

We now have the ironic situation of being able to jump right to the bottom line without reading the rest of the page... Since the degree of departure from our previous approaches and the potential of this procedure are so great, one will not be guilty of hyperbole in calling it "the New Genetics."

(David E. Comings, 1980)

Future historians will record the end of the 20th and the beginning of the 21st centuries as a time of tremendous growth and revelation in the field of human genetics. It is now clear that genetic factors play a fundamental role in human health and development, and genetic research continues to have a growing impact on nearly every medical specialty. Advances in our ability to analyze gene structure have led to a barrage of new diagnostic tests, as well as the tantalizing prospect of gene therapy for inherited diseases. When considering AIDS, cancer, Alzheimer's disease, and many other common conditions, our current knowledge is due in large part to recent technological advances in the study of genetics.

THE FOUNDATION FROM THE PAST

Although the genetic discoveries of the past three decades are unprecedented, human fascination with reproduction and heredity is centuries old. On the basis of early observations, ancient civilizations were able to selectively breed both animals and plants. The Hindu caste system is based on the flawed premise that children always inherit parents' traits and can never escape their genetic destiny. In contrast, in Medieval Europe, people believed in *spontaneous generation,* the idea that living organisms could spontaneously arise from nonliving matter.

Our current understanding of heredity, however, can be traced to the formal study of animal and plant genetics in the 19th century. In the 1860s, the Austrian monk Gregor Mendel demonstrated specific patterns governing the inheritance of physical traits in garden pea plants. Although his conclusions were widely ignored at the time, their rediscovery in the early 1900s marked the start of intense scientific and public interest in human genetics. By then, too, it was known that genes—the factors that determined physical traits—were inherited in mammals through structures called chromosomes contained in egg and sperm cells. Although chromosomes could be readily seen with a microscope, the genes they contained were abstractions to early scientists, who even as recently as the first half of the 20th century had little clue as to their structure and function.

Even for most of the modern history of the human genetics field, scientists have only been able to study genes indirectly, by analyzing the *consequences* of gene change. These scientists therefore documented patterns of physical and behavioral symptoms; these ultimately formed the basis of clinical syndromes. Early geneticists also recorded family histories (pedigrees), which offered clues as to the inheritance of certain traits, and looked for common biological threads among the symptoms of known syndromes to gain insights into mechanisms of gene action.

The New Genetics

Using these methods, traditional genetic approaches accurately identified and delineated hundreds of syndromes and conditions. For example, long before a specific genetic defect was found to cause Marfan syndrome, its symptoms of nearsightedness, tall and lanky body build, and cardiovascular problems all pointed toward an underlying abnormality in the body's connective tissue. Family history studies showed the specific inheritance pattern by which Marfan syndrome was passed down from one generation to the next, and much was known about its prognosis and variability. But it was only in 1991 that the Marfan gene mutation, which causes an abnormality in a connective tissue protein called *fibrillin,* was finally detected, adding a fundamental piece to the Marfan puzzle (Dietz et al., 1991). This ability to analyze genes directly at the *molecular* rather than merely at the *consequence* level, prompted

Dr. David Comings in 1980 to distinguish our era of research as the "New Genetics."

Though Comings coined this term much later, the new genetics actually grew out of discoveries made in the 1960s. These discoveries gave researchers the technological tools they needed to break the genetic code and to apply objective laboratory measures to the study of heredity. The new genetics, then, adds technological refinements to a surprisingly accurate foundation. To this day, departures from Mendel's laws remain the exception, while his theories of inheritance continue to hold up and form the backbone of genetic counseling. Decades-old descriptions of obscure clinical syndromes are receiving new interest in light of objective laboratory studies. Direct DNA (deoxyribonucleic acid) analysis is leading to a better understanding of disorders with unusual inheritance patterns and poorly defined clinical symptoms. And just as Mendel's original theories of inheritance had a profound impact on the understanding of mental retardation, so the new genetics is revolutionizing the way we classify, diagnose, and treat developmental disabilities.

> *The new genetics, then, adds technological refinements to a surprisingly accurate foundation.*

GENETIC CAUSES OF DEVELOPMENTAL DISABILITIES

Efforts to categorize and quantify the causes of mental retardation have met with as many methodological and philosophical debates as have attempts at definition. Current research acknowledges the important contribution of both genetic and environmental factors (Thapar, Gottesman, Owen, O'Donovan, & McGuffin, 1994), although the relative influence and malleability of each remain unclear.

Genetics and the Brain

Although the notion of an intelligence gene sometimes makes its way into the popular press, such a concept is extremely simplistic. Physiologically, many diverse factors affect brain development and functioning throughout the life span. Certain genes dictate the formation of brain structures during pre- and postnatal development; different genes are involved in the production of brain chemicals, such as neurotransmitters; still other genes drive the brain's regulatory processes, such as normal cell death associated with aging. Even those genes not directly involved in brain development can produce body chemicals that affect its functioning, such as the genes that regulate body hormones. Some genes are "turned on" all the time, whereas others have a time-limited function, such as those that play a brief but critical role in embryonic brain development.

Because of this complexity, myriad possible factors, without even counting the environmental ones, can result in abnormal brain functioning. Consider the following three examples: 1) One of the associated features of fragile X syndrome is an underdevelopment of the area of the brain known as the *cerebellar vermis;* 2) in Miller-Dieker syndrome, a specific missing section of chromosome 17 results in the failure of a growing embryo to develop the characteristic curves of the brain's surface; and 3) individuals with phenylketonuria (PKU) have an abnormal buildup of the body chemical phenylalanine, which damages their structurally normal brains. In just these few examples, we see how different genes on three different chromosomes result in mental retardation through entirely different mechanisms.

Even before the advent of new diagnostic technologies, the role of organic factors in the etiology of moderate to profound mental retardation was well recognized. Many genetic syndromes were first described decades ago among those institutionalized with severe disabilities. As such, these disorders became inexorably linked with a poor prognosis. Conversely, these syndromes were only looked for and diagnosed among people with severe disabilities. Because severe impairments account for less than 20% of all occurences of mental retardation, these early descriptions linking genetic disorders and severe impairments reinforced the notion that genetic syndromes played only a minor role in the overall causation of developmental disabilities. Recent technological advances, along with a renewed, if cautious, willingness by mental retardation professionals to reconsider etiology (see Chapter 1) have begun to challenge this long-standing assertion.

Most people with mental retardation have mild intellectual impairments resulting from a multitude of diverse causes, both congenital and acquired. Many have "nonpathological" functional deficits that may simply represent the lower end of the normal IQ distribution (so-called sociocultural–familial retardation). By definition, this common type of mental retardation includes both genetic and environmental components. Until recently, both genetic and environmental factors involved in this type of retardation remained murky, although with new genetic techniques it may be possible to identify numerous individual genes, each of which slightly affects one's intellectual abilities (Chorney et al., 1998). In any case, the prevalence rates of sociocultural–

familial mental retardation may not be anywhere near the 75% figure widely held from the late 1960s (Zigler, 1967). Instead, the actual prevalence of true sociocultural–familial mental retardation seems likely to be significantly lower, as people with even the mildest degrees of intellectual impairment are increasingly being diagnosed with specific genetic syndromes (Rutter, Simonoff, & Plomin, 1996). A majority of people with Prader-Willi, Williams, and Klinefelter syndromes, as well as people with many other genetic conditions, function within the mild range of mental retardation or higher, as do most females with fragile X syndrome, now known to be the most common inherited cause of mental retardation. Thus, the formerly clear-cut linking of "lower IQ–organic" and "higher IQ–environmental" retardation is no longer so straightforward.

Prevalence Studies

Institutional surveys provide some insight as to the numbers of people affected by genetic causes of developmental disabilities. A 1993 study of 400 institutionalized people with mental retardation in Kuwait revealed 50.75% had a "constitutional" disorder (i.e., a recognizable syndrome of primarily genetic origin; Farag et al., 1993). A similar Belgian survey of 158 institutionalized people in 1988 found 45.6% had constitutional disorders (Dereymaeker, Fryns, Haegeman, Deroover, & Van den Berghe, 1988).

However, results of institutional surveys can vary dramatically, even from one center to another. Institutional surveys also cannot claim to be representative of the majority of people with mental retardation who are mildly affected and not institutionalized. Although only a handful of studies have looked at the prevalence of genetic factors in people with mild mental retardation, the results are surprisingly similar to those just cited. In a Finnish population-based study in 1995, Matalainen, Airaksinen, Mononen, Launiala, & Kaarianen found prenatal, primarily genetic, etiologies in 41% of 151 people with mental retardation ranging from mild to severe. A survey of 91 Swedish school children with IQ scores between 50 and 70 found that constitutional syndromes and/or polygenic causes accounted for almost half of these disabilities (Hagberg & Kyllerman, 1983). Similarly, a 1988 British study concluded that 42% of 169 children with mild mental retardation had medical and genetic factors that directly contributed to their disabilities (Lamont & Dennis, 1988). Neither of these studies from the 1980s included fragile X testing and other recent DNA technologies developed after that time, which would have further increased the number of genetic diagnoses.

Much more work remains to document the genetic causes of developmental disabilities. Even now, however, few can argue against the fact that genetic factors play a significant role in the etiology of mental retardation at all IQ levels. With the current exponential growth in genetic information, it is possible that our understanding of the causes, treatment, and prevention of developmental disabilities will grow in tandem.

UNDERSTANDING BASIC GENETIC CONCEPTS

Although an in-depth understanding of the highly technical aspects of genetics is not necessary for the purposes of this book, an appreciation of basic concepts is helpful in orienting the nongeneticist.

Genes and Chromosomes

Inside the nucleus of most body cells, tiny, stick-like structures called *chromosomes* are visible with an ordinary light microscope. The chromosomes are composed of highly condensed coils of DNA, a chemical string that serves as the blueprint for how a body develops and functions, from conception until death. Genes are specific sections along this DNA string, much like closely spaced knots along a rope. Each chromosome represents a continuous double chain of DNA (the rope), containing hundreds to thousands of distinct genes (the knots).

Chromosomes, and the genes they contain, are found in pairs within the body's cells: One member of each chromosome pair is inherited from a person's mother and the other one from his or her father, at the time of conception. Specific chromosomes can be distinguished from one another based on their size and banding (stripe) patterns. Most people have 46 chromosomes (23 pairs). The first 22 pairs are called *autosomes* and are similar in both males and females. The chromosomes making up the 23rd pair are called the *sex chromosomes* because they determine a person's gender. In females, both sex chromosomes are alike and are called X chromosomes, while males have one X and one Y sex chromosome. (Figure 2.1 provides examples of karyotypes of a female and a male showing the differences in the sex chromosomes).

Each chromosome appears to have a "waist," a pinched-in section called the *centromere*, which allows the delineation of two subsections: The smaller area above the centromere is called the chromosome's *p* arm (so named for the French *petite*); the area below the centromere is known as the *q* arm (see Figure 2.2). Within these two subsections, specific regions, which correspond to the chromosome's visible bands (stripes), are identified using a numerical mapping system. For example, Prader-Willi syndrome is most often associated with a missing

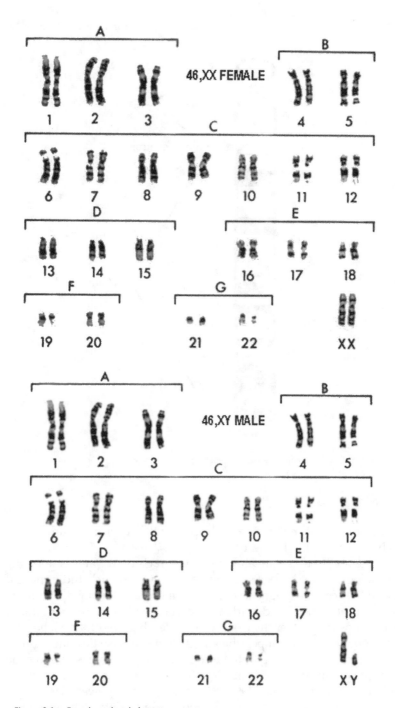

Figure 2.1.   Female and male karyotypes.

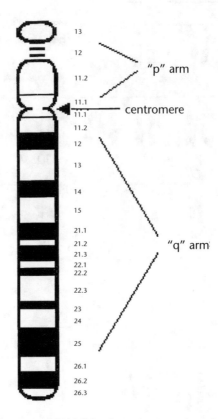

Figure 2.2. Idiogram of chromosome 15 identifying the centromere and p and q arms.

section of genetic material from the part of the "q" arm of chromosome 15 between bands q11 and q13.

The ability to isolate and view human chromosomes is not a new technology. Since the 1960s, chromosome (cytogenetic) studies have allowed the accurate diagnosis of Down syndrome, Klinefelter syndrome, and a number of other disorders associated with an abnormal number of chromosomes. Over the past two decades, high-resolution laboratory techniques have made it possible to visibly distinguish tiny subsegments of chromosomes, leading to the recognition of syndromes due to subtle gaps (deletions) or other visible differences in a person's chromosomal makeup (Punnett & Zakai, 1990). Still, even the most powerful techniques for viewing chromosomes are far too crude to detect changes at the DNA level.

From DNA to "Gene Product"

More than 100,000 genes, referred to in total as the *human genome,* are contained within the 22 autosomes and 2 sex chromosomes in humans. Two copies of each of these genes are packed into the paired chromosomes within the nucleus of each body cell. Although chromosomes are large enough to be seen using a microscope, the individual genes that form them are not, so visually studying a person's chromosomes can provide only a superficial glimpse of the human genome. The major impact of new genetic advances is the ability, using molecular techniques, to detect and analyze these submicroscopic genes and the DNA from which they are made.

The major impact of new genetic advances is the ability, using molecular techniques, to detect and analyze these submicroscopic genes and the DNA from which they are made.

Genes provide the blueprint for the production of proteins, the so-called "gene products" that drive the body's chemical reactions and serve as building blocks for its various structures. Genes are made of DNA, which in turn is composed of molecules known as *nucleotides.* Each nucleotide contains a component called a base, of which there are four variant forms, designated by the letters A, C, G, and T—for adenine (A), cytosine (C), guanine (G), and thymine (T). A gene is essentially a long double chain of nucleotides, arranged in a specific order that the cell can read, three "letters" (bases) at a time, in groups called triplets (e.g., AAG CGG TAG).

Each three-letter triplet, in turn, codes for a corresponding amino acid. Using the DNA triplet sequence as a template, the cell links together strings of amino acids to form proteins. For example, part of a gene sequence might read: AGT AAC GTG GGA. These four triplets correspond to the amino acids serine, leucine, histidine, and proline, which the cell can link together in exactly this order to form part of a specific protein. A different triplet sequence would necessarily result in a different protein. This basic pathway, from DNA to protein, provides the fundamental mechanism that allows genes to determine body structure and biochemistry. Through the inheritance of DNA, this code is preserved and human traits are passed down from one generation to the next.

Detecting Changes in the Genetic Code

Molecular diagnostic technology takes advantage of the fact that DNA is actually a double-stranded chemical string, made up of two parallel sequences of nucleotides, linked together much like the two sides of a zipper. As in a zipper, the two DNA strands are not identical but *complementary;* that is, they can only fit together if their nucleotide bases are matched in a certain way: Adenine (A) must always be paired on its corresponding strand with thymine (T), whereas guanine (G) pairs with cytosine (C). Thus, a triplet sequence of ATG CCG TAA on one of the two DNA strands would be paired to a complementary sequence of TAC GGC ATT on the other.

In the laboratory, a sample of DNA can be manipulated to force its two strands to come apart. The resulting single-stranded DNA can then be chopped up into billions of short snippets of DNA, using chemicals that cleave the strands at very specific points along the DNA sequence. Trying to find and analyze a single gene sequence among this vast pile of chopped DNA is akin to searching for a needle in a haystack or, more aptly, trying to locate the corresponding half of a particular zipper among a mountain of different zipper halves. Fortunately, scientists have developed techniques using molecular probes that allow them to hone in on the exact genes they wish to analyze.

A molecular probe is a short piece of DNA with a known sequence that can be reproduced (cloned) in the laboratory. Specific DNA probes are now available for hundreds of different genes, and can be used in the diagnosis of certain genetic disorders. A known DNA probe can be used to search for its complementary sequence among an unrelated sample of single-stranded DNA that is being analyzed. The laboratory probe will seek out and combine with its complementary DNA sequence if it finds it among the DNA pieces being studied. In order to distinguish the laboratory probe from the DNA under study, the probe is "labeled" by being tagged with radioactive or fluorescent chemicals that give off a detectable signal. By analyzing how or if a known molecular probe pairs with sequences in the sample DNA, one can determine if an abnormality exists in that particular gene.

The unraveling of the DNA code has ultimately led to powerful new diagnostic tools aimed at detecting the genetic changes that cause inherited disorders. Such tests can zero in on specific stretches of DNA and determine whether the sequence of nucleotides in a specific individual differs from the expected code. Some genetic disorders result from a change in just a single nucleotide base, while others are due to the absence or duplication of a long series of nucleotides. For most inherited disorders, the genes involved have not yet been determined, so direct DNA testing is not available. But each year, more and more genes for inherited conditions are discovered, allowing highly accurate detection of affected individuals and gene carriers.

Direct DNA Analysis

Once the specific genetic abnormality underlying an inherited condition is known, direct DNA analysis can definitively check for the presence of that gene change in DNA obtained from blood, amniotic fluid, or other body tissues. This type of analysis is not dependent on blood samples from multiple family members, nor does it necessarily require that the person tested have a family history of the disorder. Although a particular probe may be highly reliable for the specific gene change it is designed to detect, it may not pick up different changes that can result in the same disorder. For example, certain molecular probes for the elastin gene detect a specific abnormality in more than 95% of people with Williams syndrome (Ewart et al., 1993); in the remainder, the disorder may be due to a different mutation of the elastin gene, requiring other types of probes. Direct DNA analysis is currently available for many genetic conditions, including myotonic dystrophy, Huntington's disease, fragile X syndrome, and cystic fibrosis.

Linkage Analysis

Linkage analysis is a technique used in the diagnosis of disorders for which a specific gene change has not yet been identified. It is the genetic equivalent of circumstantial evidence, in that it relies on the analysis of DNA near—but not at—the suspected gene mutation. By comparing genetic variations between affected and unaffected relatives in the same family, linkage studies can sometimes allow researchers to track a gene's transmission without directly analyzing it. In some families, linkage analysis can provide accurate carrier and prenatal testing for certain genetic disorders. But because it requires DNA samples from both affected and unaffected family members, it is often costly, time-consuming, and impractical. In many cases, linkage studies eventually lead to the discovery of specific disease genes. For example, prior to 1991, many families underwent linkage analysis for fragile X syndrome; these studies ultimately led to the development of direct DNA testing for fragile X (Oberle et al., 1991), which has now made linkage analysis for this syndrome obsolete.

FISH

The laboratory techniques that allow one to view and analyze chromosomes are usually quite distinct from those employed by scientists studying genes at the molecular level. Recently, however, these two areas of study have begun to overlap. *Fluorescent in situ hybridization,* otherwise known as FISH, represents the interface between cytogenetic and molecular technologies. FISH is a diagnostic technique whereby a specific molecular probe, labeled with a bright fluorescent chemical tag, is added to a chromosome preparation. Not only does this allow one to see whether the probe finds its sequence-specific match at the molecular level, but it can also show the chromosomal location of that sequence.

A good example of how FISH works involves testing for Smith-Magenis syndrome. To test for Smith-Magenis, a FISH probe is used that contains part of the nucleotide sequence of chromosome 17p11.2 (i.e., at section 11.2 of the small arm of chromosome number 17) (Juyal et al., 1995). If a normal chromosome preparation is FISHed with this probe, two bright lights (signals) show up, one for each of the two intact number 17 chromosomes. In a person with Smith-Magenis syndrome, however, only one signal appears, because the second chromosome 17 is missing a section of DNA specific to that FISH probe. FISH is particularly useful in the diagnosis of this and other deletion syndromes associated with missing small (often, submicroscopic) sections of genetic material.

CATEGORIES OF HUMAN GENETIC DISORDERS

Most genetic conditions are caused by the disruption of just one gene (single-gene disorders), or by the combined effects of several genes acting in concert, with or without an environmental influence (polygenic or multifactorial disorders). Visible abnormalities of the chromosomes (cytogenetic disorders) constitute a small but yet important class of genetic conditions, which has particular relevance for the study of developmental disabilities.

Visible abnormalities of the chromosomes (cytogenetic disorders) constitute a small but yet important class of genetic conditions, which has particular relevance for the study of developmental disabilities.

Cytogenetic Syndromes

The visualization and study of human chromosomes is called *cytogenetics.* Because tens of thousands of genes are packaged into just 23 chromosome pairs, a visible abnormality involving a whole chromosome or even just a small section of one disrupts many different genes. In chromosome disorders, clinical symptoms are the consequences of either a lack or an excess of genes and their corresponding proteins. Cytogenetic syndromes almost invariably include mental retardation as a characteristic feature. Thus, although cytogenetic syndromes account for only a small fraction of all human genetic disorders, they represent a major cause of developmental disabilities. Between 15% and 20% of all mental retardation can be traced to a specific cytogenetic abnormality involving a difference in either the number or the structure of chromosomes (Matilainen et al., 1995).

Numerical Chromosomal Abnormalities

Numerical chromosomal abnormalities are those in which a person has either more or fewer than the usual number of chromosomes found in body cells.

   Trisomies   The term *trisomy* indicates the presence of a third copy of a chromosome (instead of just two), and may involve either an autosome or a sex chromosome. Because the inclusion of an extra chromosome into a fertilized cell at conception is usually an accidental occurrence, disorders due to chromosomal trisomies are generally one-time events that do not run in families. Although babies with trisomic chromosomal abnormalities can be born to women of any age, the chance of conceiving such a child increases as a woman gets older (see Table 2.1). Due to this increased risk of trisomies, pregnant women older than 34 are routinely asked to consider prenatal diagnostic procedures, such as amniocentesis and chorionic villus sampling (CVS). Such procedures allow analysis of fetal chromosomes to check for trisomies and other obvious visible abnormalities. It is important to note, however, that these tests do not rule out all, or even most, genetic disorders.

   The most common autosomal trisomy is Down syndrome, which occurs on average in approximately 1 in 700–1,000 births. The technical name for Down syndrome is trisomy 21, because most people with this condition possess an extra copy of chromosome number 21. (See Figure 2.3.) Less common are the disorders called trisomy 13 and trisomy 18. In contrast to Down syndrome, these two disorders have a poorer prognosis, often resulting in severe disability and early death related to congenital malformations.

   Trisomies involving either of the sex chromosomes (as opposed to the autosomal chromosomes) generally result in milder disabilities and a more variable picture. A boy born with an extra X sex chromosome (having two Xs and one Y, or XXY) is said to have Klinefelter syndrome. In addition to hormonal imbalances and infertility, males with Klinefelter syndrome typically have learning difficulties, with verbal skills disproportionately affected as compared with nonverbal abilities. A different condition, known as XYY syndrome, occurs when a boy is

Table 2.1. Incidence of chromosomal abnormalities, including Down syndrome, among infants born to mothers of various ages

Maternal age	Incidence of Down syndrome among liveborn infants	Incidence of all chromosomal abnormalities
21	1 in 1,500	1 in 500
27	1 in 1,000	1 in 450
33	1 in 600	1 in 300
34	1 in 450	1 in 250
35	1 in 400	1 in 200
36	1 in 300	1 in 150
37	1 in 220	1 in 125
38	1 in 175	1 in 100
39	1 in 140	1 in 80
40	1 in 100	1 in 60
41	1 in 80	1 in 50
42	1 in 60	1 in 40
43	1 in 50	1 in 30
44	1 in 40	1 in 25
45	1 in 30	1 in 20

Adapted from Schreinmachers, Cross, & Hook, 1982.

conceived with an extra Y sex chromosome. Boys and men with XYY are often completely asymptomatic but may have educational or behavioral differences related to their extra Y chromosome. Females with the so-called triple X syndrome (XXX) are conceived with a third X chromosome. Many women with triple X are diagnosed when they seek treatment for infertility in adulthood. Some have learning disabilities or mental retardation, but an unknown number may go through life undetected, without significant educational or medical difficulties.

   Monosomies   Just as any of the 23 pairs can have a third chromosome, so too can one have only one of a pair. *Monosomy,* or the absence of one of the two chromosomes in a pair, occurs far less frequently than trisomy. Monosomies involving the autosomes are exceedingly rare. However, Turner syndrome (XO), in which a child (always female) is conceived with only one X chromosome, is relatively common among live-born girls. Turner syndrome is also the most frequently identified chromosomal abnormality in miscarried pregnancies. In addition to short stature, infertility, and learning disabilities, females with Turner syndrome may have a variety of congenital malformations, including heart and kidney defects and webbing of the neck.

Structural Chromosomal Abnormalities

Structural chromosomal abnormalities are those in which there is a loss or gain of a portion of chromosomal material, or a difference in the expected arrangement of material on the chromosomes. A *deletion* is the loss of a segment of a chromosome, either from its tip (terminal deletion) or from within the body of the chromosome (interstitial deletion). The clinical signs and symptoms associated with a deletion depend on the exact piece deleted. For example, most people with cri-du-chat syndrome, so called because of the characteristic cat-like cry in affected infants, are missing a section of chromosome 5 between bands p14 and p15 (thus, the syndrome's other name, 5p- syndrome). Those individuals missing a section from the p11.2 band of chromosome 17 have a completely unrelated condition, with different physical and behavioral features, known as Smith-Magenis syndrome. Thus, as we describe later in this book, many physical and behavioral differences exist even from one deletion syndrome to another.

Deletions   In recent years, many different syndromes caused by chromosomal deletions have been identified. These have come to be known as *contiguous gene deletion syndromes* because the deleted segment involves several different genes lying contiguously (next to each other) along the chromosome. By studying the different genes that are deleted in contiguous gene syndromes, researchers hope to better understand specific clinical symptoms and treatment strategies.

Technically, cytogenetic deletion disorders are those in which a chromosomal deletion is microscopically visible. However, several conditions can often be seen using high-powered microscopes, but not in every case. Thus, many syndromes that were originally associated with cytogenetic deletions are now also being diagnosed at the molecular level in subsets of affected individuals who have normal-appearing chromosomes. Using FISH, molecular probes that encompass short stretches of DNA can be used to detect *microdeletions*, which are invisible at the microscopic level. For example, a deletion of chromosome 15q (i.e., the long arm of chromosome 15) can be visibly detected in approximately 65% of all individuals with Prader-Willi syndrome. But in an additional 10% of people with this syndrome the chromosomes appear normal; a smaller deletion within the same 15q area can be detected only by using molecular probes (Mascari et al., 1992). Likewise, Angelman, Smith-Magenis, and a few other genetic syndromes can be associated with either a specific, visible chromosome deletion or a smaller, "invisible" microdeletion at the same site.

Translocations   In addition to deletions, another important structural chromosome abnormality involves *translocations*. In a translocation, a section of one chromosome is rearranged so that it becomes attached to a different chromosome. Thus, a part of chromosome 11 might "switch" with a part of chromosome 22. Some of these rearrangements do not result in any net loss or gain of genetic material within the cell, as when two chromosomes simply trade parts or become attached to each other. Such rearrangements do not usually cause any symptoms, and are known as *balanced* translocations.

Balanced translocations in asymptomatic parents can lead to different consequences in their offspring. Because of the way chromosomes divide during the process of egg and sperm formation, balanced translocation carriers are at risk for conceiving children with *unbalanced* translocations. In this type of translocation, there is a loss or gain of genetic material. Many fetuses conceived with unbalanced translocations are miscarried, but those who come to term may have a variety of developmental and physical differences, depending on which chromosomes are involved in the translocation. As such, often a person first learns that he or she is a balanced translocation carrier after having a child with an unbalanced form of the translocation or after a series of unexplained pregnancy losses.

For example, a person may unknowingly have a balanced translocation whereby his or her two number 21 chromosomes are attached to each other at the "p" (or short) arms. The person has no symptoms as there is no missing or extra genetic material. But every time that person conceives, the child will inherit both 21s (because they are joined together), in addition to a free 21 from his or her other parent. All their children will effectively have three number 21 chromosomes, giving them Down syndrome. Clinically, children with this rare, 21-21 translocation type of Down syndrome are no different from those who have the "usual" type of trisomy 21. There are, however, different genetic implications for their parents. Parents of children with trisomy 21 have a relatively low risk of recurrence in future pregnancies, whereas a balanced 21-21 translocation carrier faces a 100% recurrence risk.

Fortunately, most balanced translocations do not result in such a dramatically high risk for chromosomal abnormalities in the next generation. And many unbalanced translocations arise for the first time, accidentally, in an affected child whose parents are not carriers. But any person known to have a translocation or other unusual rearrangement of chromosomal material should have careful genetic family studies done to determine its origin.

Mosaicism   Chromosomal abnormalities usually begin in either the egg or sperm, which goes on to conceive an affected child. As a result, every one of the child's cells, having grown from that original fertilized egg, shows the same pattern of abnormality. Occasionally, however, a

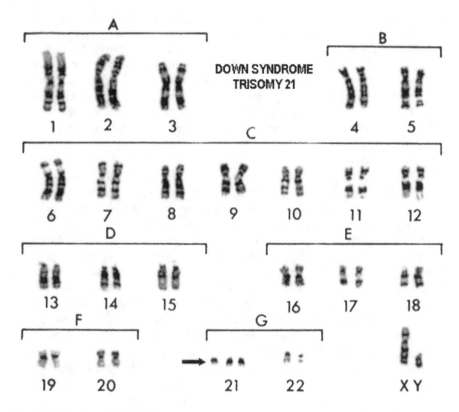

Figure 2.3. Karyotype of trisomy 21.

situation occurs such that not every one of the individual's cells shows the chromosomal abnormality. This pattern is referred to as a *mosaicism.*

In the development of a person with mosaicism, the baby is conceived with the normally expected chromosome pattern (i.e., 23 pairs of chromosomes). But somewhere during the very early process of embryonic cell division, a chromosome abnormality accidentally occurs in one of the dividing cells. Several different populations of body cells then develop. All of the subsequent cells growing from the one with the abnormality will themselves also have the abnormality. In contrast, the other cells (i.e., the ones without the abnormality) continue to produce cells with a typical chromosome number and arrangement. The child is then born with two different populations of body cells, some with a chromosome abnormality and some without.

An individual with mosaicism typically has at least one group of body cells with a normal chromosome pattern (although there are exceptions, particularly with the sex chromosome disorders). As such, a person with a mosaic type of chromosome abnormality is often less affected by the syndrome's disabling symptoms. For example, compared with children with "full" (nonmosaic) trisomy 21, groups of children with the rare mosaic form of Down syndrome tend to achieve higher levels of functioning and to have fewer physical differences (Fishler, Koch, & Donnell, 1976). Similarly, the vast majority of living children with trisomy 8 (an extra copy of the number 8 chromosome) have mosaicism (Riccardi, 1977); those conceived with the extra chromosome in all of their body cells are almost always miscarried or stillborn.

Despite this relatively milder course, however, a wide range of disability exists among people with chromosomal mosaicism. This variability is presumably due to variations in both the size and the location of the abnormal cell population. All other things being equal, individuals with larger percentages of abnormal cells are generally more affected. But the proportion of chromosomally normal versus abnormal cells in the same person can vary widely from one body tissue to another. Moreover, even if a person's blood analysis shows relatively few abnormal cells, his or her brain cells could potentially have a much higher percentage with a chromosome abnormality. Thus, for any individual infant or child with a mosaic chromosome abnormality, one cannot necessarily predict a better prognosis. Some people with mosaicism (affecting only some of their body's cells) are as affected as those who have the abnormality in every body cell.

Conditions Related to Parental Imprinting

Until recently, it was universally assumed that the effect of any given gene was the same regardless of whether it was on the chromosome (of each pair) that the person received from the mother or the father. Hence, any deletion or other genetic abnormality on any one chromosome of a chromosomal pair should cause the same problem. But in the late 1980s, researchers discovered a surprising contradiction to this basic law.

This exception was first discovered in two genetic mental retardation disorders, Prader-Willi syndrome and Angelman syndrome (Mascari et al., 1992). Prader-Willi syndrome is a condition characterized by mild intellectual impairment, severe infantile hypotonia (poor muscle tone), and an obsessive eating disorder (see Chapter 6). In contrast, Angelman syndrome is a clinically different condition in which individuals who have it exhibit severe to profound mental retardation; an unsteady gait; and frequent, unprovoked laughter (and no eating disorders).

Although the clinical characteristics of Prader-Willi and Angelman syndromes vary widely, new molecular techniques turned up a curious finding. Using techniques that allow one to determine the parental origin of genes and chromosomes, researchers discovered that, in people with Prader-Willi syndrome due to a deletion of chromosome 15q11–13, it was always the *paternal* copy of chromosome 15 that was deleted. Even more surprising, those born with a similar deletion in the *maternal* copy of chromosome 15 had symptoms of Angelman syndrome. Essentially, the same chromosome deletion caused a different clinical picture depending on whether it was passed down through a mother's egg or a father's sperm. It was concluded that certain genes in the chromosomal region 15q11–13 become chemically altered (imprinted) during the process of egg or sperm formation, so that they behave differently according to their parental imprint.

This finding soon led to a further revelation: In virtually all people with Prader-Willi syndrome for whom no deletion could be detected, studies showed that both of their copies of chromosome 15 had come from their mothers. Thus, these individuals had two chromosome 15s from their mothers and none from their fathers, as opposed to the usual situation in which one copy of each chromosome pair comes from a person's mother and the other from his or her father. Even though these individuals with Prader-Willi syndrome had chromosomes that were neither numerically nor structurally abnormal, they were affected by the syndrome because they did not inherit a paternally imprinted copy of number 15. Likewise, a small proportion of people with Angelman syndrome were shown to have inherited two intact paternal copies of chromosome 15, leaving them with no maternal contribution. In order for imprinted gene pairs to function properly, both a maternal and a paternal copy of the gene are required.

This phenomenon, in which a disorder results from unequal parental inheritance of chromosomes containing imprinted genes, is known as *uniparental disomy* (one parent, both chromosomes). So far, only a few specific genes in addition to those on chromosome 15q have been shown to be affected by parental imprinting. For most genes, their parental origin is inconsequential. However, the unexpected finding of uniparental disomy

However, the unexpected finding of uniparental disomy and imprinting effects in Prader-Willi and Angelman syndromes has opened up avenues of research that may ultimately yield new approaches to the diagnosis and treatment of many genetic disorders.

and imprinting effects in Prader-Willi and Angelman syndromes has opened up avenues of research that may ultimately yield new approaches to the diagnosis and treatment of many genetic disorders.

Single-Gene Disorders

Only a small percentage of genetic disorders are associated with the types of chromosomal abnormalities described in the previous section. Instead, most genetic conditions involve changes at the submicroscopic, molecular level. These disorders, then, cannot be seen under a microscope. They occur when one or both copies of a specific gene pair undergoes a change (mutation) that alters its function.

Some genetic disorders, such as neurofibromatosis (once referred to as "elephant man disease"), frequently arise as the result of new mutations. That is, the gene change occurs accidentally in a person with no prior family history of the condition. Other genetic disorders rarely or never result from new mutations, and all known cases of the disorder are familial. The genetic mutation that causes fragile X syndrome, for example, has been present in affected families for as many generations as researchers can test.

Today, most single-gene disorders are still diagnosed indirectly, based on a recognizable pattern of symptoms and family history findings. Most of what we know about single-gene disorders comes from the study of these indirect consequences of gene mutation. Abnormalities in single genes are not detectable by a visual chromosome study, although increasingly, molecular laboratory probes to directly analyze specific genes are becoming available for more and more syndromes.

Several different mechanisms underlie the thousands of known single-gene disorders and traits in humans. For example, the change of simply one nucleotide base, from an A to a T, in the genetic code for hemoglobin, causes a difference in its structure that is associated with sickle cell disease, a blood disorder common among people of African ancestry. In one form of Charcot-Marie-Tooth disease, a progressive neurological condition, a gene is duplicated, resulting in clinical symptoms due to the overproduction of its protein product (Lupski & Garcia, 1992). Williams syndrome, a well-described cause of developmental disabilities (see Chapter 4), is associated with a missing section of the genetic code for elastin, an important component of the body's connective tissue (Ewart et al., 1993).

Triplet Repeat Expansions   One recently discovered class of gene mutations involves the unstable expansion of specific triplet sequences within the genetic code. This phenomenon, known as *trinucleotide (triplet) repeat expansion*, was first identified in 1991 as the underlying cause of fragile X syndrome. Since the early 1990s, such triplet repeat expansions have been implicated in several other hereditary conditions, including Huntington's disease and myotonic dystrophy. In fragile X, the nucleotide triplet CGG, which is on the X chromosome and is usually repeated as many as 50 times in a row, is repeated hundreds of times. As a result, the normal gene is inactivated, resulting in the symptoms of the syndrome (Oberle et al., 1991). The presence or absence of symptoms in1 people with fragile X mutations is closely correlated with the number of repeats a person inherits. Current fragile X research aims to better understand this correlation as well as ways to prevent or reverse gene inactivation. Table 2.2 presents some of the chromosomal causes of developmental disabilities as well as their associated conditions and clinical features.

Table 2.2.   A few of the many chromosomal causes of developmental disabilities

Condition	Chromosomal basis	Associated clinical features
Down syndrome	Extra copy of chromosome 21	Upslanting eyes, underdeveloped midface, congenital heart defects, variable mental retardation
Klinefelter syndrome	Male with an extra X chromosome	Small testes, infertility, failure to develop secondary sex characteristics, learning disabilities
Turner syndrome	Female with a single X chromosome	Short stature, webbing of the neck, chromosome infertility, failure to develop secondary sex characteristics, learning disabilities
Trisomy 8 syndrome	Extra copy of chromosome 8, usually not in all cells	Deep creases on sole of foot, joint contractures, variable mental retardation
Inverted duplication 15	Extra chromosome having duplicated material from 15p and 15q	Poor muscle tone, seizures, autistic features, variable mental retardation
Cri-du-chat syndrome	Deletion 5p14–15	Cat-like cry in infancy, wide-spaced eyes, severe mental retardation typical
Smith-Magenis syndrome	Missing section of 17p11.2	Underdeveloped midface, prominent jaw, self-injurious behaviors, sleep disturbance, variable mental retardation
Prader-Willi syndrome	Missing section of paternal 15q11–13	Poor muscle tone, underdeveloped genitalia, obsessive eating disorder, mild mental retardation typical
Angelman syndrome	Missing section of maternal 15q11–13	Wide-based, awkward walking gait; seizures; frequent laughter/smiling; severe mental retardation typical
18q- syndrome	Missing section of 18q12	Underdeveloped midface, growth retardation, hearing impairment, behavior disorders, variable mental retardation

PATTERNS OF INHERITANCE

Regardless of the mechanism by which a chromosome abnormality or single-gene mutation first occurs, its presence in an individual has the potential of being transmitted to the next generation. Thus, there are families in which specific disorders, such as fragile X syndrome, can be traced back over many generations. However, some genetic conditions may never affect more than one member of a family if the person with the condition does not reproduce. Many of the contiguous gene syndromes, as well as genetic disorders such as Rett, Williams, and Down syndromes, are usually sporadic—that is, occurring only once in a family. They are clearly genetic, but because they arise for the first time in an affected individual who is not likely to reproduce, they begin and end as genetic disorders confined to that one person. Although it seems like a contradiction in terms, a condition can indeed be genetic but not necessarily familial.

As discussed previously, Mendel's original observations again form the basis for understanding human inheritance patterns. From intensive study of his pea plants, Mendel realized that inheritance works on the concept that genes come in pairs, one from each parent. A father's sperm cells and a mother's egg cells each contain only one copy of each chromosome, so that at conception, a baby's first cell contains two copies of each. For single-gene disorders, then, specific patterns of inheritance are apparent depending on the type of gene involved, and its location on either an autosome or a sex chromosome.

Autosomal Dominant Inheritance

In autosomal dominant inheritance, the presence of a mutation in just one of the two copies of a gene pair is enough to cause symptoms of the disorder. By definition, these dominant genes are found on the autosomes and not on the sex chromosomes. As a result, these disorders generally affect males and females equally. For dominant conditions that do not significantly impair a person's ability to reproduce, such as dominantly inherited adult-onset colon cancer, an affected person has a 50% chance of passing on the dominant gene each time he or she conceives a child. As such, autosomal dominant conditions often illustrate "vertical" transmission—that is, inheritance from parents to children over many generations of a family tree.

Sometimes, an autosomal dominant gene mutation accidentally occurs for the first time when a child is conceived. In such families, neither parent is affected and the disorder seems to arise "out of the blue." Although the parents' chance of having another child with the same new mutation is very low, the affected child will have a 50% chance of passing on the changed gene each time he or she conceives a child. In these cases, the dominant disorder arose for the first time in that one child but now has the potential to become familial in successive generations.

Autosomal dominant conditions are notoriously variable from one person to another. Even within the same family, a dominant gene may cause severe disability in one person but mild effects in another. For example, a child with tuberous sclerosis may have mental retardation, a seizure disorder, and benign tumors in various body organs. Although it may initially appear that the child's disorder resulted from a new mutation, one of his or her "unaffected" parents may be found to have mild characteristics, such as white skin spots, which confirm that the parent also has the tuberous sclerosis gene. For such a couple, the chance of having another child with tuberous sclerosis is 50%, as opposed to a very low risk for recurrence if neither parent had been affected.

Autosomal Recessive Inheritance

In contrast to dominant inheritance, in some genetic disorders if at least one gene in a pair is working properly, a change in the other copy will not cause any symptoms. Only when *both* copies in the pair are changed will a child be born with the disorder. Such gene mutations, which need to be present in both gene copies before having an effect, are known as autosomal recessive.

Typically, each parent of a child with an autosomal recessive disorder is an unaffected, "silent" carrier of one copy of the recessive gene. However, each time these parents conceive a child, there is a 25% chance that their child will inherit two copies (one from each parent) of the gene, and will be affected by the recessive condition. If only one of the two parents is a gene carrier, there is virtually no chance of their conceiving an affected child, although some of their offspring may be gene carriers like the carrier parent.

Autosomal recessive disorders typically show a "horizontal" inheritance pattern. That is, recurrences happen within one generation, but not from one generation to the next. Multiple siblings may be affected, but not their parents, their offspring, or other family members. The reason for this is simple: Although a single recessive gene may get passed on through many generations of a family, it will only show its effects when a gene carrier conceives a child with someone who also happens to carry the same exact recessive gene. But most recessive disorders are rare enough that the chance of encountering such a person outside one's own family is small.

Such transmission patterns also demonstrate why many societies have come to ban marriages among close relatives. Each of us, regardless of family history, is thought to silently carry five or more recessive genes that have the potential to cause genetic disorders in the next generation. But the chance of conceiving a child with a recessive disorder is low because most unrelated couples do not carry the exact same recessive genes. Conversely, because members of one's immediate or extended family share a similar genetic makeup, it becomes easier for two autosomal recessive genes to match up to cause a particular disorder. Thus, children conceived by parents who are related to each other are at higher than average risk for being affected by autosomal recessive disorders. And in certain cultures in which marriages between relatives are the norm or in which many people preferentially choose partners with the same inherited trait (e.g., a marriage between two people with deafness), recessive conditions occur more commonly than expected.

X-Linked Inheritance

Because they have only one X chromosome, males are susceptible to a number of genetic conditions that only rarely affect females. The genes for color blindness, Duchenne muscular dystrophy, and hemophilia are all X-linked recessive, that is, caused by recessive genes located on the X chromosome. As males have only one X chromosome, a recessive X-linked disorder cannot be "buffered" by the other X chromosome (as in females); X-linked recessive disorders, then, almost exclusively affect males.

The situation in females is slightly more complicated. A female who inherits a gene for an X-linked recessive disorder shows few or no symptoms. Even though one of her X chromosomes has a gene for the disorder, she has another X chromosome that in most cases is normally functioning. Thus, because the disorder is recessive, the woman herself remains unaffected. Such women are, however, at high risk for having affected sons. These sons, with only one X chromosome, would have no additional X chromosome (as would the woman's daughters) to buffer them from the disease gene's harmful effects.

X-linked genes play an important role in causing developmental disabilities, and they partly explain why many more males are affected by mental retardation than females. More than 70 different X-linked causes of developmental disabilities have now been identified; as a group, X-linked genes are thought to account for more than 25% of mental retardation in males (Glass, 1991). One example is Lesch-Nyhan syndrome, a rare X-linked recessive mental retardation syndrome whose hallmark behavioral feature is severe self-mutilation of the fingers and lips (see Chapter 7). Unaffected female carriers of the Lesch-Nyhan gene are at high risk for having affected sons. Another example is aqueductal stenosis, an X-linked form of hydrocephalus ("water on the brain") that is easily distinguishable through brain imaging (computed tomography/magnetic resonance imaging or MRI scan) from noninherited forms of hydrocephalus.

A few X-linked conditions are also thought to be caused by dominant genes, that is, genes that result in symptoms regardless of the presence of a second, functioning gene copy on the other X chromosome. In contrast to the disorders mentioned previously, X-linked dominant conditions appear to primarily affect females. Why females are more often affected than males is unclear, but it is theorized that males conceived with certain X-linked dominant disorders cannot develop and may be miscarried shortly after conception. But females, because of their second, normally functioning X chromosome, are spared the most severe consequences of these genes—they can survive. These girls are, however, born with or develop symptoms of the disorder. One such disorder is Rett syndrome, a neurodevelopmental disorder characterized by stereotypic hand-wringing movements and severe to profound mental retardation. Rett syndrome is virtually always diagnosed in females and is thought to be caused by an X-linked dominant gene that is lethal in the male offspring who inherit it (Moser & Naidu, 1986).

A final category of X-linkage shows neither a typical recessive nor dominant inheritance pattern. The best example here is fragile X syndrome (see Chapter 4). Although fragile X syndrome primarily affects males, it can result in significant disability among females as well. The syndrome is by far the most common X-linked cause of mental retardation, resulting from a newly discovered genetic mechanism involving trinucleotide repeat expansion. Few can disagree that the discovery of fragile X syndrome represents the most important genetic breakthrough of the past two decades in our search to understand the causes of mental retardation. See Table 2.3 for a listing of single-gene disorders and their inheritance patterns.

Multifactorial Inheritance

As its name implies, multifactorial inheritance depends on both genetic and nongenetic factors. In order for a multifactorial condition to occur, a number of different genes working in concert (polygenic) are necessary, as are nongenetic (environmental) influences. Such conditions often cluster in families, but with a less predictable pattern than seen in single-gene disorders. Several common medical conditions in adults, such as heart disease and diabetes, clearly result from a combination of familial and lifestyle factors that can vary from one person to the next.

Table 2.3. Some single-gene disorders and their inheritance patterns

Condition	Inheritance pattern	Asociated clinical features
Myotonic dystrophy (congenital form)	Autosomal dominant	Facial muscle weakness, cataracts, mental retardation
Neurofibromatosis	Autosomal dominant	Cafe-au-lait spots and benign nodules (neurofibromas) on skin, mental retardation
Tuberous sclerosis	Autosomal dominant	White spots/rough patches on skin, wart-like lesions over bridge of nose, brain calcifications, mental retardation
Smith-Lemli-Opitz syndrome	Autosomal recessive	Abnormal genitalia, webbing between the second and third toes, low blood cholesterol level, mental retardation
Phenylketonuria (PKU)	Autosomal recessive	Excess phenylalanine in blood and urine, early progressive neurologic impairment, seizures, mental retardation
Homocystinuria	Autosomal recessive	Dislocation of the eye lens; tall, lanky body build; vascular abnormalities; excess homocystine in blood and urine; mental retardation
Hunter syndrome	X-linked recessive	Buildup of mucopolysaccharide leads to progressive coarsening of physical features, neurological impairment, early death, primarily in males
Fragile X syndrome	Unusual X-linked pattern related to trinucleotide repeat expansion	Long, narrow face; large testes; autism-like features; mental retardation, primarily in males but can also affect females
Aicardi syndrome	X-linked dominant	Agenesis of the corpus callosum (absence of the brain structure that connects the brain's two hemispheres); eye abnormalities; mental retardation, primarily in females

Many psychiatric conditions, as well as alcoholism and other substance abuse disorders, are now considered to involve an underlying inherited predisposition triggered by significant environmental stressors.

Because multiple genes are involved in addition to variable non-genetic influences, the exact mechanism of multifactorial inheritance remains poorly understood. At this time, no definitive laboratory tests exist that can predict with certainty whether a person will develop a late-onset multifactorial disorder such as alcoholism. In many cases, however, knowing about an inherited tendency can allow a person to manipulate nongenetic influences. Thus, individuals with a family history of heart disease can pay special attention to their diet and exercise, as well as receive frequent medical checkups.

Several common birth defects often occur alone as multifactorial traits and tend to cluster within families. Most common among these defects are spina bifida, cleft lip, congenital heart problems, and club foot. These conditions may also be found along with other physical anomalies as part of single-gene or chromosomal syndromes. In addition, certain prenatal environmental exposures can result in an increased incidence of one or more of these birth defects, as in the high rate of congenital heart defects among babies with fetal alcohol syndrome.

This complex interaction between genetic and nongenetic factors is well illustrated by the example of spina bifida, a medical condition in which a baby's spine fails to close early in embryonic life. Certain families and ethnic groups, including people of Irish descent, display a higher than usual prevalence of spina bifida. But research shows that a woman who has had one child with spina bifida can substantially reduce her chance of having a second affected baby by taking supplements of folic acid (one of the B vitamins) before and during early pregnancy (Milunsky et al., 1989). Thus, a genetic predisposition to spina bifida can, in many cases, be averted due to an environmental manipulation (in this case, the mother's taking folic acid).

Implications for People with Mental Retardation

A significant proportion of mild mental retardation appears to be multifactorial, with an inherited tendency toward low IQ being compounded by environmental deprivation in early life. Again, recognizing and intervening to prevent environmental deprivation can significantly improve the developmental outcomes of these children. In fact, given the variability and complexity of the genetic factors involved, the most rational approach to effectively preventing multifactorial mental retardation is to place a strong emphasis on environmental interventions.

A significant proportion of mild mental retardation appears to be multifactorial, with an inherited tendency toward low IQ being compounded by environmental deprivation in early life.

GENETICS AS A MEDICAL SUBSPECIALTY

Over the past two decades, genetics has expanded out of the research laboratory and well into the mainstream of American medicine, where it has immediate benefits for affected individuals and their families. As never before, in diseases ranging from AIDS, to diabetes, to rare metabolic syndromes, our understanding of genetics is guiding rational approaches to treatment and prevention. Such practical, everyday medical benefits are being seen throughout the nation. Clinical genetics centers exist in every state, generally affiliated with major university medical centers. Many centers also support satellite clinics to serve families in more remote areas.

Despite a lingering perception of genetics as a research-based subspecialty, genetic services now constitute standard medical practice and encompass a variety of services including genetic counseling, evaluation, and diagnosis, described in the next section. In recent years, most genetic and metabolic laboratory tests are no longer considered experimental, and physician and genetic counseling fees are paid for by most insurance plans, including managed care and state Medicaid programs.

Genetic Counseling

Genetic counseling is a process whereby families concerned about genetic conditions receive understandable information and nonjudgmental support. Such information and support allows families to make informed reproductive decisions and to maximize the health and functioning of affected family members.

Families concerned with developmental disabilities seek genetic evaluation and counseling for many different reasons. A child with a developmental delay may be referred in order to identify a specific cause that could help determine the child's prognosis. Expectant couples with a family history of mental retardation may be interested primarily in learning about reproductive risks and prenatal diagnoses. An adult with mental retardation could be evaluated for the possibility of a genetic syndrome that might explain a pattern of challenging behaviors. The caregivers of a person with a genetic diagnosis may seek practical information about medical and educational recommendations for this specific syndrome. All of these are valid reasons to see a genetic counselor; each also underscores the wide scope of purposes served by a genetic evaluation.

In the United States, several different professionals—with somewhat different training—can be involved in the process of genetic counseling. Most genetic counselors have a master's degree in human genetics or genetic counseling. Some master's-level counselors are called genetic associates. The term geneticist usually refers to physicians or doctoral-level scientists who make clinical and laboratory diagnoses, and who are also involved in the genetic-counseling process.

Genetic counselors typically serve as the main contact with individuals and families regarding the findings of their genetic evaluation. They obtain and provide information, and coordinate testing and follow-up. Genetic counselors also help families to recognize and deal with the many painful and distressing emotions that go along with finding out about a genetic diagnosis.

Diagnostic Genetic Evaluation

A clinical genetics evaluation refers to the medical workup of an individual or family with a potential or known genetic condition. For the child or adult with mental retardation, a main goal of the genetic workup is to identify, if possible, the underlying etiology of the disability. Once the cause is understood, the genetic, medical, and functional implications of the diagnosis can be specifically addressed. If no etiological diagnosis is reached, the individual and family can still benefit from a discussion of the findings, including the correction of any misconceptions about the cause as well as a review of the estimated chance of recurrence in future generations.

The comprehensive genetic evaluation of a person with developmental disabilities typically involves a detailed physical examination; appropriate laboratory studies; and a review of available prenatal, developmental, behavioral, and family histories. Although some pediatricians and other specialists now include chromosome and fragile X laboratory studies as part of their assessments of children with developmental delay, these tests alone do not constitute a complete genetic workup. As mentioned previously, most genetic disorders cannot be detected cytogenetically, so even a person with seemingly "normal" chromosomes may well have a diagnosable genetic condition.

Clinical Diagnosis Certain combinations of physical and behavioral features occur together often enough to be recognizable as syndromes. Most nongeneticists, for example, can identify the characteristic pattern of facial and physical features of Down syndrome. Likewise, genetics specialists can routinely recognize hundreds of other syndromes that are little known outside the genetics field. These syndromes are not restricted to severe disabilities, and many result in only mild cognitive impairment.

Many syndrome diagnoses are made solely on the basis of a person's physical, behavioral, developmental, and family history findings; at present, no known laboratory marker exists for these syndromes. When made by a qualified physician geneticist, however, such "clinical diagnoses" are highly accurate and valid; again and again, the reliability of clinical diagnoses has been upheld as new genes for many disorders have been discovered. One example is Williams syndrome, a condition associated with subtle but recognizable facial differences, congenital heart abnormalities, mild mental retardation, and a characteristic behavior and learning profile (see Chapter 4). Since the 1960s, hundreds of individuals have been diagnosed with Williams syndrome on the basis of clinical evidence alone. Then, in 1993, a specific microdeletion was found in the gene for elastin on the q arm of chromosome 7 in a person with Williams syndrome (Ewart et al., 1993). Subsequent molecular testing has confirmed the microdeletion in more than 95% of all people with this clinical diagnosis. Although Williams syndrome can now be included among syndromes for which there are laboratory diagnoses, many other disorders, such as Cornelia de Lange and Rett syndromes, can still only be diagnosed clinically.

Laboratory Diagnosis The comprehensive genetic workup of a person with mental retardation almost always includes some laboratory studies. These lab studies can confirm or rule out suspected diagnoses. Chromosome studies are routinely recommended to check for cytogenetic abnormalities in people having mental retardation, even when a specific syndrome is not clinically obvious. Cytogenetic abnormalities account for a significant percentage of all mental retardation, and many different numerical and structural abnormalities can be detected by this one type of study. Likewise, molecular fragile X analysis should be considered for all males and females with mental retardation of unknown etiology, because this a common condition that has far-reaching implications for families.

Apart from these two examples, tests for genetic disorders are most often done only when a person shows physical or behavioral symptoms suggesting a specific diagnosis. For example, the molecular FISH study needed to detect a microdeletion of chromosome 7q would usually be done only if a child or adult shows some clinical features of Williams syndrome. A different individual who has neuromuscular features suggesting myotonic dystrophy might have blood drawn to check for the trinucleotide repeat expansion associated with that disorder. In each case, a thorough clinical evaluation by a geneticist is crucial in specifying which genetic laboratory studies are indicated.

In addition to laboratory tests to detect chromosomal or molecular changes in the genetic material itself, many studies are available to check for biochemical differences that result from gene changes, as in the measurement of phenylalanine in people with PKU. Although technically not "genetic" studies (because they do not involve analysis of chromosomes or DNA), these tests can aid in the diagnosis of a genetic condition by measuring the biochemical consequences of a potential disorder. One example is Smith-Lemli-Opitz (S-L-O) syndrome, a recessive condition resulting in a recognizable pattern of birth defects and mental retardation. Although direct gene testing for S-L-O is not yet available, recent research has determined that children with S-L-O have abnormally low levels of cholesterol in their blood due to a genetic defect involving cholesterol metabolism (Tint et al., 1994). By measuring cholesterol and related compounds in people with clinical symptoms of S-L-O, the diagnosis can be confirmed. Sophisticated biochemical studies can now detect more than 200 inherited metabolic disorders, only a handful of which, like PKU, are routinely screened for at birth. Diagnosis of this group of genetic metabolic disorders is particularly crucial because, in many such conditions, dietary treatment can prevent or lessen mental retardation.

> *Diagnosis of this group of genetic metabolic disorders is particularly crucial because, in many such conditions, dietary treatment can prevent or lessen mental retardation.*

Unfortunately, these potentially treatable disorders are also greatly underdiagnosed at the present time. In 1994, metabolic screening of 58 individuals with selected developmental disabilities diagnosed 5 people (8%) with a previously unrecognized inherited metabolic disorder (Kurtz et al. 1994). Sadly, had the diagnoses been possible when these individuals were younger, dietary therapy might have lessened or even prevented the disabilities resulting from these conditions.

Prenatal Diagnosis   Many chromosomal disorders, including Down syndrome, can be definitively diagnosed during pregnancy by chromosome analysis of cells obtained by either amniocentesis or chronic villus sampling (CVS). Amniocentesis involves the extraction of a small amount of amniotic fluid from around a developing fetus at 16–20 weeks' gestation. The amniotic fluid contains fetal cells that can be grown in the laboratory for genetic analysis. CVS can be performed earlier in pregnancy (9–11 weeks). CVS is accomplished by obtaining minute amounts of placental tissue that has the same genetic constitution as the developing embryo. Both procedures are associated with small but significant risks to the pregnancy; currently in the United

States, only women ages 34 or 35 and older are routinely offered these prenatal diagnostic options.

As opposed to the diagnostic studies described previously, all pregnant women in the United States receiving prenatal care, regardless of age, are now being offered a less invasive, but also less sensitive, test called *multiple marker screening*. This blood test can identify pregnancies at higher-than-average risk for birth defects, including Down syndrome. Multiple marker screening refers to the analysis of specific body chemicals that, if present in either higher or lower than expected amounts in maternal blood during pregnancy, can sometimes reflect an underlying fetal abnormality.

One common form of marker screening is called a *triple screen*. A triple screen checks three different body chemicals to identify pregnancies at risk for Down syndrome, spina bifida, and a few other genetic conditions. Ultimately, the babies of most women with abnormal triple screen results do not have Down syndrome or other disorders. An abnormal triple screen result does, however, identify those women who should be offered more definitive testing. For example, a 29-year-old pregnant woman with no family history of inherited conditions would usually not be offered the option of prenatal diagnosis for Down syndrome because her chance of having an affected child is far lower than her risk of losing the pregnancy due to amniocentesis or CVS. At about 15 weeks of pregnancy, however, she could decide to have a blood test for multiple marker screening. A normal (i.e., negative) test result would not rule out the possibility of Down syndrome in her child, but would indicate a very low risk. But in contrast, an abnormal result could indicate a higher risk than that of most women her age for this pregnancy, so that her chance of carrying a baby with Down syndrome might actually be similar to that of a 37-year-old woman. This woman would then be offered the option of amniocentesis, which would definitively show whether the infant was affected.

Underdiagnosis of Genetic Mental Retardation Syndromes

Alone or in combination with environmental influences, genetic factors are major contributors to the causes of mental retardation. Yet most genetic syndromes remain underdiagnosed among people with developmental disabilities. Indeed, the majority of people with mental retardation have never been assessed using current genetic technology, nor even had relatively routine forms of testing such as chromosome and fragile X analyses. Consequently, many professionals in the developmental disabilities field only rarely work with people who have been *diagnosed* with specific syndromes, reinforcing their perception that genetic etiologies have little bearing on the people they serve.

Underdiagnosis also has some important consequences for families and individuals. In some disorders, genetic diagnoses may have far-reaching hereditary implications, as in fragile X syndrome. Even though fragile X is the most common inherited cause of mental retardation, as many as 80% of those affected have not been diagnosed (National Fragile X Foundation, 1994). Families of such individuals thus remain unaware of the potential for this condition to recur in future generations.

Even for disorders that do not usually run in families, the failure to accurately diagnose often leads to uncertainty, misplaced guilt, and misdiagnosis. To give but one example, although Rett syndrome is easily recognized because of its characteristic behavioral regression and hand-wringing behaviors, only a fraction of females with Rett syndrome have been diagnosed (Moser & Naidu, 1986). Families of undiagnosed girls and women often receive no explanation for the dramatic loss of skills in their young daughters, and are unable to gain access to the wealth of support and information available to them through organizations such as the International Rett Syndrome Association.

Increasingly, underdiagnosis can also mean failure to provide syndrome-specific educational, behavioral, medical, and pharmaceutical interventions. Undiagnosed children and adults with Williams syndrome may not receive medical monitoring for the known health conditions related to this disorder, whereas undiagnosed children with S-L-O syndrome are missing out on promising new findings regarding dietary therapy. In future years, specific educational interventions may also prove effective for children with some of these genetic syndromes (Hodapp & Fidler, 1999).

Genetic syndromes are underdiagnosed due to several factors. First, many types of genetic tests are relatively new. As a result, many of these tests have not yet been used on many people with different genetic disorders. Equally important, however, is the pervasive lack of awareness of genetic syndromes by both medical and nonmedical professionals outside the genetics field. As a result, families and individuals cannot take advantage of needed genetic services; if neither medical nor nonmedical professionals inform families about genetic evaluation and counseling, families cannot benefit. Unfortunately, however, those professionals who are most in a position to influence the services parents and affected individuals receive are often unaware of the benefits of clinical genetic services and the indications for referral.

We seem increasingly faced, then, with a gap between those services that parents and individuals could obtain versus those that they do, in fact, receive. With each passing year, effective medical therapies are discovered for many syndromes, as a barrage of new laboratory tools are developed to diagnose them. But without the full participation of teachers, psychologists, therapists, physicians, and others outside the genetics field, these many practical applications of genetic research can neither be implemented nor expanded on. One aim of this book is to bring to such professionals genetic and behavioral information about a variety of genetic mental retardation disorders.

We seem increasingly faced, then, with a gap between those services that parents and individuals could obtain versus those that they do, in fact, receive.

II

GENETIC DISORDERS

3

Down Syndrome

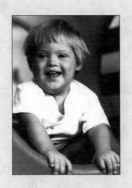

For many reasons, Down syndrome stands apart from all other mental retardation syndromes. Although researchers often view Down syndrome as a "stand-in" for mental retardation in general, Down syndrome actually features its own distinctive patterns of behavioral strengths and weakness. And even though most people can easily recognize the typical facial characteristics of inidviduals with Down syndrome, they generally know very little about the intricacies of this disorder. This chapter describes in depth commonly and not-so-commonly known facts about Down syndrome. For example, Down syndrome

- Is the most prevalent chromosomal cause of mental retardation

- Has a 130-year history and rich tradition of behavioral research

- Enjoys as many behavioral studies as all 750 other genetic mental retardation syndromes combined

- Is characterized by an average life span that, although shorter than average, has *quintupled* over the course of the 20th century

- Is the subject of popular television shows and books
- Has distinctive cognitive, linguistic, and behavioral profiles
- Elicits positive reactions from others
- Results in successful functioning in more integrated school, living, and work environments

HISTORICAL BACKGROUND

Down syndrome was first described in 1866 by H. Langdon Down, a British physician working in an asylum in Earlswood, England. In his brief article detailing this condition (excerpted in Dunn, 1991), Down described these individuals' characteristic epicanthal folds (i.e., folds of skin around the eyes), broad face, thick tongues, language problems, shortened life expectancy, and "humorous" personalities. He even noted the tendency of many individuals who had this condition to show fluctuations in development—gains followed by losses. He wrote, "whatever advance is made intellectually in the summer, some amount of retrogression may be expected in the winter" (Dunn, 1991, p. 828).

By way of explanation, Down felt that people with this syndrome showed a "retrogression" of European stock into the lower Mongolian race (Scheerenberger, 1983; Zellweger, 1977). He therefore designated people with this condition as having a "Mongolian type of idiocy," based on their facial similarities to people of Mongolian ancestry. Although in recent years the term has been replaced by the less offensive *Down's syndrome* and, now, *Down syndrome* (without the possessive), the term *mongolism* persisted in both the professional and public domains for more than 100 years. Although such racial typologies demonstrate the not-so-subtle racism of Victorian-era Britain (Gould, 1980), Down was nevertheless a careful observer of the syndrome that today bears his name.

The history of Down syndrome also reflects the many changes that have occurred in the mental retardation field over the past century. In 1933, Lionel Penrose estimated that the average person with this disorder lived 9 years; by the mid-1990s, the average life expectancies of people with Down syndrome were estimated to be about 60 years (Rasore-Quartino & Cominetti, 1995).

The syndrome shows societal changes in other ways too. Besides being the impetus behind several nationally prominent parent groups—including the National Down Syndrome Society and the National Down Syndrome Congress—Down syndrome is the first mental retardation disorder to reach widespread public consciousness. In the early

1990s, the television show *Life Goes On* featured a family with an adolescent with Down syndrome. The show's star, Chris Burke, has become an inspiration to other individuals with the syndrome and their families. Other prominent individuals with Down syndrome include Jason Kingsley and Mitchell Levitz, two young men who have written a book, *Count Us In* (1991), describing their successful lives in politics and in the entertainment industry.

A Tradition of Overgeneralization

A less positive outgrowth of such popularity is the widely accepted idea that Down syndrome constitutes the prototypical mental retardation disorder. To many researchers and members of the general public, Down syndrome is thought to be synonymous with mental retardation in general. In many studies, children and adults with Down syndrome serve as the control or contrast group to other individuals with other disabilities. Although such a practice may be understandable given the syndrome's prevalence and longstanding research tradition, Down syndrome should not be considered a stand-in for mental retardation at large. In actuality, this syndrome features its own genetic, physical, and behavioral characteristics.

Although such a practice may be understandable given the syndrome's prevalence and longstanding research tradition, Down syndrome should not be considered a stand-in for mental retardation at large.

GENETIC AND PHYSICAL ISSUES

Etiology

Down syndrome is the most common congenital disorder associated with mental retardation. Occurring in an average of 1 out of every 700–1,000 births, it affects both males and females of all ethnic and socioeconomic backgrounds. Unlike individuals with many other genetic syndromes, the vast majority of individuals with this condition in the United States are correctly diagnosed in infancy.

The characteristic facial features of Down syndrome include a small head with a flat-looking face, small ears and mouth, protruding tongue, broad neck, and an upward slant to the eyes, with epicanthal

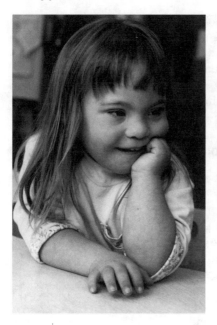 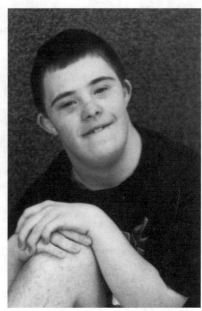

Figure 3.1.   A child and a young adult with Down syndrome.

folds at the inner corners. Many people would recognize the photographs in Figure 3.1 as a child and a young adult with Down syndrome.

Down syndrome is caused by the presence of all or part of an extra copy of chromosome 21 (see Chapter 2). Full trisomy 21, the presence of an extra chromosome 21 in all body cells, accounts for more than 92% of all occurrences of Down syndrome in live-born infants. But this group represents only a fraction of the total conceived because as many as 75% of trisomy 21 conceptions result in miscarriage or stillbirth. Between 2% and 3% of people with Down syndrome have a mosaic form of trisomy 21, meaning that only some of their cells show the trisomy 21 pattern. Down syndrome is caused by an unbalanced translocation involving chromosome 21 in 3%–5% of cases, some of which may be familial (see Chapter 2). The remaining small group of people with Down syndrome have unusual chromosomal differences, all related to chromosome 21, such as an extra ring-shaped 21 or the presence of a small extra piece of 21 (partial trisomy 21). Most occurrences of Down syndrome are not familial, and parents have a relatively low chance of conceiving a second child with the syndrome. But, as described in Chapter 2, there is a much higher chance for recurrence in the small percentage of cases associated with a familial chromosome translocation. Although a child with Down syndrome can be born to parents of any age, the chance of this occurring increases as a woman gets older (see Table 2.1).

Still, more than 80% of all babies with Down syndrome are born to women *younger* than 35. This seeming contradiction can be explained by the fact that younger women have many more babies than do older women. Thus, even though women younger than 35 have a lower chance of conceiving babies with Down syndrome, as a group their total number of pregnancies greatly outnumber those of women older than 35. Also, and contrary to popular belief, a woman having a first pregnancy at an older age is at no greater risk for having a child with Down syndrome, or any other genetic disorder, than a woman of the same age who has had previous children.

Health Issues

Individuals with Down syndrome are at higher-than-normal risk for a number of associated medical conditions. These are summarized in Table 3.1.

Congenital heart defects are present in as many as 50% of newborns with Down syndrome; fortunately, most of these are either mild or can be surgically corrected. Increased rates are also found of hearing and vision impairments; gastrointestinal, thyroid, and dental problems; and instability of the neck bones (see Roizen, 1996, for a review). Furthermore, many people with Down syndrome are prone to being overweight or obese (Prasher, 1995), which may be related to the lower resting metabolism of many with the disorder (Chad, Jobling, & Frail,

Table 3.1.   Salient medical concerns in people with Down syndrome

Medical concern	Percentage affected
Congenital heart defects	50
Hearing loss	66–89
Ophthalmic conditions (e.g., strabismus, refractive errors)	60
Gastrointestinal conditions	5
Endocrine conditions (e.g., hypothyroidism)	50–90
Dental conditions (e.g., crowding, periodontal disease)	60–100
Orthopedic anomalies (e.g., subclinical atlanoaxial subluxation)	15
Obesity	50–60
Skin conditions (e.g., eczema, dry skin)	50
Seizure disorders	6–13
Leukemia	0.6

1990). Other likely contributing factors are the sedentary lifestyle and lack of regular exercise among many with Down syndrome, as well as hypotonia (poor muscle tone), poor eating habits, and endocrine anomalies such as hypothyroidism.

Given these many medical complications, the American Academy of Pediatrics (1994) has developed specific guidelines for monitoring the health of children with this disorder. These include regular cardiac, vision, hearing, and thyroid examinations beginning in early infancy; neck radiography after age 3 to check for atlantoaxial instability; and preventative dental care and weight management (see Cooley & Graham, 1991, and Roizen, 1996, for details).

Fertility   With only rare exceptions, males with Down syndrome are infertile due to decreased production of sperm. Women with Down syndrome have decreased fertility, but some have been known to reproduce. Pregnant women with Down syndrome do, however, have a higher-than-average risk for having children with Down syndrome. Still, in most cases, these women give birth to unaffected babies.

Life Span   Although advances in medicine have dramatically increased the survival of people with Down syndrome born since the 1950s, the condition is still associated with a reduced life span as compared both with the general population and with other people who have mental retardation. Approximately 80% of babies with Down syndrome born without heart defects will now live to at least age 30 (Baird & Sadovnick, 1987). An extra copy of genes on chromosome 21 predisposes adults to Alzheimer's disease. Older adults with Down syndrome are at a particularly high risk for developing Alzheimer's characteristic "plaques and tangles" in brain tissue; indeed, virtually all adults with Down syndrome older than 35 develop these brain changes (Devenny et al., 1996). Far fewer, however, exhibit the actual clinical symptoms of Alzheimer's disease, an issue that we discuss in more detail later in this chapter.

COGNITIVE AND LINGUISTIC FUNCTIONING

Although IQ levels vary from individual to individual, most people with Down syndrome function in the moderate range of mental retardation, with mean IQ scores in the fifties (Connolly, 1978; Gibson, 1978). Overall IQ scores, however, must be qualified by trajectories of intellectual development (defined in the next section) and cognitive-linguistic strengths and weaknesses. This chapter first discusses these issues in terms of the childhood years, then examines special issues relevant to adults with Down syndrome.

Trajectories of Intellectual Development

Although any one child with mental retardation may speed up or slow down in cognitive development over the childhood years, as a group, people with mixed etiologies of mental retardation show a constant, stable rate of development. This constant rate of development can be seen in both cross-sectional and longitudinal studies, at all points over the childhood years. In Down syndrome, however, a clear decline occurs in rates of intellectual development over the childhood years. Almost invariably, the highest IQ (or developmental quotient; DQ) scores are noted in infancy, with lower IQ scores evident as the child gets older (see Hodapp, Evans, & Gray, 1999, for a review). This decline in IQ score does not indicate that the child with Down syndrome has stopped developing, only that development becomes progressively slower over the childhood years. Table 3.2 describes IQ changes in children with Down syndrome compared with those in groups of children with heterogeneous causes of mental retardation. Several factors are implicated in the slowing developmental trajectories of children with Down syndrome.

> *This decline in IQ score does not indicate that the child with Down syndrome has stopped developing, only that development becomes progressively slower over the childhood years.*

Task-Related Slowing The first involves difficulties in accomplishing one or more developmental tasks (Hodapp & Zigler, 1990). Even early on, children with Down syndrome have difficulty in mastering new developmental skills. For example, Dunst (1988, 1990) noted that infants with Down syndrome slow in their development in several Piagetian sensorimotor tasks, exhibiting particular difficulties developing from Piaget's sensorimotor Stage III to Stage IV and from Stage IV to Stage V.

In the same way, these children show marked difficulties in developing certain language skills. As Fowler, Gelman, and Gleitman (1994) noted, many children with Down syndrome have difficulties in attaining Brown's (1973) Stage III grammar. Stage III grammar is characterized by sentence lengths (i.e., mean length of utterances, or MLUs) of approximately 2.50 to 3.25 morphemes per sentence; this stage usually appears at 30–36 months in typically developing children. Stage III features longer sentences; the correct usage of many grammatical morphemes (*-ed* for past tense, *-ing* for progressive tense); the beginnings of

Table 3.2. IQ changes with age in children with Down syndrome versus children with mixed etiologies

Study	N	Chronological age (in years)							
		<3	3–5	5–7	7–9	9–11	11–13	13–15	15+
		IQ scores							
Children with Down syndrome									
Cross-sectional									
Melyn & White, 1973	642	56.9	51.8	46.9	44.8	42.7	35.9	37.7	
Morgan, 1979	217	65.8	45.9	41.0	38.3	33.4	26.8		
Hodapp, Evans, & Gray, 2000	52			50.7	41.0	38.7	39.6	37.7	41.3
Longitudinal									
Carr, 1995	54	80	45						
Cunningham, 1987	181	70.9	58.7				37.2		41.9
Children with mixed etiologies (all studies are longitudinal)									
Bernheimer & Keogh, 1988	34–37	67.1		71.3		70.3			
Bernheimer, Keogh, & Guthrie, 1997	82		72.2	69.6			66.1		
Silverstein et al., 1982	101					65.7	66.4	64.0	
Stavrou, 1990 (mild mental retardation)	60				64.7			63.5	63.1

Adapted from Hodapp, Evans, & Gray, 1999.

negatives, *wh-* questions, (e.g. "who," "what," "when," and "where") and yes/no questions; and overgeneralizations such as "feets" and "goed." Children with Down syndrome seem to remain at Stage III for many years. Rondal, Ghiotto, Bredart, and Bachelet (1988) found no correlation between increasing chronological age and grammatical levels once children had reached Stage III grammar. For children with Down syndrome, then, Stage III grammar seems particularly problematic. Moreover, "the slowdown at Stage III . . . raises the possibility that linguistic factors are one important determinant in explaining a child's failure to progress [in other areas]" (Fowler et al., 1994, p. 135).

Age-Related Slowing A second source of slowed development is associated with the child's chronological age. Fowler (1988) noted that several individuals with Down syndrome in her study simply did not develop in grammar from approximately age 6–11 years. Before and after this time, children did develop, but they showed a plateau in development during these middle childhood years. Although less intensively studied, such plateaus in development—at roughly the same age periods—may also occur in overall intelligence (Gibson, 1966) and in adaptive behavior (Dykens, Hodapp, & Evans, 1994). Joined with these children's difficulties in performing certain developmental tasks (task-related slowings, e.g., learning Stage III grammar), such age-related slowing may further affect rates of development in these children as they get older.

Strengths and Weaknesses

Cognitive Profiles Although relatively few studies have examined the cognitive profiles of people with Down syndrome, findings to date are remarkably consistent. Early researchers, working with large numbers of children and adults with Down syndrome in institutions, noted that these individuals performed much better on visual-spatial tasks than on verbal or auditory tasks (e.g., Haxby, 1989; Rohr & Burr, 1978; Silverstein, Legutki, Friedman, & Takayama, 1982; Thase, Tigner, Smeltzer, & Liss, 1984).

These patterns are seen as well in studies of noninstitutionalized children who were assessed with newer IQ tests. Using the Kaufman Assessment Battery for Children (K-ABC; Kaufman & Kaufman, 1983), for example, several researchers found that children with Down syndrome do not exhibit striking differences between their scores in sequential processing (solving problems bit by bit in serial or temporal order), simultaneous processing (using a holistic, gestalt-like approach), and achievement (learned information, reading, math) (Hodapp et al.,

1992; Powell, Houghton, & Douglas, 1997; Pueschel, Gallagher, Zartler, & Pezzullo, 1987).

Relative strengths are found, however, in K-ABC performance on specific subtests. Reminiscent of early research, children with Down syndrome exhibit strengths in tasks assessing visual as opposed to auditory processing. As shown in Table 3.3, children with Down syndrome are better able to repeat a series of hand movements presented visually by the examiner as opposed to a series of numbers that are presented verbally. Similar examples of strengths in visual as opposed to auditory memory occur on other IQ tests as well (Hodapp, et al., 1999).

Even infants and toddlers with Down syndrome seem to show a proclivity for remembering hand movements and other visual gestures. Comparing infants with Down syndrome with those with Williams syndrome, Harris, Bellugi, Bates, Jones, and Rossen (1997) found that those with Down syndrome showed higher levels in early gesturing. As discussed later, strengths in visual-motor skills, visual memory, and gesturing bode well for interventions such as sign language (Hodapp et al., 1992) and reading—the visual understanding of language (Buckley, 1995).

Linguistic Profiles   Language is perhaps the most well-researched behavioral domain in Down syndrome. Many carefully done studies have identified the intricacies of grammar, expressive language, phonology, and articulation as areas of particular difficulty for individuals with Down syndrome.

Grammar   As noted previously, people with Down syndrome seem particularly impaired in their grammatical abilities, with many individuals not progressing beyond the 3-year-old level (Fowler, 1990). Children with Down syndrome seem to have particular difficulties in acquiring adult formations for negatives, *wh-* questions; irregular past tense (went, said); embedded sentences ("I see that John is coming"); passives; and other, more complicated sentence types. Even when they become adults, these individuals rarely reach mature levels of communication, which typically developing children routinely attain by about age 5.

Expressive Language   A second area of linguistic weakness concerns expressive language. Beginning during the earliest years, children with Down syndrome display expressive language that is behind receptive levels. Miller (1988, 1992) found that 64% of preschoolers with Down syndrome showed receptive abilities (and mental ages) that were 3 or more months above expressive levels. Furthermore, such strength in receptive skills (or weakness in expressive skills) became evident in a growing number of children as they developed. While 54%–61% of children (depending on the testing session) showed the

Table 3.3. Performance of visual versus auditory processing tasks in Down Syndrome

Auditory tasks	Visual tasks			
	Hand movements	Gestalt closure	Number recall	Word order
K-ABC				
Peuschel et al., 1987 (scaled)	3.15 (scaled score)	4.55	2.35	1.70
Hodapp et al., 1992 (age equivalents)	5.58 (years)	5.40	3.18	3.75
Powell et al., 1997	5.81 (years)	5.41	4.16	4.38
Stanford-Binet IV	*Bead memory*		*Memory for sentences*	
Hodapp et al., 1999	3.89 (years)		3.08	

Adapted from Hodapp et al., 1999.

weakness in expressive abilities when their MAs were below 24 months, 83%–100% showed the receptive over-expressive pattern when MAs were above 25 months.

Pronunication and Articulation   Finally, these children have particularly impaired *pronunciation.* Articulation problems are commonly noted (Miller, Leddy, Miolo, & Sedey, 1995), and almost all parents (95%) report at least occasional difficulties in understanding their children with Down syndrome (Kumin, 1994). Such difficulties relate to deviant or impaired articulation, as well as to disfluencies involving sound prolongations; pauses; and repetitions of sounds, syllables, parts of words, and whole words (Leddy, 1999). Even during adolescence, those with Down syndrome (compared with a mixed etiological group) articulated fewer consonants correctly on the Goldman–Fristoe Test of Articulation (Rosin, Swift, Bless, & Vetter, 1988).

Contributing Factors in Language Impairment   Both hearing and oral structure abnormalities contribute to such language difficulties. From 60% to 80% of children with Down syndrome have inner-ear involvement (Pueschel, 1990), including peripheral, conductive hearing loss due to stenotic ear canals, a small nasopharynx, dysfunctional eustachian tubes, and adenoid and tonsil hypertrophy (Roizen, Walters, Nicol, & Blondes, 1993). Oral problems are also common, including abnormalities of the tongue, oral cavity, and facial muscles (Bersu, 1981). Such articulation difficulties undoubtedly relate to difficulties in expressive language.

Articulation difficulties may also be linked to difficulties in grammatical development. Several linguists have hypothesized that grammar and articulation constitute a single computational linguistic capacity (Rondal, 1995). This system may be separable from semantics (the meaning relations of words and sentences) and from pragmatics (the uses of language). As such, language itself seems separable into various semi-independent "modules," and individuals with Down syndrome may illustrate such linguistic modularity. Grammar and articulation are both relatively poor in this syndrome and seem to form a single package that functions separately from semantics and pragmatics. Semantics and pragmatics, in turn, seem more tied to overall MA levels (see Rosenberg & Abbeduto, 1993, for a review).

Consider, for example, the semantic, or vocabulary, development of these children. Although children with Down syndrome produce fewer vocabulary words than young, typically developing children at the same MA, their vocabularies generally increase with advancing mental age (Miller et al., 1995). In addition, children with Down syndrome produce similar words as children without mental retardation in their first word utterances. Like typically developing children, children with Down syndrome also realize that a mother's earliest object words to the child usually refer to entire objects (that when mother points out an object and says "car," she refers to the entire automobile, not to the car's wheels or windows). Furthermore, in the context of a simple hiding game, children with Down syndrome acquire object labels after a single exposure—or "fast-map" labels onto objects—with similar degrees of success as MA-matched children without mental retardation (Chapman, Kay-Raining Bird, & Schwartz, 1990).

In pragmatics, or the uses of language, children with Down syndrome also show performance levels that are tied to MA. Like children without mental retardation, children with Down syndrome use language for the same communicative functions (Owens & MacDonald, 1982). They answer and ask questions, name objects, make declarations, and suggest or command actions. Although the study of linguistic pragmatics is complicated by a variety of methodological issues (see Rosenberg & Abbeduto, 1993), most developmental psycholinguists consider the pragmatics of children with Down syndrome as more tied to overall cognitive levels and less impaired than functioning in other areas of language (Rondal, 1996). In brief, grammar, expressive language, and phonology are particularly affected in Down syndrome, whereas semantics and pragmatics are more consistent with MA expectations.

In brief, grammar, expressive language, and phonology are particularly affected in Down syndrome, whereas semantics and pragmatics are more consistent with MA expectations.

Neurological Correlates

Recent research on the brain, both magnetic resonance imaging (MRI) and neuropathological studies, shed new light on the cognitive and linguistic profiles seen in individuals with Down syndrome. Based on the MRIs of 15 adolescents—6 with Down syndrome and 9 with Williams syndrome—Jernigan, Bellugi, Sowell, Doherty, and Hesselink (1993) found that both groups had reduced total cerebral volumes. Unlike their counterparts with Williams syndrome, however, those with Down syndrome had reduced proportional size of the temporal limbic cortex. Furthermore, neuropathological studies in Down syndrome find hypoplasia (underdevelopment) in the temporal lobe regions (Golden & Hyman, 1994). Taken together, these temporal lobe anomalies may be implicated in the difficulties that many people with Down syndrome have with auditory short-term memory. At the same time, Jernigan et al. (1993) observed that the posterior cortical volume of individuals with Down syndrome was relatively preserved, and this may be related to the relative strengths in visual-motor tasks seen in many with this syndrome.

Wang, Doherty, Hesselink, and Bellugi (1992) found decreased width in a specific area of the corpus callosum of subjects with Down syndrome. This observation, along with the frontal lobe hypoplasia, may be related to the linguistic difficulties that characterize Down syndrome, especially problems with expressive language and verbal fluency tasks that require the coordinated work of the two frontal regions of the brain (see Wang, 1996, for a review). Further work is needed to follow up these observations, especially in younger individuals who do not yet show the behavioral and neurological complications of dementia.

ADULT ISSUES

Two additional cognitive-linguistic issues also arise as people with Down syndrome enter their late childhood and adult years.

Development of Intelligence

The first concerns whether these individuals can develop intellectually during late adolescence and early adulthood. In most people without mental retardation, development of intelligence stops somewhere between 16 and 18 years of age, at least as defined by IQ tests. Thus, although we expect a 15-year-old to be more intelligent than a 10-year-old, we do not necessarily expect a 40-year-old to be more intelligent than a 35-year-old.

In the field of mental retardation however, Fisher and Zeaman (1970) first suggested that people with mental retardation (of any etiology) might continue developing into the early adult years. To date, the possibility of a longer age-span of development in Down syndrome seems supported for at least some domains of functioning. In a longitudinal study of British teens and young adults with Down syndrome, adolescents continued developing, albeit at slowed rates, until their early twenties in their vocabulary, some aspects of early language, and social competence (Shepperdson, 1995; see also Berry, Groeneweg, Gibson, & Brown, 1984). Moreover, by far the best predictor of continued development was a good environment. Those adolescents and young adults who experienced more stimulating environments—who regularly participated in family outings, club memberships, vacations, and other age-appropriate activities—performed better than did individuals from less stimulating environments.

In other areas, however, it seems possible that development may gradually come to a halt during the early teen years. Although controversial, grammar may be one area in which such a critical or sensitive period exists. Evidence from deaf individuals learning sign language and from those learning a second language (Newport, 1990), as well as from exceptional cases of children first exposed to language after puberty (Curtiss, 1977), all suggest that certain aspects of grammar develop mainly during the prepubertal years (Hodapp, 1998). After approximately 13–14 years of age, development in linguistic grammar may be more difficult. Late learners of a language, then, can become reasonably proficient in that language, but they generally find it extremely difficult to acquire the more subtle aspects of grammar.

Although most psycholinguists feel that a sensitive period exists for linguistic grammar, such may not be the case in Down syndrome. Chapman, Seung, Schwartz, and Kay-Raining Bird (1998), for example, have recently examined the critical age issue cross-sectionally, comparing individuals with Down syndrome who were 5–8 years old, 9–12 years old, 13–16 years old, and 16.5–20 years old. Analyzing both conversational speech and narratives (e.g., the person's story about a favorite television show or other experience), these researchers found no evidence of a critical period for grammar. MLUs (a common measure of grammatical complexity) were 2.00 and 2.46 morphemes per utterance for the children in the 5- to 8- and 9- to 12-year groups, respectively, and continued rising—to 3.15 and 4.47—for the 13- to 16- and 16.5- to 20-year-old groups. Although longitudinal work is needed, this study does cast doubt on whether grammatical development really does stop or slow dramatically after early puberty in individuals with Down syndrome.

Intellectual Declines

A second issue concerns *intellectual declines* as one ages in adulthood. Individuals without mental retardation show small, gradual intellectual declines as they age, although such aging effects differ by the type of intellectual task one performs. The most pronounced, age-related declines occur in tasks involving cognitive/perceptual speed, spatial orientation, reasoning, and memory, whereas the smallest declines occur in verbal and number abilities (Horn & Hofer, 1992). And, like adults with Down syndrome, adults without mental retardation who enjoy stimulating environments and who continue to engage in intellectual tasks throughout their lives show less severe declines. Like most human abilities, one either "uses or loses" intellectual abilities as one ages.

High Risk of Alzheimer's Disease   In Down syndrome, the issue becomes complicated due to the presence of Alzheimer's disease. Alzheimer's disease, which occurs in 127 per 100,000 typical adults older than age 60, is found in exceptionally high percentages of people with Down syndrome (Zigman, Schupf, Zigman, & Silverman, 1993). This increased risk may be associated with the presence on chromosome 21 of two genes that are implicated in Alzheimer's disease (an amyloid precursor protein and a superoxide dismutase) (Korenberg, 1995). As mentioned previously, most studies indicate that after age 30 the brains of nearly all people with Down syndrome show the plaques and tangles characteristic of Alzheimer neuropatholgy (Wisniewski, Wisniewski, & Wen, 1985).

Yet in Down syndrome, the Alzheimer neuropathology does not reliably relate to the behavioral changes associated with dementia. Although findings vary by study, only 15%–40% of adults older than 40 with Down syndrome show the behavioral signs and symptoms of Alzheimer's disease (Dalton & Crapper-McLachlan, 1984; Thase, Liss, Smeltzer, & Maloon, 1982). In essence, the brain changes that usually directly relate to impaired functioning in older people without mental retardation are not so tightly connected in Down syndrome. This disconnection between brain changes and Alzheimer's dementia continues to puzzle researchers. Some speculate that this lag is associated with certain shifts in the brains of people with Down syndrome, specifically an increase

In essence, the brain changes that usually directly relate to impaired functioning in older people without mental retardation are not so tightly connected in Down syndrome. This disconnection between brain changes and Alzheimer's dementia continues to puzzle researchers.

after 50 years of age of "neuritic" or malignant, fibrillized plaques as opposed to more benign, diffuse plaques (see Zigman, Silverman, & Wisniewski, 1996, for a review).

Given this state of affairs, it is difficult to examine the typical cognitive and linguistic changes associated with aging in individuals with Down syndrome. In this vein, Devenny et al. (1996) followed 91 adults with Down syndrome over a 6-year period, and found an early but normal aging pattern in all but four individuals, who showed substantial declines. Any sample of aging adults with Down syndrome will undoubtedly contain many—perhaps all—individuals who have the neuropathology of Alzheimer's disease, as well as a third or more of individuals who experience Alzheimer's behavioral effects. Findings from Devenny et al. (1996) thus called into question the idea of widespread cognitive declines among older people with Down syndrome. Importantly, although certain intellectual tasks may help indicate the behavioral effects of Alzheimer's (e.g., Brugge et al., 1994), memory and cognitive loss may ultimately prove less sensitive indicators of dementia than are certain noncognitive tasks (Zigman et al., 1993).

ADAPTIVE AND PERSONALITY FUNCTIONING

In order to look at the entire spectrum of behavior as it relates to individuals with Down syndrome, we now turn to noncognitive measures of adaptive and maladaptive functioning.

Adaptive Functioning

Adaptive Trajectories   A first issue concerns trajectories of adaptive behavior. As in intellectual development and, possibly, in grammar as well, children with Down syndrome slow in their adaptive development as they get older (Brown, Greer, Aylward, & Hunt, 1990; Cornwell & Birch, 1969; Morgan, 1979). But when and why these slowings occur remains unclear. Using the Vineland Adaptive Behavior Scales (Sparrow, Balla, & Cicchetti, 1984), Loveland and Kelley (1988, 1991) did not find declines in cross-sectional samples examined over either the preschool or the adolescent years. In both studies, however, a restricted age range was considered, and standard scores from preschool to adolescence did show declines. Preschoolers showed standard scores from 60 to 73 across different domains, whereas adolescents and young adults had standard scores from 50 to 60.

In contrast, Carr (1988) found significant declines before age 4, but not from ages 4 to 11. In one additional study, Dykens et al. (1994) found declines in standard scores and a plateauing of age-equivalent levels of adaptive development from approximately 6 to 11 years in a cross-sectional sample examined over the 1- to 12-year period. Although various researchers have found different points and possible reasons for adaptive slowings, some slowings occur during the childhood years. Again, these are slowings—not ceasings—of development.

Importance of Stimulation   Possibly to an even greater extent than in other domains, adaptive development can continue over the adolescent and even adult years. The salient element seems to be a stimulating environment. Adolescents with Down syndrome who have stimulating environments and appropriate supports often continue developing in adaptive behavior into the early adult years (Hodapp, 1997a; Shepperdson, 1995). In addition, greater adaptive advances may be made by children who have higher MAs, and who have mothers who enjoy greater amounts of social support and a more active style of coping (i.e., a more problem-solving as opposed to an avoidant style) with their children's problems (Sloper & Turner, 1996).

Aging and Adaptive Behavior   In addition to the many studies of increasing performance during childhood and early adulthood, recent years have also seen a focus on aging. Again, Alzheimer's disease and its effects are of primary interest. Indeed, several studies have found that, relative to cognition, adaptive behavior is a more sensitive indicator of Alzheimer's-related declines. In a large-scale study comparing more than 2,000 adults with Down syndrome with 4,000 adults without Down syndrome, Zigman, Schupf, Lubin, and Silverman (1987) found that activities of daily living differentiated the two groups over different age periods. Whereas individuals with Down syndrome performed better than the non-Down syndrome group when adults were 20–50 years old, the groups performed identically by ages 50–59. After age 60, the group with Down syndrome performed much worse in daily living skills. This decline after age 60 in people with Down syndrome was also noted in their cognitive abilities, albeit to a much less striking degree.

In another study of large numbers of adults with Down syndrome, Collacott (1992) also found deterioration in most adaptive skills beginning at age 50; by age 60, these adults scored lower on virtually every aspect of adaptive behavior than did younger adults with Down syndrome. Adaptive behavior therefore provides an effective indicator of aging—and Alzheimer's-related—declines in adults with Down syndrome. Despite aggressive research efforts, it remains unclear why the neuropathological changes noted by ages 30–40 years do not manifest themselves in Alzheimer's dementia until almost 20 years later.

Adaptive Strengths and Weaknesses   In general, children with Down syndrome show higher levels of adaptive behavior (e.g., eating, grooming, following rules, getting along with others) than of intelligence. Comparing performance on the Vineland Social Maturity Scale (Doll, 1953) and Stanford-Binet Intelligence Scale (Terman & Merrill, 1960), Cornwell and Birch (1969) found that IQs generally were lower than SQs (social quotients) throughout the childhood years. Furthermore, the decline in IQ was more marked than in SQ as children got older. More recently, Loveland and Kelley (1988, 1991), using the Vineland Adaptive Behavior Scales (Sparrow et al. 1984), compared children with Down syndrome and children with autism. At both preschool and adolescent years, adaptive age-equivalent scores were generally higher than were mental age scores. Adaptive behavior therefore seems a relative strength for children with Down syndrome.

All areas, however, may not be equally high. Dykens et al. (1994) found that Vineland communication age-equivalent scores of children with Down syndrome fell below age-equivalent scores in daily living and socialization. Loveland and Kelley (1988, 1991) found similar, albeit nonsignificant, weaknesses in communicative skills relative to daily living skills and socialization (but Rodrigue, Morgan, & Geffken, 1991, did not). Although the Vineland provides only a general measure of communication, it, too, may indicate the linguistic weaknesses found by language development researchers.

Affect and Personality

From Down's (1866) original observations researchers have argued about the existence of a "Down syndrome personality." Reviewing this literature in 1978, Gibson noted that the stereotype included five aspects: an amiable nature, some obstinancy, a keen sense of the ridiculous, a facility for imitation, and an excellent memory. Research has called into question the latter three components, and whether these individuals as a group have a pleasant disposition (but with some obstinacy) continues to be debated.

These personality traits touch on larger issues of affect and social relating—how people with Down syndrome express their emotions and relate to others. Here, data are somewhat mixed, perhaps as a function of development. Infants with Down syndrome appear to have muted affect. These infants smile when babies without mental retardation might laugh, or show a down-turned face when others might whimper or cry. In addition, affective expressions seem tied to cognitive abilities, such that infants with Down syndrome show similar (though more muted) emotional reactions, but at later ages. Babies without delay will laugh at intrusive stimuli (e.g., being tickled) before 6 months and at cognitively incongruous displays (e.g., mother making a funny face) at 1 year. Infants with Down syndrome traverse the same sequence, but at later chronological ages (CAs) (Cicchetti & Sroufe, 1976).

At later ages, infant and toddler temperament has been examined, although no clear conclusions can be drawn (see Cicchetti & Ganiban, 1990, for a review). Using parent-report temperament questionnaires, these studies compare children who have Down syndrome to subjects matched on CA or MA. Although children with Down syndrome may show less persistence at a task, a higher threshold for frustration, and a positive mood, such differences are not always apparent.

Sociability   In interactions with their mothers or primary care-givers during the toddler years, these children more clearly exhibit be-haviors that might be considered as social. For example, many children with Down syndrome look longer at faces than at objects or other events (Kasari, Freeman, Mundy, & Sigman, 1995; Kasari, Sigman, Mundy, & Yirmiya, 1990; Ruskin, Kasari, Mundy, & Sigman, 1994). In addition, some (not all) studies find that young children with Down syndrome display the same or more positive affect compared to MA-matched comparison groups (sometimes consisting of premature in-fants, sometimes of typically developing toddlers).

Part of the difficulty in judging affect may be due to qualitative differences among the groups. In contrast to MA-matched typically de-veloping children, children with Down syndrome exhibited signifi-cantly more "slight smiles," including smiles that did not involve the entire face or that were briefer in duration (Kasari et al., 1995; Kasari, Mundy, Yirmiya, & Sigman, 1990). Relative to others, then, children with Down syndrome more often look to adults and briefly "half-smile" to them.

Even at later ages, personality and affect issues remain complex, but lend at least some support to the "sociability" of children with Down syndrome. Most interesting here is the fact that whereas some studies were designed to debunk the idea of a "stereotypic" Down syndrome personal-ity, they actually provide unintentional support for such a personality. In one study, for example, Wishart and John-ston (1990) developed a rating scale of the "stereotypical Down syndrome per-sonality." Parents, teachers, and medical students each rated children with Down syndrome on 23 items from 1 (*least stereo-typical*) to 5 (*most stereotypical*). When all groups' ratings were tallied, including mothers of children without mental re-tardation, teachers in mainstream versus inclusive class, and medical students, these children scored above the midpoint stereotypical score of 3.0, with scores ranging from 3.30 to 4.17. Mothers of children with Down syn-drome were most instructive. These mothers generally eschewed the presence of a Down syndrome personality when rating children with Down syndrome in general, but they exhibited the highest scores of all, 4.22 on a 5-point scale, when rating their own child with the syndrome.

> *Most interesting here is the fact that whereas some studies were de-signed to debunk the idea of a "stereotypic" Down syndrome personality, they actually provide uninten-tional support for such a personality.*

Although the meaning of these findings can be debated, one would expect mothers to be the best judges of their own child's personalities.

In a similar vein, Hornby (1995) interviewed 90 fathers of 7- to 14-year-old children with Down syndrome and found that nearly one half (46%) of fathers spontaneously commented on their children's cheerful personalities. An additional one third referred to their children as being lovable, and nearly a quarter described their offspring as sociable or friendly (see also Carr, 1995). Regardless of whether children with Down syndrome possess a "Down syndrome personality," these children are perceived as being pleasant and sociable by their parents and others.

Motivation A related issue concerns motivation and its connection to children's personality (and even to cognitive development). In a series of studies, Wishart (1995) and her colleagues have discovered that children with Down syndrome differ in their motivations to succeed at intellectual tasks. In object permanence tasks given from birth until almost 3 years of age, infants and toddlers with the syndrome generally showed the same sequences of development, albeit at a slower pace and with more instability, as demonstrated by children without mental retardation. These infants were much more likely to show a particular high-level behavior on one testing session, but then to fail the identical item a few weeks later (see Dunst, 1988, 1990). As Down (1866; cited in Dunn, 1991) noted, then, these children were indeed more likely to show advances in summer and retrogressions in winter.

Yet why such instability occurs is unclear. As suggested by their lesser degrees of task persistence from parent temperament ratings, children with Down syndrome often engage in off-task behavior when faced with a difficult task. But such off-task behavior often seems social in nature. Pitcairn and Wishart thus noted

> The Down syndrome children were not simply more social. It was rather in their response to failure that they differed. They exploited their social skills, producing a variety of distracting behaviors that focussed attention (their own and that of the experimenter) away from the task at hand. (1994, p. 489)

Such exploitation of their social skills—which Pitcairn and Wishart called "party tricks"—seem related to personality and to problem-solving styles. Such socially based behaviors also seem to involve the convergence of personality, motivation, and cognitive development.

MALADAPTIVE BEHAVIOR—PSYCHOPATHOLOGY

Relative to others with mental retardation, people with Down syndrome exhibit serious maladaptive behavior or psychopathology less often and less severely. Collacott, Cooper, and McGrother (1992), for example, found that 26% of adults with Down syndrome showed psychiatric disorders, while 38% of the contrast group did so. Similarly, Dykens and Kasari (1997) reported clinically elevated Child Behavior Checklist (Achenbach, 1991) scores in 23% of 43 children and adolescents with Down syndrome versus 39% of those with nonspecific mental retardation. Table 3.4 summarizes other studies of psychopathology in Down syndrome.

Yet lower rates of serious psychopathology do not mean that children or adults with Down syndrome are problem free. Among children, high percentages are found for certain maladaptive behaviors, and these may or may not reach clinically significant levels. Approximately 15%–25% of children and adolescents with Down syndrome have behavioral or emotional problems that lead to adaptive impairment or interference with learning (Dykens & Kasari, 1997; Gath & Gumley, 1986; Meyers & Pueschel, 1991; Pueschel, Bernier, & Pezzullo, 1991). Primary problems include disruptive disorders such as attention-deficit/hyperactivity disorder (ADHD), oppositional defiant disorder, and conduct disorder; less frequently, anxiety disorders are seen. Interestingly, autism is rarely found in children with Down syndrome; a review of prevalence studies revealed only a 1%–2% overlap between the two disorders (Dykens & Volkmar, 1997).

Externalizing types of problems thus predominate in childhood, and these observations are seen as well on the Child Behavior Checklist, which we administered to parents of 155 children and adolescents with Down syndrome (Dykens, Shah, King, & Rosner, 1999). Table 3.5 presents those maladaptive behaviors seen in 40% or more of the sample. Although 60%–75% of these individuals had difficulties concentrating and were disobedient, stubborn, and argumentative, only 30%–35% were hyperactive or had temper tantrums.

Certain maladaptive problems appear to shift over the course of development (Dykens et al., 1999). Although based on cross-sectional data, we found robust declines across the childhood years of day- and night-time wetting, and overactivity. In contrast, remarkable stability was seen in disobedience at home, impulsiveness, stubbornness, attention-seeking, and difficulty in concentrating. Finally, two types of problems seemed to emerge from younger to older age groups: underactivity and a proneness for being overweight; and withdrawal, lability, irritability, sulking, whining, and obsessive thinking.

Depression　　Age-related increases in internalizing symptoms may be harbingers of later-onset depression (see also Dykens & Kasari, 1997). Indeed, unlike the externalizing difficulties of childhood, adults with Down syndrome seem most prone to depressive disorders (Collacott,

Table 3.4. Main studies of psychopathology in Down syndrome

Study	N	Ages	% Psychopathology	Main Problems
Children				
Gath & Gumley, 1986	193	6–17 years	34%	Conduct disorder = 10.9%; childhood psychosis = 8.8%; hyperkinetic conduct disorder = 7.25%; mixed conduct/emotional disorder = 4.6%
Meyers & Pueschel, 1991	261	<20 years	17.6%	Attention deficit disorder = 6.1%; aggression = 6.5%; conduct or oppositional deficit disorder = 5.4%; stereotypies = 2.7%
Adults				
Collacott, Cooper, & McGrother, 1992	378	>16 years	25.9%	Depression = 11.3%; conduct disorder = 6.2% pre-senile dementia = 4.3%
Meyers & Pueschel, 1991	164	>20 years	25.6%	Major depressive episode = 6.1; aggression = 6.1%; stereotypies = 4.3%; Attention deficit disorder = 2.4%

Table 3.5.　Percentages of 155 children and adults with Down syndrome (mean age = 10 years) showing maladaptive behavior on the Child Behavior Checklist

Behavior	Percentage
Speech problems	90
Stubborn	75
Disobedient at home	73
Can't concentrate	66
Disobedient at school	62
Argues a lot	62
Prefers playing with younger kids	53
Demands attention	52
Impulsive	50
Would rather be alone than with others	48
Shy, timid	45
Clumsy	45
Daydreams	40

From Dykens, Shah, King, & Rosner, 1999.

et al. 1992; Meyers & Pueschel, 1991; Warren, Holroyd, & Folstein, 1989). Prevalence rates of depression in adults with Down syndrome range from 6% to 11%, many times higher than the rates found in people with mental retardation in general (Collacott et al., 1992; Meyers & Pueschel, 1991).

Depression in Down syndrome is often characterized by passivity, apathy, withdrawal, disorganized thinking, and mutism. Curiously, unipolar depression predominantes, and bipolar disorder, or alternating periods of depression and mania, is rarely ever seen. Down syndrome may even confer some protective advantage against mania (Craddock & Owen, 1994; Sovner, Hurley, & Labrie, 1985). Although more research is needed, it is noteworthy that, in a syndrome in which 10% of adults suffer from affective disorders, very few present with mania.

Although more research is needed, it is noteworthy that, in a syndrome in which 10% of adults suffer from affective disorders, very few present with mania.

Dementia　Given the clinical overlap between depression and dementia, difficulties often arise in distinguishing these two disorders. In some cases, depression and dementia may co-exist, while in others those diagnosed with depression may actually be showing early signs of dementia (e.g., Pary, 1992; Szymanski & Biederman, 1984). In still other individuals, diagnoses of dementia may overshadow a depressive condition. Indeed, Warren et al. (1989) reported five cases in which adults with Down syndrome were referred for apparent dementia but were instead successfully treated for depression.

To improve differential diagnoses, more accurate criteria are needed for adults with mental retardation and depression versus dementia, in all of its phases of decline. This recommendation becomes even more daunting in light of new findings on behavioral differences in older adults with dementia and Down syndrome compared to adults with dementia and mental retardation due to other causes (Cooper & Prasher, 1998). Adults with dementia and Down syndrome were more apt to have a depressed mood, auditory hallucinations, sleep disturbance, and restlessness; and although they were more uncooperative, they showed less aggression than their counterparts. These depression-like symptoms among Down syndrome adults with dementia underscore the difficulties in teasing apart the symptoms of these two disorders.

INTERACTIONAL AND FAMILY ISSUES

Much of the literature on interactions and families in the mental retardation field has focused on Down syndrome. The preponderance of family studies on Down syndrome may be another indicator that this particular syndrome, more than any other, has come to represent all children with mental retardation in the minds of both researchers and laypeople alike.

Mother–Child Interactions

Two traditions underlie work in the area of mother–child interactions. The first begins with Solnit and Stark's (1961) view that mothers of children with disabilities mourn the loss of the perfect baby. According to this view, mothers of children with disabilities differ from mothers of typically developing children. They may be more intrusive, didactic, directive, and concerned about giving their infant every possible chance to develop intellectually. Mothers of infants without mental retardation, in contrast, are much less worried, and as a result, they tend to be more playful and less didactic.

In general, such stylistic differences have been noted in most mother–infant interactional studies. Compared with mothers of children without mental retardation, mothers of children who have Down syndrome take interactive turns that are longer and more frequent (Tannock, 1988). Similarly, these mothers clash—or speak at the same time as—their infants more frequently than do mothers of infants without mental retardation (Vietze, Abernathy, Ashe, & Faulstich, 1978). Mothers of children with Down syndrome (and with other developmental disabilities) thus engage in asymmetrical patterns of interaction, themselves performing more of the actions—and allowing their infants less chance to initiate. As one mother of a child with Down syndrome noted: "It's sit him on your knee and talk to him, that's the main object. Play with him, speak to the child, teach him something" (Jones, 1980, p. 221). But a second tradition does not find differences between mothers of children with and without Down syndrome. Specifically, once matched to children without mental retardation on overall levels of language (e.g., MLU), mothers of children with Down syndrome provide appropriate levels of input language (Rondal, 1977). The length of the mother's utterances, their complexity, informational content, and other, more structural aspects all seem appropriate to the child's levels of language.

How, then, can one reconcile these conflicting reports of interactions between mothers and their young children with Down syndrome? Although seemingly contradictory, both may apply to mother–child interactions (Hodapp, 1995). Styles of communication indeed differ, as mothers of children with Down syndrome are generally more didactic, intrusive, and directive. At the same time, however, these mothers also provide appropriate levels of language input to their children.

An additional question concerns the effects of such a "same but different" interactive pattern. Whereas several professionals have developed interventions designed to help mothers of children with disabilities to become less directive (e.g., Mahoney, 1988), others question the degree to which "directiveness" is a unitary construct (Marfo, 1990, 1992). Harris, Kasari, and Sigman (1996) found that fewer maternal directive behaviors within a particular context at one session predicted their young child with Down syndrome's language levels at a second session 13 months later. Mothers who maintained their child's attention to a toy had children with higher receptive language ages than did the children of mothers who redirected their child's attention from one toy to another. Indeed, the importance of joint attention—of both the child and mothers attending to the same object or event—seems particularly important for the language development of children with Down syndrome (Harris et al. 1996). Emphasizing the specific context surrounding a maternal behavior, not just the behavior itself, seems an important consideration that is only now being examined.

Families

Since the mid-1980s, research on the families of children with disabilities has exploded (see Hodapp, 1995, for a review). Although a complete overview of family research is beyond the scope of this chapter, one aspect—the effects of the child's characteristics on family functioning—deserves our attention. In short, are families of children with Down syndrome—compared with families of children with mental retardation or with disabilities more generally—differently affected? If so, what aspects of the child with Down syndrome relate to parental and family reactions?

Coping As Table 3.6 illustrates, many studies find that families of children with Down syndrome cope better than do families of children with other disabilities. Such studies span a variety of age groups and comparison groups: younger (Kasari & Sigman, 1997) or older (Holroyd & MacArthur, 1976) children with autism, young children with other types of developmental disabilities (Erikson & Upshure, 1989), adolescents with emotional disturbance (Thomas & Olsen, 1993), and adults with other types of mental retardation (Seltzer, Krauss, & Tsunematsu, 1993). Additional studies find other advantages. In fact, Mink, Nihira, and Meyers (1983) found that almost two thirds of "cohesive harmonious" families—their most desirable family type—included children with Down syndrome, a much larger percentage than in the sample as a whole.

Yet another area of family research involves the siblings of children with Down syndrome. In two large-scale studies, siblings were found to have few interpersonal problems with their brothers or sisters with Down syndrome (Byrne, Cunningham, & Sloper, 1988; Carr, 1995). In her study, Carr compared quarrels in sibling dyads when the index child (the child with Down syndrome versus the typically developing child) was 11 years of age. She noted that 37% of the siblings with Down syndrome had no quarrels and 44% had some quarrels; these compare with 18% of control siblings with no quarrels and 54% with some quarrels. "The picture is then of quite harmonious relationships between the young people with Down's syndrome and their sibs" (Carr, 1995, p. 122).

A Down Syndrome Advantage? Why do parents, families, and siblings appear to react well to children with Down syndrome? One set of explanations may rest in factors that surround the syndrome. Down syndrome is prevalent, is widely recognized by the public, and is the focus of many successful parent support groups. Furthermore, although in total more Down syndrome births occur to younger (i.e., less

Table 3.6. Studies of families of offspring with Down syndrome

Study	Groups examined	Offspring ages	Findings
Erikson & Upshure, 1989	Down syndrome, motor-impaired, and developmentally delayed	<2 years	DS mothers: greater satisfaction with support from friends and community groups
Kasari & Sigman, 1997	DS, autism, mental retardation, and controls— all mental age-matched	3–5 years	DS = controls; both show less parental stress than autistic or MR
Holroyd & MacArthur, 1976	DS, autism and outpatient	3–12 years	Less parental stress in DS versus others
Mink, Nihira, & Meyers, 1983	Severe to profound mental retardation	12 years	Two-thirds of families in DS groups were "cohesive-harmonious"
Thomas & Olsen, 1993	Emotionally disturbed	13–18 years	DS identical to controls on family coherence, adaptibility, and communication (better than 2 emotionally disturbed groups)
Seltzer, Krauss & Tsunematsu, 1993	MR	35 years	mothers of DS (vs. other MR) = less caregiving stress and burden, less family conflict, more satisfying social networks

From Hodapp, R. M. [1996]. Down syndrome: Developmental, psychiatric, and management issues. *Child and Adolescent Psychiatric Clinics of North America, 5*, p.887; reprinted by permission.

than 35 years) than older mothers, it may be that some mothers of children with Down syndrome are "older and wiser," and more financially stable, than are mothers of children with other types of disabilities (Cahill & Glidden, 1996). Cultural familiarity, support, and more mature mothers may thus partly account for the Down syndrome advantage.

Another set of reasons why families of children with Down syndrome cope so well rests in the children themselves. Such child-related characteristics would be in line with the indirect effects of genetic disorders that we have discussed in Chapter 1. Three distinct qualities of these children likely contribute to improved family functioning. First, as previously discussed, many children with Down syndrome have a sociable orientation and upbeat, if not "charming" personality. In particular, as mentioned previously in this chapter, children with Down syndrome look to others more than to objects, "half-smile" more often, and use their sociable "party tricks" to avoid performing difficult tasks. Furthermore, they are generally perceived by others as cheerful and lovable. Second, also as noted previously, children with Down syndrome have fewer maladaptive behaviors than do others, as well as less serious psychopathology. These children are more apt to show attention problems, disobedience, and a stubborn streak than severe psychopathology (e.g., autism) or acting-out behaviors such as temper tantrums.

A final possible explanation for the Down syndrome advantage is that children with Down syndrome may also possess a less mature, baby-like facial appearance. Such faces, called "babyfaces," generally involve a more pug-like nose (with a "sunken bridge"), a rounder face, lower placements of features on the face (due to a larger forehead), and smaller features (Zebrowitz, 1997). Most children with Down syndrome have such faces. Allanson, O'Hara, Farkas, and Nair (1993) found that compared with the faces of age- and sex-matched typically developing children, the faces of Down syndrome children characteristically show 1) a striking negative nasal protrusion (akin to Zebrowitz's "sunken bridge"), 2) reduced ear length (i.e., "smaller features"), 3) reduced mouth width (i.e., "smaller mouth"), and 4) a head length shorter than the width (i.e., "rounder face").

More importantly than the face itself, however, are the many traits that adult observers attributed to people with babyfaces. This "baby-face overgeneralization" yields positive reactions to "individuals whose appearance merely resembles" an infant in some way (Zebrowitz, 1997, p. 56). Across numerous studies, observers attributed higher ratings of warmth, weakness, and naiveté to pictures of adult faces with babylike features (Zebrowitz & Montepare, 1992). When individuals have these features, others perceive them as dependent and give them warm and protective responses (Zebrowitz, Kendall-Tackett, & Fafel, 1991).

One study showed that adults react to faces of children with Down syndrome as they would to faces of younger children. Fidler and Hodapp (1999) showed college undergraduates three sets of faces: one of children with Down syndrome, one of children with 5p- syndrome (who generally have longer, more angular, adult-like faces), and one of typically developing children. Each set consisted of one 8-year-old, one 10-year-old, and one 12-year-old. Respondents rated each face on the degree to which the face appeared physically babylike, was likely to have babylike traits (warmth, naïveté, kindness, honesty), and was likely to display babylike behaviors (someone who would cuddle with his or her mother, be compliant to others, or believe a far-fetched story).

Respondents rated the Down syndrome faces as younger looking, more dependent, and more likely to engage in immature behaviors. At every age, raters judged faces of children with Down syndrome as more immature in both traits and behaviors. Combining across the three ages, Figure 3.2 shows the degree to which raters considered children with Down syndrome (compared to typical children or children with 5p- syndrome) as being warmer, kinder, more honest, and more naïve. Although this study needs to be extended to more "real-world" settings, the degree to which children with Down syndrome appear babyfaced seems to readily influence the reactions and perceptions of others.

Although this study needs to be extended to more "real-world" settings, the degree to which children with Down syndrome appear babyfaced seems to readily influence the reactions and perceptions of others.

INTERVENTION IMPLICATIONS

Education

The first important educational issue involves the "what" of intervention. What strategies have or should be attempted with these children, and to what effect? In addition to more standard intervention services, recent interest in Down syndrome has revolved around sign language training during the early years, and reading instruction during the school-age period.

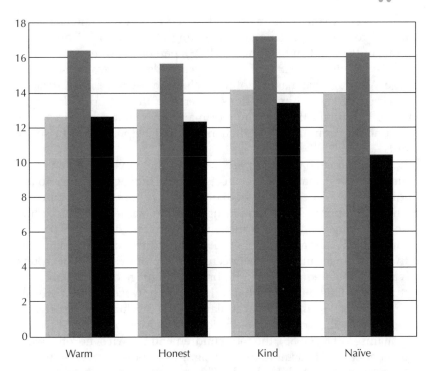

Figure 3.2. Trait ratings of faces of children with 5p- syndrome, Down syndrome, and same-age typical children. (Key: ▨ = 5p- syndrome, ▨ = Down syndrome, ■ = same-age typical children.)

Sign Language Because children with Down syndrome eventually speak, it may seem strange to teach sign language. Yet sign language—or, more precisely, *total communication* (signing and using speech simultaneously)—may prove especially helpful given the linguistic difficulties experienced by children with this disorder. If articulation and verbal expression both are problematic for these children, manual signs may prove easier to acquire. Moreover, Harris et al. (1997) found that children with Down syndrome were at the 75th–80th percentile in gestural-symbolic behaviors relative to typical children of the same language age. Thus, manual signs may provide a bridge into verbal language, especially for children with Down syndrome. (Abrahamsen, Cavallo, & McCluer, 1985).

> *Thus, manual signs may provide a bridge into verbal language, especially for children with Down syndrome.*

In recent years, then, many early intervention programs have attempted to teach sign language to young children with Down syndrome. In Pueschel and Hopmann (1993), parents reported that 56% of 1- to 3-year-olds and 43% of 4- to 6-year-olds are learning sign language. Although the majority of these children use fewer than 10 signs in their everyday communications, parents further reported that signing was helpful for their children, primarily by making them less frustrated about communicating their needs and helping them to speak words.

In addition to parental reports, a few studies have attempted to examine more systematically the effects of sign language training. So far, findings show some, though not conclusive, support for a total communication approach. In comparing children with Down syndrome who were taught orally with those who were taught with total communication, Weller and Mahoney (1983) found few differences in cognitive or linguistic measures between the two groups, with both groups advancing about equally in cognition and language over the 5 months of the study. One difference that did emerge, however, was an advantage in the total number of vocabulary words produced (either signed or spoken) by the total communication group. Moreover, in a study by Abrahamsen et al. (1985), the four children with Down syndrome were much better able to acquire manual signs as opposed to verbal words among their earliest object labels. This pattern of sign over word acquisition was in contrast to that observed in children with other types of disabilities (mainly prematurity and hydrocephaly); the sign advantage also occurred even though interventionists generally spoke more than they signed, providing an imbalance in favor of speech in the adult linguistic input.

Sign language training, then, does not hinder children with Down syndrome and may slightly help their entrance into spoken language. Indeed, Weller and Mahoney (1983) described several children who first signed a word, then provided a sign plus the spoken word, then the spoken word alone. Although not a panacea for the expressive speech and grammatical problems of young children with Down syndrome, sign language training may still constitute an important addition to the interventionist's repertoire (Abrahamsen, Lamb, Brown-Williams, & McCarthy, 1991).

Reading Until recently, the entire literacy issue could not be examined, as few school-age children with Down syndrome were provided reading instruction. Now, however, many of these children are being taught to read. Parents report that almost half of 11- to 21-year-olds can read more than 50 words; most of these adolescents read sentences and short books and enjoy the experience of reading (Pueschel

& Hopmann, 1993). Furthermore, in a study of 24 children with Down syndrome who were being taught to read, Byrne, Buckley, MacDonald, and Bird (1995) found that reading abilities of these children were significantly ahead of abilities in other aspects of language (e.g., grammar), short-term memory, and numerical skills. Although children with Down syndrome rarely read above third- or fourth-grade levels, many accomplish the beginnings of reading ability.

A second issue pertains to *how* children with Down syndrome read. Reading (and instruction in reading) generally involves both the ability to sound out letters phonetically and to read at a glance entire words (so-called *logographic skills*). Most likely, both come into play for the accomplished reader, as one sounds out novel words (e.g., the word "logographic"), while at the same time reading as a single chunk most common words. Children may even advance from recognizing individual words, to sounding out words letter by letter, to recognizing most individual words on sight, but also sounding out words when necessary (Frith, 1985). Moreover, in typical children, use of phonetic decoding is a strong predictor of both first- and third-grade reading skills (McGuinness, 1997).

To what extent can children with Down syndrome sound out words, and to what extent are these children whole word readers? Cossu, Rossini, and Marshall (1993b) reported that children with Down syndrome can read at 7- to 8-year-old levels in the absence of phonological awareness. Such awareness involves being able to rhyme words, say how many syllables are in a word, and repeat a spoken word while deleting the first syllable. However, Cossu et al.'s claim has been challenged by several reading researchers (see Bertelson, 1993; Byrne, 1993; Morton & Frith, 1993; then Cossu et al.'s, 1993a, reply).

Part of the issue may concern the levels of reading that have been studied (Hodapp & Ly, in press). When children with Down syndrome of both lower and higher reading levels are examined, the role of phonological awareness becomes clearer. Fowler, Doherty, and Boynton (1995) examined 33 adolescents and young adults with Down syndrome whose reading ranged from kindergarten to twelfth-grade levels. In addition to general cognitive measures such as the K-ABC (Kaufman & Kaufman, 1983) and the Peabody Picture Vocabulary Test-Revised (PPVT–R; Dunn & Dunn, 1981), Fowler et al. also gave their subjects the Woodcock Reading Mastery Tests–Revised (Woodcock, 1987), as well as tests of phonemic awareness, verbal memory span, word retrieval, visual memory, and auditory comprehension of language.

In contrast to the findings of Cossu et al. (1993b), Fowler et al. (1995) found clear relationships between reading abilities and several other measures. Even after accounting for general levels of ability (using the K-ABC and PPVT–R), these researchers found that phonemic awareness accounts for high percentages of the variance in reading tasks such as word recognition (49% of variance) and decoding (36%). In addition, both visual short-term memory and digit span (i.e., auditory short-term memory) also correlated with higher levels of reading. In a similar study using nonword repetition as the phonemic task for children ages 5–18 years, Laws (1998) found a similar relationship between nonword repetition and reading ability (the K-ABC's reading-decoding subtest). Again, more than 30% of the variance was accounted for by the phonemic test, even after controlling for the children's ages and nonverbal abilities.

Moreover, the relationship between phonemic awareness and reading may constitute a "necessary but not sufficient" condition. As Fowler et al. noted, "No person in our study achieved decoding skills beyond the first-grade level without answering at least 10 items correctly [from among 40] on our phoneme awareness measure" (1995, p. 191). Similarly, "No one achieved beyond the third-grade decoding level without responding correctly to at least half of the phonemic awareness items" (p. 192).

Although the issue of reading in Down syndrome has devolved into a highly technical argument among reading researchers, all agree that many children with Down syndrome can achieve preliminary levels in reading. Less clear is how far children with Down syndrome can progress in reading, how best to teach it, and how reading skills (at both lower and higher levels) relate to these children's generally poor phonological skills. Despite such unresolved issues, instruction in reading constitutes an important intervention for school-age children with Down syndrome.

What Is the Best Educational Setting?   In addition to the "what" of intervention, additional questions revolve around the placement, or where intervention takes place. In recent years, this "where" question has dominated American special education, possibly to the detriment of the more important issues of what takes place within any setting.

In Down syndrome, preliminary evidence suggests that these children may indeed perform better when in inclusive schools versus more restrictive placements. Sloper, Cunningham, Turner, and Knussen (1990) examined the academic performance of 123 British 6- to 14-year-olds with Down syndrome. Although MA was by far the best predictor of academic performance (accounting for more than 60% of the variance), other factors were also important. Chief among these was whether the child attended an inclusive classroom or a special, segregated school. Even after accounting for MA, a small but significant amount of the variance (about 6%) was attributable to general education class placement. In addition, girls performed better than did boys academically, and academic achievement was also affected slightly by the fathers' more internal locus of control (i.e., fathers' sense that their successes and failures were under their own control).

In considering where children with Down syndrome receive their education, few studies yet exist on parental desires. Only one, by Freeman, Kasari, and Alkin (1999), asked parents directly about their educational preferences for their preschool and school-age children. Parents overwhelmingly preferred a fully inclusive classroom for their child with Down syndrome but at the same time a classroom that provided their child with additional help as needed. Compared with children with Prader-Willi syndrome, parents of children with Down syndrome were also much more concerned about their children attending the local school (Hodapp, Freeman, & Kasari, 1998). Furthermore, parents less enthusiastically supported full inclusion as their children got older; it may indeed be that parents increasingly feel that their child's academic needs require more intensive educational interventions.

Recreation and Friendships

Optimizing the recreation and leisure options of people with mental retardation is of keen interest to many interventionists, particularly with respect to increased choice, inclusion, and self-determination. Despite these conceptual advances, surprisingly few studies have documented exactly how people with Down syndrome make use of leisure time, develop hobbies or interests, or make friends.

Despite these conceptual advances, surprisingly few studies have documented exactly how people with Down syndrome make use of leisure time, develop hobbies or interests, or make friends.

Comparing social competence in 32 children with Down syndrome versus Williams syndrome, we found elevated scores in the Down syndrome group on both the activity and social domains of the Child Behavior Checklist (Hodapp et al., 2000). As a group, children with Down syndrome were more likely than their counterparts were to perform well in diverse jobs or chores, to participate in clubs or organizations, to engage in pretend play, and to get along with their peers. Examining friendships, Freeman and Kasari (1999) found that while most children with Down syndrome had at least one friend, the quality of these friendships was best among dyads of a similar age, gender, and MA level. Furthermore, we found that the maladaptive behavior of children with Down syndrome more adversely affected their social relationships than other recreational activities (Hodapp et al., 2000).

Compared with even a decade ago, more diverse avenues exist for promoting friendships, recreation, and social competence of people with mental retardation, from enrolling in community-based arts programs to attending the movies. For those with sports interests, Special Olympics International provides a wealth of options, from sport and play readiness programs for young children, to competitive sports involving people with or without mental retardation, to more low-key, age-appropriate sports for elderly athletes.

Special Olympics is the largest volunteer sports program for people with mental retardation in the world, and on two fronts, it is of particular relevance for those with Down syndrome. First, as previously reviewed, people with Down syndrome are particularly prone to obesity, and physicians consistently recommend that people with this syndrome both watch their diet and engage in a sustained program of regular exercise or physical activity (e.g., Roizen, Luke, Sutton, & Schoeller, 1995). To this aim, Special Olympics has a long and successful history of meeting the physical fitness needs of athletes with Down syndrome (Songster, Smith, Evans, Munson, & Behen, 1997). Second, we found that participation in Special Olympics is associated with improved social competence in jobs, chores, peer relations, and other nonsports activities, as well as with enhanced self-esteem (Dykens & Cohen, 1996). For both improved physical fitness and psychosocial adjustment, then, many children and adults with Down syndrome benefit from enrollment in Special Olympics. The enthusiasm, determination, and joy of these athletes are aptly demonstrated in Figure 3.3.

Employment and Residential Issues

Few studies have specifically examined the working and living arrangements of adults with Down syndrome; however, a general sense persists that these adults do well in more community-based settings. Even casual observers note the presence of adults with Down syndrome working in a variety of unskilled or semiskilled jobs, such as at fast-food restaurants or as custodians. Similarly, as a group, people with this disorder may do well in more community-based residences.

Although most studies focus only on mixed groups, Carr (1994) summarized three large-scale British studies that examined the life outcomes of adults with Down syndrome. She noted that from 70% to 90% of adults with Down syndrome attend adult centers (i.e., sheltered work-

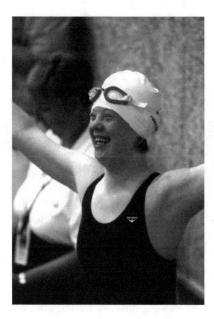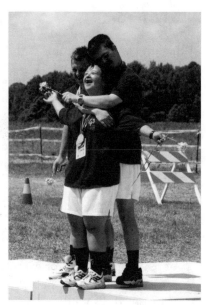

Figure 3.3. Athletes with Down syndrome participating in Special Olympics.

shops), with relatively small numbers (a quarter or less) participating in full- or part-time paid jobs in the private sector. Further, Lane (1985) noted that these adults have difficulties securing employment due to their appearance, slowness or lack of skills, difficulties in using public transportation to get to their jobs, and a general discrimination on the part of some employers to hire people with disabilities. Compared with even a decade or so ago, many of these impediments may be changing, with better adaptive and vocational training and more enlightened public attitudes allowing greater numbers of adults with Down syndrome to become productive employees.

In the same way, the residential situation may also be improving. Although Carr's (1994) review showed that from two thirds to three fourths of teens or young adults with Down syndrome live in their family homes, the percentages living in other, more independent placements may grow in coming years. Thus, although the employment and residential pictures may not be as encouraging as sometimes portrayed, adults with Down syndrome are increasingly taking active, productive roles in their communities. Such trends are expected to continue in future years.

NEXT STEPS

Although Down syndrome is the focus of almost as many behavioral studies as all other genetic disorders combined, we still do not know much about many aspects of behavior in this syndrome. These issues, which promise to be the focus of sustained research more than the next few years, include the following:

- Is there a critical or sensitive period for the development of grammar in this population? If not, can high-level grammatical abilities be taught to teens or young adults?
- Is there a "Down syndrome personality"? What percentages of individuals might have this personality, and does this characteristic personality change with age?
- In what ways do children's characteristics such as personality, lack of psychopathology, or even facial characteristics influence others, and what are the repercussions of such effects on others' behaviors?
- Why do adults with Down syndrome show the Alzheimer's neurological plaques and tangles by age 30 or 35 but not the dementia that generally accompanies such brain changes in Alzheimer's adults without mental retardation?
- Are interventions in reading and in total communication more effective in the education of children with Down syndrome than other, non–visually-based approaches?

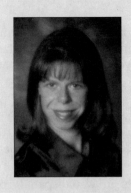

4

Williams Syndrome

Remarkable progress has been made to further our understanding of the genetic and neurological correlates of many of Williams syndrome's physical and behavioral features.

Relative to other syndromes featured in this book, Williams syndrome leads the way as the one receiving the most scrutiny from cognitive scientists, linguists, and neuropsychologists. In a flurry of recent papers on Williams syndrome, professionals in these disciplines have described it has having an unusual cognitive-linguistic profile, initially thought to involve impairments in visual-spatial functioning and *spared*, or near-typical, expressive language, even in the face of global mental retardation. Although the details of this cognitive-linguistic profile are now under considerable debate, researchers generally agree that people with Williams syndrome show unique areas of strength and impairment.

In contrast to cognitive and linguistic functioning, relatively few studies have examined the adaptive and maladaptive features of Williams syndrome or the syndrome's characteristic over-friendly personality. This extreme sociability was first observed some 35 years ago by cardiologist Alois Beuren, one of the first to discover the syndrome. Even so, remarkable progress has been made to further our understanding of the genetic and neurological correlates of many of Williams syndrome's physical and behavioral features. As described in this chapter, we now know that many people with Williams syndrome

- Show a proclivity for musical talent and an increased interest in music
- Have strengths in the ability to recognize faces and express themselves verbally
- Typically show pronounced impairments in visual-spatial construction tasks
- Have a paradoxical set of social findings—a friendly or even empathic approach to others on one hand and marked difficulty making and keeping friends on the other hand
- Exhibit very high rates of anxiety, fears, and phobias

After reviewing the genetic, diagnostic, and physical features of Williams syndrome, this chapter examines these and other complexities of the Williams syndrome behavioral phenotype.

HISTORICAL BACKGROUND

Williams syndrome was first identified in the 1960s by two independent teams of physicians: Williams, Barrett-Boyes, and Lowe (1961) in New Zealand and Beuren, Apitz, and Harmjanz (1962) in Germany. Collectively, these physicians described a small group of individuals who showed mental retardation, distinctive facial features, and a cardiac anomaly called supravalvular aortic stenosis (SVAS)—a narrowing of the arteries that reduces blood flow. Most of the early studies of Williams-Beuren syndrome—now commonly referred to as Williams syndrome in the United States—focused on its medical manifestations, including cardiac disease and other problems such as infantile hypercalcemia, or elevated blood calcium levels. Yet, even some of these early medical researchers informally observed that many individuals with Williams syndrome were highly verbal, loquacious, and overly friendly (e.g., Jones & Smith, 1975; Von Armin & Engel, 1964).

The genetic etiology of Williams syndrome remained unknown until the early 1990s, when several key discoveries were made. First, several families were described by Morris, Thomas, and Greenberg (1993) as having parent-to-child transmission of Williams syndrome. These families showed an autosomal dominant pattern, meaning that the parents had a 50% chance of transmitting the disorder to their offspring. Although the presence of Williams syndrome in parents in these families went undetected until their children were diagnosed, additional cases have now been identified of both men and women with known diagnoses of Williams syndrome who have transmitted the syndrome to their offspring.

Another atypical family, described by Morris, Locker, Ensing, and Stock in 1993, helped narrow the search for the possible genetic cause of Williams syndrome. This family had SVAS due to a translocation involving chromosome 7 that resulted in a disruption of the gene for elastin, or ELN (see Chapter 2). As SVAS is common in Williams syndrome, anomalies in ELN emerged as a promising etiological hypothesis in this disorder. Subsequently, Ewart and colleagues (1993) found that individuals with Williams syndrome invariably had a micro-deletion on the long arm of one of their chromosome 7s, at 7q11.23, which included the gene for elastin.

GENETICS AND PHYSICAL FEATURES

Elastin is a connective tissue protein that provides strength and elasticity to the skin, blood vessels, and the walls of organs and arteries. Deletion of the elastin gene on one of the chromosome 7s is now thought to be responsible for the SVAS and other cardiovascular diseases in individuals with Williams syndrome (Tassabehji et al., 1999). Insufficiency of elastin may also be implicated in other medical or physical features and conditions, such as premature aging of the skin, a hoarse voice, full cheeks, and a tendency to develop hernias and bladder diverticulae.

Willams syndrome is now considered a contiguous gene deletion syndrome, meaning that many adjacent genes deleted in the critical region on chromosome 7 contribute to the Williams syndrome phenotype. To date, 13 genes have been identified in the relatively large region (1.5 megabases) of chromosome 7 that is missing in people with Williams syndrome (see Bellugi, Lichtenberger, Mills, Galaburda, & Korenberg, 1999, for a review). Aside from ELN, the phenotypic significance of these other genes, then, is still unknown.

> *Willams syndrome is now considered a contiguous gene deletion syndrome, meaning that many adjacent genes deleted in the critical region on chromosome 7 contribute to the Williams syndrome phenotype.*

One of these genes, however, called LIM-kinase 1 (LIMK1), has generated considerable debate as to its role in the Williams syndrome cognitive phenotype. LIMK1 encodes a protein, kinase, that is expressed in the developing brain. In 1996, Frangiskakis et al. reported two individuals with rare so-called partial Williams syndrome deletions. These individuals had SVAS and impaired visual-spatial construction abilities, but no other features of Williams syndrome, such as mental retardation or hypercalcemia. Genetically, these individuals were missing the elastin gene and LIMK1, and, as best as the researchers could determine, no other genes. Hemizygosity of LIMK1 (i.e., having just one LIMK1 gene) emerged as a promising hypothesis to explain the specific impairments in visual-spatial construction in Williams syndrome.

In contrast, however, Tassabehji et al. (1999) found no such association in three individuals with partial deletions in the Williams syndrome region. These individuals showed deletions of variable sizes that included ELN and LIMK1, and although all had SVAS, none showed weaknesses in their visual-spatial construction abilities, nor did they manifest other features of the Williams syndrome cognitive profile. These authors concluded that the LIMK1 deletion may be unrelated to the Williams syndrome cognitive profile or that the deletion of this gene is a necessary but not sufficient condition for the Williams syndrome cognitive profile. It will prove challenging for researchers to clarify these conflicting reports, as cases with partial Williams syndrome deletions are quite rare.

Diagnosis

Williams syndrome occurs in approximately 1 per 20,000 people; it is equally prevalent in males as in females and in all races and cultures of the world. Unlike other disorders, such as Prader-Willi or Angelman syndromes, Williams syndrome does not have a parent-of-origin effect; the deletion on chromosome 7 is just as likely to be transmitted through the mother or father. Furthermore, the risk that a healthy couple without Williams syndrome would have more than one child with Williams syndrome is low because Williams syndrome occurs sporadically in the general population. As previously noted, however, there is a 50% chance that a male or female with Williams syndrome could transmit the disorder to his or her offspring.

Children with Williams syndrome are typically identified as a result of their SVAS or other cardiac problems, developmental delay, and infantile hypercalcemia as well as a characteristic facial appearance that becomes more obvious with age. Increasingly, older children are also referred for a Williams syndrome evaluation as a result of their behavioral features, primarily their cognitive profile and their tendency to be overfriendly.

Once a diagnosis is suspected, a fluorescent in situ hybridization, or FISH, test is typically performed. As described in Chapter 2, a FISH test can detect submicroscopic deletions that are too small to be picked up with more standard cytogenetic procedures. With the FISH technique, the ELN gene is marked with a fluorescent probe; in Williams syndrome just one of the chromosome 7s "lights up" or shows the florescent ELN marker. By examining FISH results from hundreds of people, it is now known that the ELN deletion is found in virtually all (97%) individuals with classic Williams syndrome (e.g., Lowery et al., 1995). Laboratory testing for the ELN deletion is widely available, and it is also more objective than a clinical diagnosis alone. As a result, children with Williams syndrome are likely to be accurately diagnosed at younger ages, allowing their families to take better advantage of available treatments and supports.

Facial Features

Although the facial features in Williams syndrome are distinctive, they are not readily apparent in infants until approximately 6 months of age

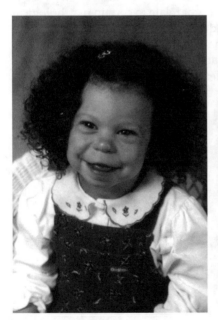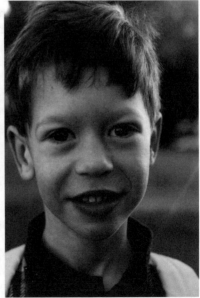

Figure 4.1. Facial features of two children with Williams syndrome.

(Morris, Demsey, Leonard, Dilts, & Blackburn, 1988). As shown in Figure 4.1, children with Williams syndrome typically have a short, upturned nose; long philtrum (groove under the nose); broad forehead with bitemporal narrowing; full cheeks; puffiness under the eyes; and prominent earlobes. In previous years, many workers described the face as "elfin-like," and this disorder was even nicknamed the "Elfin-Facies" syndrome. Yet, this reference to a mythical character is now considered out-dated as well as pejorative.

Instead, the faces of children with Williams syndrome seem better characterized as very appealing and cute. Indeed, the appealing faces of children with Williams syndrome may contribute to their ability to elicit positive social interactions from others. As demonstrated in Figure 4.2, as people with Williams syndrome age, their facial features generally coarsen—their faces become more narrow; the neck appears longer; dental malocclusion or crowding is more prominent; and the tip of the nose becomes more bulbous (Morris et al., 1988; Morris, Leonard, & Dilts, 1990).

Medical Features

Williams syndrome is a "multisystem" disorder with several severe medical complications. We highlight here some of these medical concerns; later, how medical problems might relate to certain psychological issues in people with Williams syndrome.

Cardiac SVAS is seen in as many as 60% of people with Williams syndrome and may co-occur with another cardiac problem, peripheral pulmonary stenosis. Wessel and colleagues (1994) found that the severity

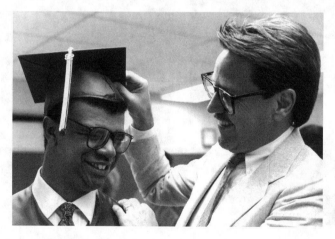

Figure 4.2. Facial features of an adolescent with Williams syndrome.

of peripheral pulmonary disease decreases over time, whereas the course of SVAS appears more variable. Severe cardiac disease, seen in approximately 30% of children with Williams syndrome, may worsen with time, with severe disease often manifesting before a child is 10 years of age (Bockoven, Kaplan, Namey, & Gleasal, 1997). Because of the prevalence of these conditions, all people with Williams syndrome should be monitored by a cardiologist over their life span (Lashkari, Smith, & Graham, 1999).

Increased risks of hypertension have also been observed; in one study as many as 40% of 140 children and adults with Williams syndrome showed hypertension (Wessel, Pankau, Berdau, & Leons, 1997). Others, however, suggest that high blood pressure may be artificially inflated due to rigidity of the arterial walls (Broder, Reinhardt, Lifton, Timborlane, & Pober, 1995). Some individuals may also show "white-coat hypertension," or elevated blood pressure readings as a result of medically related fears; indeed, medical fears are seen in as many as 90% of individuals with Williams syndrome (Dykens, 2000). One study, however, circumvented possible white-coat hypertension by using 24-hour ambulatory blood pressure monitoring in 20 individuals with Williams syndrome (Broder et al., 1999). Still, compared with healthy controls, those with Williams syndrome were more likely to show hypertension, and such differences were particularly striking among children. Approximately half of children with Williams syndrome had hypertension as opposed to 6% of typical children. Broder et al. (1999) cautioned that elevated blood pressure readings in the office setting should not be dismissed as a by-product of medical anxiety. Hypertension needs to be carefully monitored in individuals with Williams syndrome over the long term.

Musculoskeletal Many infants and young children with Williams syndrome show hyperextensible joints, as well as decreased muscle tone; these conditions may be associated with delays in walking. Older children and adults often show increased muscle tone (Chapman, De Plessis, & Pober, 1996), and both children and adults are prone to joint contractures (permanent muscular contractions) in the wrist, elbows, hands, hips, knees, and ankles (Chapman et al., 1996; Kaplan, Kirschner, Watters, & Costa, 1989). Such problems are likely associated with leg pain and cramping as well as with gait abnormalities and difficulties with fine and gross motor coordination. Clumsiness and gait and coordination problems have been observed in from 50% to 85% of different samples of individuals with Williams syndrome (Chapman et al., 1996; Kaplan et al., 1989).

Gastrointestinal/Renal Although Williams syndrome was once termed "idiopathic hypercalcemia" disease, elevated blood calcium levels are seen in only 15% of infants and young children with Williams sydrome (Morris et al., 1988). When present, however, hypercalcemia is associated with constipation and abdominal pain, and a low-calcium diet is often warranted (Martin, Snodgrass, & Cohen, 1984). As many as 70% of infants with Williams syndrome show colic, feeding difficulties, reflux, and vomiting, which is often associated with a period of failure to thrive. Adults are prone to abdominal pain, which may be related to chronic constipation, peptic ulcers, or diverticulitis (Nicholson & Hockey, 1993). Abdominal pain should be thoroughly assessed, as appropriate treatment often provides symptomatic relief.

Renal problems are seen in approximately 18% of people with Williams syndrome. Common problems include bladder diverticula, renal hypoplasia, renal artery stenosis, and urinary tract infections, especially among adults (Pankau, Partsch, Winter, Gosch, & Wessel, 1996; Pober et al., 1993). Further, urinary frequency and enuresis are seen in 50% or more of children with Williams syndrome (Morris et al., 1988). Routine renal ultrasounds and urinary analyses are recommended at regular intervals for children and adults (Lashkari et al., 1999).

Growth   Although infants often have lower-than-expected birth weights and smaller head circumferences, they often catch up to the low–typical range by middle childhood (Morris et al., 1988). Even so, short stature is seen in about 50% of people with Williams syndrome, with many adults ending up in the lower end of the typical range for height. Unlike individuals with other disorders, such as Prader-Willi syndrome, individuals with Williams syndrome do not appear to have growth hormone deficiencies (Partsch, Pankau, Blum, Gosch, & Wessel, 1994). Weight may also lag behind in the early years due to infantile failure to thrive, but most adolescents and adults are of typical weight. As with other syndromes (e.g., fragile X, Down, Prader-Willi), growth curves are now available based exclusively on children with Williams syndrome (Partsch et al., 1999).

Vision   Strabismus (e.g., crossed eyes) is a common problem in children with Williams syndrome. In one study, as many as 54% of 152 individuals with the syndrome had strabismus (Winter, Pankau, Amm, Gosch, & Wessel, 1996). Strabismus is treated using routine interventions such as corrective lenses, patches, or surgery. Farsightedness is also common, seen in 25%–50% of the population. As described later, visual-spatial construction tasks are quite challenging for people with Williams syndrome, yet it is unknown how these difficulties relate to visual problems. Most people with Williams syndrome—up to 75%—show a distinctive stellate iris pattern, involving a white lacy or starburst pattern (Winter et al., 1996). Although this "sparkly" look to individuals' eyes is unrelated to vision, they often increase the suspicion of a Williams syndrome diagnosis in clinical evaluations.

Auditory As many as 95% of people with Williams syndrome have hyperacusis, or hypersensitivity to sound (Van Borsel, Curfs, & Fryns, 1997). Hyperacusis may be manifested as an individual's increased startle-and-avoidance (e.g., covering ears) reaction to certain sounds, as well as his or her tendency to hear things well before others do. Leading culprits for offensive sounds include motors or engines of power saws, drills, airplanes, and vacuum cleaners, as well as sirens, firecrackers, and bells (Van Borsel et al., 1997). Also, up to 60% of children may suffer from chronic otitis media, or ear infections, which may necessitate the placement of tympanostomy tubes (Klein, Armstrong, Greer, & Brown, 1990). As with the general population, occurrences of otitis media tend to decrease with age. Furthermore, many parents observe that their children have fewer acute reactions to sound over the course of development (Klein et al., 1990; Van Borsel et al., 1997).

COGNITION AND LANGUAGE

Cognitive-Linguistic Functioning

An explosion of studies has refined the cognitive and linguistic profile associated with Williams syndrome. These studies have evolved from fairly general observations based on IQ tests to detailed analyses of specific cognitive and linguistic processes. Initial findings suggested a striking dissociation between language and cognition in Williams syndrome, adding fuel to increasingly popular concepts about the modularity of intelligence and language (for a review see Torff & Gardner, 1999). Recent findings challenge this apparent dissociation among language and cognition, and debates about these issues show no signs of letting up.

> *Initial findings suggested a striking dissociation between language and cognition in Williams syndrome, adding fuel to increasingly popular concepts about the modularity of intelligence and language.*

Cognitive Levels

On average, people with Williams syndrome function in the mild to moderate ranges of mental retardation. Across several studies, the mean

IQ score of people with Williams syndrome falls in the 50–60 range, yet many studies exclude from mean computations people who score below the test basal, typically an IQ of 40. Table 4.1 summarizes several studies reporting mean IQ scores in samples of people with Williams syndrome. A handful of individuals score in the borderline range of intelligence, with IQ scores from 70 to 85, and people with profound delays are occasionally identified (although see Plissart, Borghgraef, Volcke, Van den Berghe, & Fryns, 1994).

Cognitive Trajectories

Only a few studies have longitudinally examined changes in global IQ scores. In general, these studies suggest a stability in overall IQ scores over the course of development. Table 4.2 summarizes longitudinal findings to date. Crisco (1990) reported remarkable stability in 14 children with Williams syndrome tested 5 years apart, at average ages of 4 and 9 years old at the time of testing. But other studies show conflicting patterns. Increases in IQ scores were found in people averaging 12 years old at first testing and 21 years old at second testing, a finding that Udwin, Davies, and Howlin (1996) attributed to a shift in testing methods. Namely, for the first testing researchers used the Wechsler Intelligence Scale for Children–Revised (WISC–R; Wechsler, 1974), but for the second testing they used the Wechsler Adult Intelligence Scale–Revised (WAIS-R; Wechsler, 1981).

In contrast, Gosch and Pankau (1996) reported that children significantly declined in their scores on the German version of the Columbia Mental Maturity Scale (Bondy, Cohen, Eggert, & Luer, 1969) over a 2-year period. Error analyses of the Columbia at second testing revealed that children passed concrete items, and failed more abstract, classification items. These researchers also report stability in Draw-a-Person (DAP) (Ziler, 1971) scores over time, yet this drawing task is probably a better reflection of visual-motor functioning than intelligence (Dykens, 1996b).

Discrepant findings across studies may indeed be related to concerns with the tests themselves (e.g., the shift from WISC–R to WAIS–R; more abstract items at second testing on the Columbia). Yet another explanation is that different aspects of cognition in Williams syndrome may show variable developmental trajectories. In the next section, we touch on age-related shifts in specific cognitive and linguistic strengths and weaknesses.

Overall IQ scores, as depicted in Tables 4.1 and 4.2, mask an intriguing constellation of cognitive and linguistic "peaks and valleys." Relative strengths are often seen in certain aspects of language, as well as in

Table 4.1. Global IQ findings in Williams syndrome

Researchers	N	Test	Findings
Udwin, Yule, & Martin, 1987	44	Wechsler Intelligence Scale for Children–Revised (Wechsler, 1974)	Full-Scale Intelligence Quotient 54, Verbal Intelligence Quotient 62, Performance Intelligence Quotient 56
Udwin & Yule, 1991	20	WISC–R (Wechsler, 1974)	FSIQ 57, VIQ 66, PIQ 59
Greer, Brown, Pai, Choudry & Klein, 1997	15	Stanford-Binet Intelligence Test, Fourth Edition (Thorndike, Hagen, & Sattler, 1986)	Composite 62; Verbal 66, Abstract-Visual 70, Quantitative 70, STM 65
Crisco, Dobbs, & Mulhern, 1988	22	Stanford-Binet Form LM (Terman & Merrill, 1960)	Composite IQ 68
Davies, Howlin, & Udwin, 1997	70	Wechsler Adult Intelligence Scale–Revised (Wechsler, 1974)	FSIQ 62, VIQ 66, PIQ 62

Table 4.2. Longitudinal studies of global IQ in Williams syndrome

Researcher	N	Age (in years)	Test	Findings
Udwin, Davies, & Howlin, 1996	23	12–11	Wechsler Intelligence Scale for Children–Revised (Wechsler, 1974)	Full-Scale Intelligence Quotient 50, Verbal Intelligence Quotient 56, Performance Intelligence Quotient 52
		21–9	Wechsler Adult Intelligence Scale–Revised (Weschler, 1981)	FSIQ 61, VIQ 64, PIQ 60
Crisco, 1990	14	4	Stanford-Binet Form LM (Terman & Merrill, 1960)	IQ 67
		9	Stanford-Binet Form LM (Terman & Merrill, 1960)	IQ 66
Gosch & Pankau, 1996	18	6	Draw-a-Person task (Naglieri, 1987)	DAP 63; CMMS 77
			Columbia Mental Maturity Scale (Bondy, Cohen, Eggert, & Luer, 1969)	
		8	Draw-a-Person task (Naglieri, 1987)	DAP 65; CMMS 68
			Columbia Mental Maturity Scale (Bondy, Cohen, Eggert, & Luer, 1969)	

Table 4.3.   Profiles of cognitive-linguistic strengths and weaknesses in Williams syndrome

Strengths	Weaknesses	Strength or weakness?
Lexicon, vocabulary	Visual-spatial construction	Syntax
Linguistic affect	Perceptual planning	Semantics
Auditory short-term memory	Fine motor control	
Facial recognition and memory		
Theory of mind		
Musicality		

auditory short-term memory, facial recognition, social cognition, and music. In striking juxtaposition, salient impairments are found in visual-spatial constructive tasks, as mentioned previously. Table 4.3 summarizes these strengths and weaknesses. We take up each in turn, and conclude with emerging data on how these strengths and weaknesses relate to brain structure and function.

Relative Strengths

Although young children with Williams syndrome have typical delays of as much as 2 years in the acquisition of language (Harris, Bellugi, Bates, Jones, & Rossen, 1997), many adolescents and adults show remarkable linguistic capacities. These strengths are not necessarily reflected in the Verbal IQ scores summarized in Table 4.1, as these scores are a summary index of various skills that seem unevenly developed in people with Williams syndrome. When skills that compose the Verbal IQ are teased apart and supplemented with other language tasks, an intriguing and rather controversial picture emerges. The next section reviews those aspects of the linguistic profile in Williams syndrome that researchers agree on and hotly dispute.

Lexicon, Vocabulary   Relative to others as well as to their own overall mental ages (MA), many people with Williams syndrome excel in their lexicons, or basic vocabularies. Across many samples, researchers generally find that people with Williams syndrome show advanced skills on single-word receptive vocabulary tests including the Peabody Picture Vocabulary Test–Revised (PPVT–R; Dunn & Dunn, 1981) (Bellugi, Marks, Bihrle, & Sabo, 1988; Reilly, Klima, & Bellugi, 1991). Indeed, vocabulary in people with Williams syndrome was once thought to be spared or comparable to that of typically developing individuals. Examining a large sample of 123 children and adults with Williams syndrome, Mervis, Morris, Bertrand, and Robinson (1999) found that as many as 42% scored in the borderline to typical range on the PPVT–R. Considerable variability was seen in this cohort, however, and the average PPVT–R score was 66, indicating mild levels of delay for the group as a whole. Thus, researchers now agree that even though vocabulary is probably a relative strength for many individuals, it may still fall below chronological age (CA) expectations (e.g., Jarrold, Baddeley, & Hewes, 1998; Udwin, Yule, & Martin, 1987; see Chapter 8).

Mervis et al. (1999) also found a strong positive correlation among PPVT–R scores and advancing age in children. Indeed, it may be that relative strengths in certain language skills become more pronounced as individuals with Williams syndrome reach their late childhood or adolescent years. Jarrold et al. (1998), for example, did not find discrepancies among verbal versus nonverbal scores on the Differential Ability Scales (DAS; Elliott, 1990) until children were 8 years of age. Thus, the syndrome's characteristic linguistic strengths may not be readily apparent until later childhood or adolescence.

Linguistic Affect   Abnormally high levels of linguistic affect have been observed in some—though probably not all—people with Williams syndrome. These individuals clearly imbue their language with affect, as seen in both their prosody and liberal use of narrative enrichment techniques (e.g., Bellugi, Wang, & Jernigan, 1994; Reilly et al., 1991). People may, for example, sprinkle exclamatory or lexical devices in their conversations or stories, and all of these have the net affect of further engaging their audience. Linguistic affect and a rather effusive, "hyperverbal" conversational style (Udwin & Yule, 1990) may thus play a role in the positive social interactions of many with the disorder.

In our ongoing work, we administer people with Williams syndrome a projective storytelling task. Although some of their stories contain lexical devices such as "Ooh!," Uh-oh," or "Well, there was once this little boy," several people also use different voices or inflections to dramatize the thoughts or actions of different characters. This style suggests an ability to take the perspectives of others and to perhaps empathize with them, features discussed more fully later. One story that shows this type of role-taking is offered in Figure 4.3, as is a story from a control subject of a similar CA and with comparable PPVT-R (Dunn & Dunn, 1981) scores. In addition to its dramatic effect, the person relating the Williams syndrome story also shows rather impressive syntax and semantics.

Syntax and Semantics   These two aspects of language have recently come under keen scrutiny, and conflicting findings have formed a core issue of debate. People with Williams syndrome seem to show strengths in syntax and morphosyntactic rules, that is, in grammar (the ordering of words in a sentence) and in the use of word endings (*-s* for

---

Williams syndrome subject
Female, age 21 years, Peabody Picture Vocabulary Test–Revised (PPVT–R; Dunn & Dunn, 1981), age score = 10 years.

[sic] There is a grandpa and a son, and they are sitting together and the grandpa says, "Why am I getting so old?" The son says " I know you're getting old, but I still love you" "I think I am not going to live," "I know, but you have to live," "Am I going to have a stroke or heart attack?," "Yes, you might suffer a heart attack or stroke," "I need to see my physician right away," "I'll drive you to the doctor's office." They sit and talk some more, and the grandpa says "I know I still love you, my son," and the son says, "I know that you love me, grandpa."

Control subject
Female, age 18 years, PPVT–R age score = 12 years

He's thinking something, and she's thinking something, it looks like a girl I think. And at the end she takes her to a zoo or something.

Figure 4.3.   Projective stories from a Williams syndrome and control subject

plural, *-ed* for past tense). Bellugi and colleagues (1988; 1994) noted that the spontaneous speech of people with Williams syndrome show rather complex syntactic structures such as embedded relative clauses, full passives, and negations, as well as impressively long mean length of utterances (MLUs) that far exceed MA expectations. These researchers also found that people with Williams syndrome excelled on the Test for Reception of Grammar (TROG; Bishop, 1983), with 80%–90% of items correctly passed on tasks assessing passive sentences, sentence completions, and detecting and fixing ungrammatical sentences (Bellugi, Bihrle, Jernigan, Trauner, & Doherty, 1990; Bellugi et al., 1994, 1988).

Others, however, argue that morphosyntactic rules and grammatical comprehension are actually impaired in people with Williams syndrome. On the TROG, for example, Karmiloff-Smith et al. (1997) and Volterra, Capirci, Pezzini, Sabbadini, and Vicari (1996) found that participants with Williams syndrome scored below their CA and in some tasks even below MA expectations. In studies using English-, French-, and Italian-speaking children, specific difficulties have also been identified with gender assignment, past tense, and agreement among people and number (e.g., Capirci, Sabbadini, & Volterra, 1996; Karmiloff-Smith et al., 1997; Kataria, Goldstein, & Kushnick, 1984). In 1998, Karmiloff-Smith et al. used on-line tasks to examine both speed of understanding sentences and ability to choose among pictures that described different sentences. Particularly in this latter task, young adults with Williams syndrome performed poorly. For example, after hearing the sentence, "The clown photographs the policeman," all people were asked to choose from among drawings: the clown photographing the policeman (correct picture); the policeman photographing the clown (reverse role picture); and the clown lifting the helmet off of the policeman (distracter picture). Although no typical young adult made any errors in choosing the correct picture, individuals with Williams syndrome erred 24% of the time (usually by picking the reverse role picture). Such findings suggest that certain aspects of syntax may be impaired in Williams syndrome.

In semantics as well, data are equivocal. Semantics is concerned with the meaning and organization of words, including how people categorize members of a particular group such as animals. On word fluency tests, in which people are asked to name, for example, all of the animals that they can in 60 seconds, Bellugi et al. (1994) found that adolescents and adults with Williams syndrome produced more low-frequency or unusual words (e.g., *yak, ibex, newt, condor*) than MA-matched controls. These high rates of low-frequency words suggest an usual or atypical semantic organization in Williams syndrome.

In contrast, Volterra, Capirci, Pezzini, Sabbadini, and Vicari (1996) found no differences in word fluency test performance among children with Williams syndrome and MA-matched controls; the animals listed by both groups were fairly common. These findings are similar to those of Scott et al. (1995), who found no differences in the animal fluency task among 9- and 10-year-old children with Williams syndrome, and MA-matched typical and Down syndrome groups. In addition, Tyler et al. (1997) used an on-line semantic priming task and concluded that semantic memory and access to semantic information seem typical in Williams syndrome (see also Clahsen & Almazan, 1998).

In summary, then, researchers in Williams syndrome continue to debate whether syntax and semantics are relatively intact or impaired. This tension is seen as well in a growing literature on early language acquisition in infants with Williams syndrome. Relative to typical children, some aspects of early language in individuals with Williams syndrome seem atypical, such as the lack of pointing and other communicative gestures prior to the onset of first words, and an increased tendency to look at faces (Mervis & Bertrand, 1997). In other ways, however, language acquisition in children with Williams syndrome proceeds at a rate and in a sequence similar to typical children, as in the grammatical development that typically follows the mastery of two-word utterances (Mervis et al. 1999).

Lexical, syntactic, and semantic issues are likely to continue to be of keen interest to researchers, as findings have profound implications for understanding the modularity of cognition and language. If, as mentioned at the outset of this section, language is truly spared, then

Williams syndrome provides powerful evidence for the modularity of language, distinct from general cognitive abilities (Bellugi et al., 1994). If not, Williams syndrome may provide further evidence of connections among linguistic and non-linguistic abilities found in other groups of people (e.g., the possible connections among short-term memory and grammar). Further research is needed to settle these controversies.

Lexical, syntactic, and semantic issues are likely to continue to be of keen interest to researchers, as findings have profound implications for understanding the modularity of cognition and language.

Auditory Short-Term Memory Many children and adults with Williams syndrome excel in tasks assessing auditory short-term memory. Compared with CA- and MA-matched people with Down syndrome, for example, those with Williams syndrome can recall significantly longer strings of digits (Klein & Mervis, in press; Wang & Bellugi, 1994). Even in a more demanding digit task—in which two digits per second are presented instead of just one—children with Williams syndrome clearly do quite well (Mervis et al., 1999). In a large study of 65 children with Williams syndrome ages 4–17 years, most all with mental retardation, a full 65%, scored in the typical range on the more demanding digit recall task. Furthermore, individuals' correct responses to the digit span task were significantly correlated with advancing age (i.e., the older the person, the more correct responses he or she gave), and their rapid advances relative to other skills (see later in this chapter) may allow for more pronounced discrepancies from one area to another as these children get older.

Facial Recognition A fascination with faces, and a remarkable facility with facial recognition and recall, was one of the early hallmark observations of people with Williams syndrome (e.g., Bellugi et al., 1994; Udwin & Yule, 1991). Even infants and toddlers with Williams syndrome seem unusually attentive to the faces of others (Mervis & Bertrand, 1997). People with Williams syndrome do much better than do MA-matched controls on the Form SL Test of Facial Recognition (Benton, Hamsher, Varney, & Spreen, 1983), a fairly rigorous task in which people must match a stimulus face to several choices presented under different light and angle conditions (Pezzini, Vicari, Volterra, Milani, & Ossella, 1999). Using this task, Wang, Doherty, Rourke, and Bellugi (1995) also found that people with Williams syndrome performed on par with typical adults.

The advanced performance of people with Williams syndrome on facial recognition tasks may be facilitated by certain problem-solving styles. On one hand, these individuals seem to use a facial feature match-ing strategy as opposed to a style based on the global impression or gestalt of the face (Wang et al., 1995). Yet, people with Williams syn-drome also excel even when asked to use a gestalt (i.e., holistic) closure strategy to identify the gender and age (young, middle-aged, old) of various faces (Bellugi, Sabo, & Vaid, 1988). On the other hand, these same people perform quite poorly on gestalt closure tasks that do not use facial stimuli. Regardless of the strategy they use, people with Will-iams syndrome have uncanny facial recognition skills, and these apti-tudes seem associated with their abilities to read the expressions and states of others.

Theory of Mind   Several researchers have hypothesized that the-ory of mind may be an "island of sparing" in Williams syndrome, meaning that people with this disorder may be particularly adept at reading or interpreting the mental states of others. In one study, vari-ous theory-of-mind tasks were administered to 18 people with Williams syndrome ages 9–23 years (Karmiloff-Smith, Klima, Bellugi, Grant & Baron-Cohen, 1995). These researchers found that people with Williams syndrome performed as well as typically developing individ-uals in using the direction of eye gaze to infer the intentions and goals of others. The majority (94%) passed simple theory-of-mind tasks, cor-rectly predicting what protagonists in standard vignettes would think or do based on the character's false belief, not on their own knowledge of what happened.

In a related study, Tager-Flusberg, Boshart, and Baron-Cohen (1998) compared 13 adults with Williams syndrome to CA- and MA-matched people with Prader-Willi syndrome. Participants were administered "mentalizing" or "mind reading" tasks that assessed their ability to un-derstand various mental states depicted in eye expressions. This task avoids the complex narratives inherent in higher-order theory-of-mind tasks yet still tests the ability to attribute mental states to others. Rela-tive to those with Prader-Willi syndrome, adults with Williams syn-drome performed significantly better, though they were not as proficient as age-matched typical controls. Even so, people with Williams syn-drome appear quite skilled in inferring mental states from eyes, a find-ing that fits with their socially oriented, empathic personalities (Dykens & Rosner, 1999a; Gosch & Pankau, 1997).

Musicality   Early reports suggested that people with Williams syndrome have well-developed musical talents, including singing, play-ing instruments, and recognizing songs. It remains unknown, however, just exactly how widespread musical interests or talents are in the pop-ulation with Williams syndrome. Comparing 36 children with Williams syndrome with those with Down syndrome, Hodapp, Dykens, Fidler, and Rosner (2000) found that both groups enjoyed listening to music or singing, but that people with Williams syndrome were more apt to play an instrument.

Although most people with Williams syndrome have hyperacusis many also appear to have highly unusual responses to timbre, or the quality given to a sound by its overtones. Examples include being able to distinguish different brands or types of lawn mowers, vacuum cleaners, airplanes, or cars based solely on the sound of the engines. In our ongoing longitudinal study, for example, we interviewed a boy who could accurately distinguish among eight different kinds of helicopters based on the sounds they made flying overhead. This phenomenon, termed "hypertimbria" by Levitan and Bellugi (1998), may emerge as a possible variant of perfect pitch.

The affinity for music is not related to IQ, nor does it have a "savant" quality, in that most with the syndrome need to work hard to develop and improve their musical skills (Lenhoff, 1998). One aspect of music—rhythm—was recently assessed in an echo clapping task given to eight children and adolescents with Williams syndrome who attended a special music camp and eight typical children with at least 3 years of music lessons (Levitan & Bellugi, 1998). The two groups performed on par, with the same low rate of errors. Further, unlike the control group, when children with Williams syndrome made errors, they produced creative embellishments or extensions of the reference rhythm; in short, they improvised.

Musicality is a relatively underresearched aspect of the Williams syndrome behavioral phenotype, and more work is needed on the range and neurological correlates of musical talent in this population. Future work should also examine how making music might relate to increased self-esteem, or to improved recreation and leisure, both of which seem true of the performer depicted in Figure 4.4.

Relative Weaknesses

Visual-spatial functioning, perceptual planning, and fine motor control are all considered weaknesses characteristic of individuals with Williams syndrome.

Visual-Spatial Functioning   In contrast to the debates that surround linguistic functioning, researchers agree that people with Williams syndrome show profound impairments in visual-spatial functioning. Relative to controls, those with Williams syndrome show poor performances on both rote and long-term visual-spatial memory tasks (Vicari, Brizzolara, Carlesimo, Pezzini, & Volterra, 1996). Further, despite their advanced expressive language skills, people with Williams

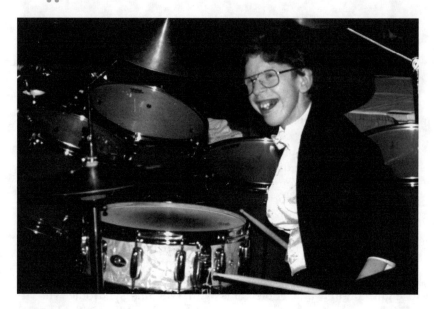

Figure 4.4. A musician in performance.

syndrome make more errors than typical children in their use of spatially oriented prepositions such as "around" or "in" (Bellugi, Lichtenberger, et al., 1999).

Most studies, however, have identified visual-spatial impairments using construction and puzzle tests as well as drawing tasks. Compared with people with Down syndrome, with mental retardation of mixed etiologies, or with typical children, people with Williams syndrome perform consistently lower on standardized tasks such as the WISC–R or WAIS–R Block Design or DAS Pattern Construction (e.g., Crisco et al., 1988; Jarrold et al., 1998; MacDonald & Roy, 1988; Mervis et al., 1999; Plissart et al., 1994; Udwin & Yule, 1991). People with Williams syndrome are less able to manipulate even two- to four-piece block sets to match a model, suggesting poor motor planning, spatial orientation, and eye–hand coordination.

Perceptual Planning and Fine Motor Control People who have Williams syndrome also show limited perceptual-motor skills on various drawing tests, such as the Developmental Test of Visual-Motor Integration (VMI; Beery, 1989). In this figure copying task, which becomes progressively more difficult, people with Williams syndrome score consistently lower than their MA- or CA-matched counterparts with or without mental retardation (Bellugi, Sabo et al., 1988; Bertrand, Mervis, & Eisenberg, 1997; Mervis et al., 1999; Wang et al., 1995). Many people with Williams syndrome also draw disorganized, disjointed depictions of objects, such as a house, an elephant, or a bicycle (Bellugi, Sabo, et al., 1988; Bellugi et al., 1994). In particular, Bellugi et al. found that drawings by children with Williams syndrome were typically unrecognizable, and although details were often present, they were not integrated into a coherent or global whole. Conversely, drawings produced by people with Down syndrome had scant internal detail but an appropriate overall gestalt. This "local–global" difference has been used to support the argument that children with Williams syndrome are deviant in the development of their drawing skills, showing impaired global, but intact local processing (Bellugi et al., 1994).

In contrast, others argue that drawing development in Williams syndrome is delayed, not deviant. Comparing MA-matched typical controls to 9- and 10-year-old children with Williams syndrome, Bertrand et al. (1997) found similar proportions of disorganized drawings across groups. Furthermore, the VMI scores of these people showed an ordinariness of items, suggesting that children with Williams syndrome follow the same developmental sequence as other children in learning to draw. On a retest 3–4 years later, a subsample of these same children showed improvements in VMI scores, and their drawings were more recognizable and organized (Bertrand & Mervis, 1996).

In one study with 30 people with Williams syndrome, researchers found a wide range of performance on the DAP test (Naglieri, 1987), from scribbles to easily recognized, well-integrated drawings (Dykens, Rosner, & Ly, 2000). People thus appear to be at different stages of drawing development, as exemplified in Figures 4.5 a–c. Using a standardized quantitative scoring system, all people with Williams syndrome had DAP age-equivalent scores that fell well-below CA expectations, but with significant age-related gains. Only two drawings showed the profound impairments in global organization previously described by Bellugi et al. Further, people with Williams syndrome earned DAP scores that were comparable to two groups of MA-matched people with mental retardation. Although preliminary these findings provide additional support for a developmental as opposed to a deviant trajectory of drawing ability in children with Williams syndrome.

NEUROLOGICAL CORRELATES

With its disparate areas of strength and impairment, Williams syndrome is particularly well-suited to neurological studies that aim to correlate brain to behavioral functioning. Using event-related potentials (ERPs), which examine the timing and organization of neural systems, unique

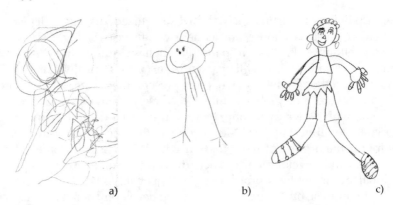

a)   b)   c)

Figure 4.5. From scribbles to person: the Draw-a-Person Task in people with Williams syndrome, a) ages 4 years, b) 9 years, and c) 19 years, respectively.

brain wave markers have now been identified for certain aspects of language functioning and for facial processing (Neville, Holcomb, & Mills, 1989; Neville, Mills, & Bellugi, 1994). These patterns of markers readily distinguished people with Williams syndrome from typical controls, suggesting that the brains of people with Williams syndrome may tap different neural systems associated with certain cognitive processes.

With its disparate areas of strength and impairment, Williams syndrome is particularly well-suited to neurological studies that aim to correlate brain to behavioral functioning.

Using structural magnetic resonance imaging (MRI), recent neuroanatomical findings shed additional light on the syndrome's cognitive-linguistic profile. Although the profound visual-spatial impairments in Williams syndrome suggest damage to the right parietal lobe, this does not appear to be the case. Indeed, there are no obvious right/left hemisphere differences in the brains of people with Williams syndrome relative to typical controls (Jernigan & Bellugi, 1994). Instead, data point to different patterns of proportions of brain volumes in people with Williams syndrome. The overall cerebral volume in individuals with Williams syndrome is smaller, at approximately 80%–85% of the volume of typical controls. Yet, the brains of people with Williams syndrome are similar to those of typical controls in their neocerebellar volumes, the volume of the frontal cortex in relationship to the posterior cortex, and in limbic structures such as the amygdala and hippocampus (Bellugi et al., 1994; Galaburda, Wang, Bellugi, & Rossen, 1994).

The relative sparing of the frontal cortex and neocerebellar structures may be associated with the linguistic competencies that characterize Williams syndrome. The limbic system and amygdala are also spared in Williams syndrome, and these structures are implicated in facial processing and affect recognition tasks (Baron-Cohen, 1995). Performance on facial recognition tasks has also been correlated with the volume of the inferior posterior medial cortex (Jones, Rossen, Hickok, Jernigan, & Bellugi, 1995). Furthermore, relative to typical controls, individuals with Williams syndrome have the same absolute volume of Heschel's gyrus, an area of the primary auditory cortex (Hickok et al., 1995). This finding may be associated with the syndrome's characteristic strengths in language, auditory short-term memory, and music.

Other findings relate to the visual-spatial impairment seen in most individuals with Williams syndrome. In particular, the relationship of visual-motor difficulties has recently been examined in dorsal versus ventral stream functioning. Dorsal stream function involves the parietal lobe and processes information about the position and action of objects, including hand control. In contrast, ventral stream function transmits information to the temporal lobe, and is involved in the recognition of objects and faces.

In a clever set of experiments by Atkinson et al. (1997), children ages 4–14 years old with Williams syndrome and CA-matched controls were asked to mail a letter in a mailbox with slots of various angles. Children in both groups were also asked to get a letter ready to be mailed by rotating a doll, letter in hand, and matching the doll's letter to the mailbox slot. Children with Williams syndrome had considerable difficulty actually mailing the letter, a task thought to tap dorsal stream function. In contrast, children with Williams syndrome performed on par with typical controls in using the doll to match the orientation of the letter to the slot, a task thought to tap ventral stream function. Findings thus imply that people with Williams syndrome have difficulties in visual-motor action or construction types of tasks (or dorsal stream functioning) as opposed to visual-spatial recognition or perception tasks (ventral stream functioning). Relatively spared ventral stream functioning may also be implicated in the ability of Williams syndrome people to recognize objects, as on the PPVT–R, and in their uncanny strength in recognizing and remembering faces.

ADAPTIVE FUNCTIONING

As with people with mental retardation in general, adaptive skills are critically important to the success and quality of life for people with Williams syndrome. Yet, unlike the numerous studies on cognition and language, only a few studies have assessed how children or adults with Williams syndrome respond to the demands of everyday living.

Children

Children with Williams syndrome show relative strengths in their adaptive communication and socialization skills and relative weaknesses in their daily living skills. When Gosch and Pankau (1994) compared Vineland Social Maturity Scale scores in nineteen 4- to 10-year old children with nonspecific mental retardation with the scores of those with Williams syndrome, lower scores were found in the Williams syndrome group. Specific problems were apparent in self-care skills such as grooming, eating, and toileting. Using the more up-to-date Vineland Adaptive Behavior Scales (VABS; Sparrow, Balla, & Cicchetti, 1984), Greer, Brown, Pai, Choudry, and Klein (1997) also identified slightly better developed communication and socialization skills in 15 children with Williams syndrome ages 4–18 years. On average, VABS scores fell slightly below IQ scores (54 versus 62, respectively), confirming moderate levels of adaptive delay for the group as a whole (Greer et al., 1997).

These adaptive profiles make sense in light of what we know about other aspects of the Williams syndrome behavioral phenotype. Children may, for example, struggle more with daily living skills such as dressing, eating, or bathing as a result of their impairments in visual-spatial functioning, motor planning, and fine and gross motor control. Strengths in socialization and communication are consistent with their socially oriented personalities and well-developed language capacities. Even so, most children with the syndrome show adaptive skills that fall well below CA and MA expectations.

Adults

Adults with Williams syndrome seem to show a pattern of adaptive skills similar to their younger counterparts. On the basis of a parental survey of 11 adults with Williams syndrome, Plissart et al. (1994) found that people performed best in communication, and worst in personal self-care. But some degree of autonomy was seen among these adults, with many showing solid skills in cooking, cleaning, and dressing (see Lopez-Rangel, Maurice, McGillivray, & Friedman, 1992).

Surveying a large sample of 119 parents of adults with Williams syndrome, Udwin (1990) found that 66% of these adults were completely independent in bathing and 61% in dressing. Though the majority, 88%, were generally self-reliant in toileting, 30% experienced daytime incontinence. Many adults (42%) took public transportation by themselves for familiar routes or trips, yet most needed supervision for longer or unfamiliar excursions (see also Lopez-Rangel et al., 1992). From 11% to 13% of the sample shopped or cooked on their own, and very few (6%) could indepedently manage their own money.

In standardized assessments of adaptive behavior as well, adults with Williams syndrome show significant delay. Interviewing 70 parents with the VABS, Davies et al. (1997) found that the overall VABS scores of adults with Williams syndrome typically lagged way behind Full-Scale IQ scores (means = 38 versus 66, respectively). In this vein, it is not so surprising that most adults with Williams syndrome live and work in supervised settings. From 75% to 80% of adults in various surveys live at home with their parents (Lopez–Rangel et al., 1992; Udwin, 1990), and most are also enrolled in supervised vocational, recreational, or continuing education programs.

Poorly developed adaptive skills in both children or adults seem surprising in light of the relatively advanced verbal skills, interest in others, and social orientation of many with Williams syndrome. Although persistent medical problems may contribute to less-than-optimal adaptive outcomes, these have not generally been implicated as an obstacle to adaptive performance (Davies et al., 1997; Lopez-Rangel et al., 1992). Instead, adaptive skills seem hampered by salient social and personality characteristics of Williams syndrome, as well as by a host of maladaptive behaviors often manifested in those with this disorder.

SOCIAL–PERSONALITY FUNCTIONING

When Beuren et al. first described individuals with Williams syndrome in the 1960s, they noted that "all have the same kind of friendly nature, they love everyone, are loved by everyone, and are very charming" (1962, p. 472). Although the "friendly and charming" label found its way into the literature and has persisted over time, it has ultimately proved a double-edged sword.

In some ways, "friendly," "charming," and "lovable" seem accurate descriptors of many with the syndrome. As shown in Table 4.4, for example, researchers found that all or most of the parents of 60 children with Williams syndrome rated them on the Reiss Personality Profiles (Reiss & Havercamp, 1998) as "caring," "kind-spirited," "forgiving," and "unselfish" (Dykens & Rosner, 1999a). These traits are likely nurtured by specific cognitive strengths of the syndrome, primarily the memory

Table 4.4.   Positive features of social interactions in 60 people with Williams syndrome

Behavior	%
Kind-spirited	100
Caring	94
Seeks company of others	90
Feels terrible when others are in pain	87
Often initiates interactions with others	87
Enjoys social activities	83
Forgiving	83
Unselfish	83
Very happy when others do well	75
Never goes unnoticed in a group	75
Strong desire to help others	66

Based on Dykens & Rosner, 1999a.

for faces; ability to identify the emotional expressions of others; and ability to "mind-read," or assume the perspectives of others.

All of these assets may set the stage for those with the syndrome to sympathize or empathize with others. Researchers found that adolescents and adults with Williams syndrome were similar to a control group in wanting to help others, and feeling happy when others do well (Dykens & Rosner, 1999a). What distinguished people with Williams syndrome from others was the finding that they were "feeling terrible when others are in pain." Further work is needed, as it is unclear from this study if people with Williams syndrome truly "feel what others feel" or are simply more reactive or agitated when others are in distress. Even so, a socially oriented, empathic streak seems quite possible in people with Williams syndrome, as demonstrated in the projective story in Figure 4.3.

However, the kind, friendly, and empathic features associated with Williams syndrome may not always be adaptive. These positive attributes also mask a more complicated personality and behavioral picture. As they have evolved over the years, these "friendly and charming" descriptors may have actually deterred researchers from examining social maladjustment or other behavior problems.

Now that researchers have begun to look behind the "charming" façade, they are indeed finding that people with Williams syndrome have salient social and behavioral vulnerabilities.

Now that researchers have begun to look behind the "charming" façade, they are indeed finding that people with Williams syndrome have salient social and behavioral vulnerabilities. Briefly, people with Williams syndrome may be

- *Too friendly:* People with Williams syndrome are actually too friendly; they are socially uninhibited and often approach others indiscriminately. Surveying 36 parents of children with Williams syndrome ages 4–10 years, Gosch and Pankau (1997) discovered that 82% were overly friendly toward strangers. Although these researchers found that adults were slightly less overfriendly (60%), Davies, Udwin, and Howlin (1998) reported that 94% of their sample of 70 adults with Williams syndrome were socially disinhibited.

- *Unable to make or keep friends:* A second concern is that despite their social orientation, many people with Williams syndrome struggle to make or keep friends. Relative to those with nonspecific mental retardation, researchers found that adults with Williams syndrome had significantly fewer friends (Dykens & Rosner, 1999a). As depicted in Table 4.5, from 76% to 96% of various samples of subjects report difficulties making or keeping friends. Part of the difficulty in making friends may stem from the tendency for some individuals with Williams syndrome to get too caught up in the melodrama of other people's lives. Although this may be related in some cases to being infatuated with others (Davies et al., 1998), for some individuals it has led to other maladaptive consequences, such as being fired from work. Researchers hypothesized as well that many people with Williams syndrome have problems making friends due to their low tolerance for frustration and teasing; their tendency toward excessive chatter and impulsivity; and, ironically, their strong desire to have friends (Dykens & Rosner, 1999a). These individuals may want friends so much that they come on way too strong with others, and then can't step back or modulate their interactions. In short, they find it hard to engage in the types of reciprocal "give-and-take" interactions commonly seen in friendships.

- *Vulnerable to exploitation:* Another salient worry is that social disinhibition, coupled with impulsivity and a strong desire for friends, render many with Williams syndrome vulnerable to exploitation or abuse (Dykens & Hodapp, 1997). Davies et al. (1998) found that 59% of adults in their sample were physically overdemonstrative, including touching, hugging, and kissing others. Further, 10% of this sample reported to the police that they had been sexually assaulted, and an additional 10% made allegations of assault that were not reported

Table 4.5. Negative features of social interaction across studies

Researchers	Behavior	%	N	Age range
Davies, Udwin, & Howlin, 1998	Problems with friends	96	70	19–39 years
Gosch & Pankau, 1994	Unreserved with strangers	79	19	4–10 years
Udwin, 1990	Solitary	71	119	16–38 years
	Overfriendly with strangers	73		
	Incessant chatter	58		
Udwin, Yule, & Martin, 1987	Solitary	84	44	6–16 years
	Not liked	30		
Dykens & Rosner, 1999a, 1999b	Few friends	76	60	4–32 years
	Highly sensitive to rejection	67		
	Low tolerance for teasing	65		
	Prefers older/younger peers	65		
	Gets teased a lot	61		
	Talks too much	53		

to the authorities. The exact rates of sexual, physical, or financial exploitation or abuse are unknown among people who have Williams syndrome. Clearly, however, these individuals' personality and behavioral features seem to place them at increased risk for being taken advantage of by others.

MALADAPTIVE BEHAVIOR—PSYCHOPATHOLOGY

In addition to social and personality concerns, salient maladaptive behaviors keep many individuals with Williams syndrome from achieving optimal adaptive outcomes. Studies to date suggest that people with Williams syndrome are prone to specific types of behavioral or psychiatric difficulties, although this is less researched than cognition or language.

Using checklists that screen for a wide variety of problems, researchers have noted difficulties associated with individuals with Williams syndrome, including externalizing problems, regulating bodily states, and internalizing types of symptoms.

Externalizing As shown in Table 4.6, high rates of externalizing problems were found in various samples of children, include hyperactivity, inattention, impulsivity, disobedience, attention-seeking, and temper tantrums. Problems with severe aggression, fighting, or destroying

Table 4.6.   Rates of maladaptive behavior across studies of people with Williams syndrome

Problem	%
Externalizing	
Inattention	91–96 [a]
Impulsivity	75
Attention-seeking	71–73
Prefers adults over peers	68–86 [a, b]
Hyperactivity	63–71 [a]
Temper tantrums	48–74
Disobedience	32–60
Fights, aggressive	25–47
State/Bodily Regulation	
Eating difficulties	45–70 [a, b, c]
Wetting self—day	27–61 [b, c]
Sleep difficulties	24–50 [b, c]
Internalizing	
Obsessions, preoccupations	70–85 [a, b]
Fears	68–73 [b]
Labile	64
Irritable	62–68
Worried	50–70 [b, c]
Anxiety	45–89 [b, c]
Somatic complaints	30–67 [b]
Feels worthless	30
Sadness, depression	10–17

Note: Percentages reported in Davies, Udwin, & Howlin, 1998; Dilts, Morris, & Leonard, 1990; Dykens & Rosner, 1999b; Einfeld, Tonge, & Florio, 1997; Gosch & Pankau, 1994, 1997; Udwin, 1990; Udwin, Yule, & Martin, 1987.

[a] Differs from controls in Einfeld et al., 1997.

[b] Differs from controls in Dykens & Rosner, 1999b.

[c] Differs from controls in Udwin, Yule, & Martin, 1987.

property are relatively less common (e.g., Gosch & Pankau, 1994; Udwin, 1990). Increased rates of overactivity, inattention, and tantrums are consistent with studies on temperament in young children with Williams syndrome. Compared with typically developing children, children with Williams syndrome show higher activity, lower rhythmicity in daily functioning, more negative moods, less persistence, lower adaptability, and greater approach to others; in short they are more "difficult" as opposed to "easy" (Tomc, Williamson, & Pauli, 1990).

Some of the externalizing behaviors noted in Table 4.6 tend to peak in childhood and are less common among adults (e.g., Gosch & Pankau, 1997; Udwin, 1990). Gosch and Pankau (1997), for example, reported difficulties sitting still in 64% of 48 children younger than 10 years of age and in only 19% of 27 adults ages 20 years and older. Unlike hyperactivity, however, difficulties sustaining attention seem to persist into the adult years, with 90% of 70 adults showing distractibility (Davies et al., 1998).

It remains unclear if problems with inattention and hyperactivity are elevated in individuals with Williams syndrome relative to those with other mental retardation syndromes. As shown in Table 4.6, Einfeld, Tonge, and Florio (1997) found significantly higher rates of inattention and hyperactivity in 70 children with Williams syndrome compared with those with heterogeneous mental retardation. We, however, found no such differences among 43 people with Williams syndrome and matched controls (Dykens & Rosner, 1999b); findings similar to Gosch and Pankau (1997), who studied 19 children with Williams syndrome and controls. Hyperactivity and inattention, then, although not necessarily more prevalent in mixed groups, still constitute difficult behaviors for many children with Williams syndrome.

Regulating Bodily Functions   Troubles regulating basic bodily functions such as toileting, sleeping, and eating have been sporadically reported in children and adults with Williams syndrome (e.g., Einfeld et al., 1997; Gosch & Pankau, 1994; Udwin et al., 1987). From 50% to 60% of children with Williams syndrome have daytime wetting; for some, this persists into the adult years (Dilts, Morris, & Leonard, 1990; Udwin, 1990; Udwin et al., 1987). Other studies show lower rates of day- or nighttime wetting (e.g., 27% and 34%, respectively; Dykens & Rosner, 1999b), which may be related to more early or intensive management of renal problems.

As many as 50% of people with Williams syndrome experience difficulties falling asleep and staying asleep, and sleep problems may be more common to individuals with Williams syndrome than they are to others with mental retardation (Dykens & Rosner, 1999b; Einfeld et al., 1997; Gosch & Pankau, 1994; Udwin et al., 1987). Finally, relative to others, individuals with Williams syndrome experience eating problems much more frequently (see Table 4.6). People with Williams syndrome are often described as being fussy, "faddy," or picky eaters, as well as eating a restricted range of food; these eating problems seem prevalent even long after the need for a low-calcium diet in infancy.

Internalizing   Many people with Williams syndrome also struggle with a host of internalizing problems. As depicted in Table 4.6, several studies find high rates of anxiety, obsessions and preoccupations, lability, somatic complaints, and fears (e.g., Davies et al., 1998; Dykens & Rosner, 1999b; Udwin, 1990). People often become obsessed with bodily aches and pains; anticipated events in the future; imagined or real disasters; other people; or fears such as helicopters, cars, or storms. The author and other researchers recently examined anxieties and fears in more depth (Dykens, 2000). On the basis of standard psychiatric interviews, 50%–57% of 51 individuals with Williams syndrome were "worriers" or were "excessively worried about the future." Moreover, 96% had marked, persistent anxiety-producing fears, and 84% avoided their fearful stimuli or endured them with great distress.

Most people studied met key diagnostic criteria for phobia, with 35% showing these along with the fear-related adaptive impairment necessary for a formal diagnosis of phobic disorder. In contrast, phobias are seen in just 0.5%–4.3% of people with mental retardation in general (Cooper, 1997; Moss, Prosser, Ibbotson, & Goldberg, 1996).

Examining fears in more detail, Dykens (2000) found more frequent and diverse fears in 46 people with Williams syndrome relative to matched controls. Using the Fear Survey Schedule (Ollendick, King, & Frary, 1989), 41 different fears were seen in 50% or more of the Williams syndrome sample; just 2 fears were seen in 50% or more of the comparison group. Table 4.7 exemplifies some of the 41 frequent fears in Williams syndrome and also depicts the 10 most intense fears shown by these people.

Some of the fears in Table 4.7 relate to specific aspects of the physical phenotype of Williams syndrome. Specifically, fears of sounds and storms, for example, likely stem from the hyperacusis that affects almost all people with this disorder. Fears of falling, high places, and carnival rides might relate to joint contractures as well as to the problems that many of these children experience with gait, balance, and gross motor coordination. Even their medical fears may be associated with the cardiac, renal, and other medical complications of the syndrome. Finally, fears of arguments, or of being teased or punished, may relate to the empathic orientation of many with the syndrome; these people may simply bristle more than others when faced with negative social interactions.

One can also hypothesize how vulnerabilities to certain physical problems might generalize as the child gets older to more widespread fears and phobias. For example, hyperacusis and anxious reactions to loud or distinctive noises may

Williams syndrome seems a model disorder to better understand the genetic, neurological, and environmental contributions to phobia in people in the general population.

Table 4.7. A sample of frequent fears in 46 individuals with Williams syndrome and controls

Fear	Williams (%)	Control (%)	Rank order of 10 most intense fears
Being teased	92	22	5
Shots, injections	90	53	1
Getting sick	89	11	
Loud sirens, noises	87	30	2
Getting punished, reprimanded	85	25	
Arguments between others	85	32	6
Fire, getting burned	82	32	9
Bee stings	79	35	3
Falling from high places	79	28	10
Being criticized	78	11	
Thunderstorms	78	36	7
Getting lost	76	14	
High places	75	45	
Roller coaster, carnival rides	75	43	4
Earthquakes	74	21	8
Having to go to the hospital	74	46	
Being left behind	73	14	
Parents getting sick	71	77	
Making mistakes	70	10	

set the stage for children to develop anxious apprehension to stimuli aside from noise. In these ways, Williams syndrome seems a model disorder to better understand the genetic, neurological, and environmental contributions to the development of phobias in people in the general population (Dykens, 2000).

Sadness and Depression   Relative to anxiety and fears, other internalizing symptoms such as sadness or depression are less routinely observed. In one study, these symptoms were seen in 17% of 43 people ages 4–21 years old, and in another they were observed in 10% of 70 adults (Davies et al., 1998; Dykens & Rosner, 1999b). Depression appears to increase with advancing age, such that adolescents and young adults may present clinically with complaints of sadness, mood swings, irritability, or feelings of worthlessness (Dykens & Rosner, 1999b; Pober & Dykens, 1996). Depressive symptoms may be masked by the syndrome's friendly and charming façade and should be carefully monitored, especially in young adults.

Other Psychopathology   Finally, rates seem low for serious psychopathology such as autism. Although six cases have been published of people with co-morbid Williams syndrome and autism (Gillberg & Rasmussen, 1994; Reiss, Feinstein, Rosenbaum, Borengasser-Caruso, & Goldsmith, 1985), this overlap is probably related to the fact that both involve mental retardation. Williams syndrome and autism actually have many features that set them apart from one another. Nonverbal reasoning is a marked weakness in Williams syndrome and a relative strength in autism; linguistic skills are advanced in Williams syndrome and weak in autism; and facial and affect recognition are well-developed in Williams syndrome, and a characteristic impairment in autism. Neuroimaging studies also suggest opposite patterns in these disorders: The neocerebellum and limbic systems are relatively spared in William syndrome and aberrant in autism (see Rumsey, 1996, for a review). Given their contrasting cognitive and neurological patterns, Williams syndrome is actually of keen interest to researchers who study autism.

INTERVENTION IMPLICATIONS

As Williams syndrome involves both physical and behavioral complexities, people with this disorder often require coordinated, long-term services from a team of interdisciplinary professionals. From the medical point of view, cardiac, gastrointestinal, renal, musculoskeletal, visual, and auditory functioning all need careful monitoring over the life span (see Lashkari et al., 1999, for specific recommendations). Other recommendations for educational, vocational, social, emotional, and family interventions stem from the syndrome's characteristic cognitive-linguistic profile, as well as from its maladaptive features.

Educational-Vocational

One set of recommendations is based on the cognitive-linguistic profile associated with Williams syndrome. To circumvent their fine motor, writing, and visual-spatial difficulties, for example, many students do best with computers, calculators, manipulatives, and audiotape recorders (Udwin, Yule, & Martin, 1987). If writing is required, students should be given ample time and extra support, and the amount of copying or writing that they do at any one time should be limited to avoid fatigue.

For tests or other anxiety-arousing situations, alternative techniques, such as use of audiotape recorders, should be considered instead of writing. Furthermore, certain adaptations can be made when children are first learning to write, such as using raised line paper or a slant board, and keeping the model to be copied on the same piece of paper (Grejtak, 1997). Occupational therapists should also be consulted for specific ideas regarding pencil grip and pressure.

In light of their linguistic and auditory processing strengths, students with Williams syndrome should be encouraged to use verbal mediation, that is, to talk through a problem as they solve it. Even visual-spatial tasks, such as copying letters, can be verbally described. Auditory strengths also have implications for teaching children to read. In particular, students with Williams syndrome may respond best to phonetic approaches to reading, with an emphasis on letter–sound associations, as opposed to visual-based approaches that require visual-spatial processing (see Grejtak, 1997, for specific phonetics curricula).

Math skills have been described as a particular weakness for many students with Williams syndrome, yet formal studies do not generally find significant weaknesses in math or in quantitative reasoning relative to reading or spelling (e.g., Jarrold et al., 1998; MacDonald & Roy, 1988). Even so, just 16% of 70 adults were able to tell time independently, and money concepts are a struggle for many individuals, with only 6% of 70 adults being able to manage their own financial affairs (Davies et al., 1997; Udwin, 1990). Indeed, we find that impulsivity, coupled with a strong desire to make friends, leads many adults to make poor financial judgments or to be financially exploited by others. (e.g., by giving their money away). Adults with Williams syndrome may thus benefit from extra supports or supervision in managing their finances.

In adulthood as well, people may benefit from vocational opportunities that minimize their weaknesses and capitalize on their strengths. Assembly-line jobs that require stacking, sorting, or visual-perceptual coordination and fine motor control are likely to invite frustration as well as fatigue. Occupational therapists may have a continuing role in helping adults gain enough fine motor control for personal grooming, dressing, and other adaptive tasks.

Of concern is that many adults with Williams syndrome find it difficult to stay productively employed, primarily because of interference from their distractibility, social disinhibition and overfriendliness, and anxiety (Davies et al., 1997). As a result, most adults need fairly high levels of supervision both on and off the job, and very few individuals live or work completely independently (Davies et al., 1997, 1998; Udwin, 1990). Once in a suitable work setting, then, most adults with

Williams syndrome require the ongoing and sustained support of job coaches; this recommendation differs from the usual approach in which job coaches are "faded" with increased time on the job. Furthermore, some adults do well with people-oriented jobs that tap their empathic streaks and interest in others; examples include working in day care centers, nursing homes, or as receptionists in offices. These work settings are usually successful only with a high level of supervision to ensure that sociability is appropriately channeled.

Maladaptive and Social-Emotional Behaviors

The following intervention strategies may help to alleviate or lessen some maladaptive and social-emotional challenges faced by people with Williams syndrome:

- *Minimize distractions:* Other recommendations for interventions take into account the maladaptive and social-personality features of Williams syndrome. As many children show high levels of inattention and distractibility, they do better in classroom settings that minimize auditory and visual distracters. Typical recommendations for students with attention-deficit/hyperactivity disorder (ADHD) are often helpful with children with Williams syndrome, such as reducing the flow of people through the class, keeping extraneous material to a minimum, and placing the desk in a cubicle or in the front of the classroom. Furthermore, findings from preliminary open and double-blind pharmacological studies are encouraging. Six children with Williams syndrome showed positive responses to methylphenidate (Ritalin); specifically, they had decreased impulsivity, irritability, inattention, and activity levels (Bawden, MacDonald, & Shea, 1997; Power, Blum, Jones, & Kaplan, 1997).

- *Manage sensitivity to sound:* In addition, some children need special help managing their heightened sensitivities to sound. If certain noises in the classroom are distressing (e.g., bell, pencil sharpener, clapping), teachers may find it helpful to comfort the student, explain the source of the sound, and have the child begin to exercise some control over the sound. For instance, the teacher could have the child clap, start up the vacuum, or audiotape the sound (Udwin & Yule, 1988). Some students may simply need to leave the classroom if sounds become too offensive.

- *Use obsessive thinking positively:* At times, the obsessive thinking about a specific topic or object shown by many people with Williams syndrome can be appropriately tapped to facilitate learning. Examples might include using time with the favored object as a reward for on-task behavior, or weaving the topic of interest into lessons to be learned (e.g., reading books about airplanes, using a worksheet cut in the shape of an airplane). Yet, for many individuals who have Williams syndrome, being fascinated by airplanes, classmates, disasters, or future events gets in the way of learning or the performance of everyday activities. In these cases, it often helps to set boundaries around the topic or activity and keep them circumscribed to a certain time of day or to a specific place.

- *Alleviate anxieties*: Individuals with anxieties and fears also respond well to containment tactics. Many children and adults become easily carried away with their fears, and seek constant reassurances from parents and teachers. Although reassurances are important, limits are often necessary so that fears and adult attention-seeking are not inadvertently rewarded. After providing a brief period of comfort and reassurance, for example, many teachers and parents find it effective to move on to another topic or activity. If anxieties and fears persist or are associated with considerable distress or adaptive impairment, pharmacotherapy or cognitive-behavioral approaches may be helpful (Dykens, 2000).

- *Assess sadness and loss*: Although depression is less common, people with Williams syndrome should be screened to ensure that the syndrome's charming façade doesn't mask underlying feelings of sadness or low self-esteem. Given their investments in people, we find that many children and adults with Williams syndrome are overly sensitive to loss, be it through experiencing the death of a relative or letting go of previous relationships with teachers, friends, or therapists. Ruminating about these losses may re-emerge in times of stress; if so, reassuring and then redirecting the individual may help him or her to dwell less on past losses.

- *Provide social skills training*: In light of their social problems (summarized in Table 4.5), many children and adults benefit from social skills training (Davies et al., 1998; Dykens & Rosner, 1999a). Although curricula vary, social skills lessons particularly relevant to people with Williams syndrome include how to make and keep friends (e.g., approaching others, taking turns, starting and ending conversations); how to be appropriately wary of strangers; and for adults, how to deal with romantic attachments. Enrollment in recreational programs such as Special Olympics is also a way to foster social skills and appropriate friendships, as seen in the two athletes with Williams syndrome participating in 1995 Summer World Games (see Figure 4.6). Using a team or "buddy" system to practice social

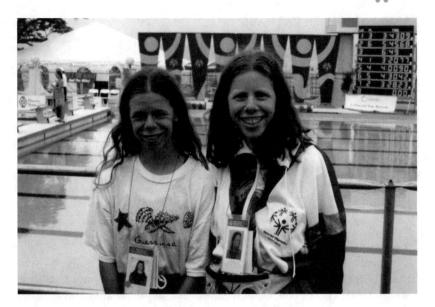

Figure 4.6. Two athletes with Williams syndrome competing in the 1995 Special Olympics Summer World Games.

skills may work in school settings, although older adolescents and adults may do well with group therapy aimed at promoting social skills and self-esteem. Although the syndrome's characteristic verbal skills and abilities to recognize others' emotions bode well for group therapies, groups may not be appropriate for people who are overly anxious or easily distracted.

- *Seek music therapy or lessons:* Finally, some individuals with Williams syndrome may respond well to music therapy or music lessons. Music therapy takes advantage of a variety of musical strategies to promote nonmusical cognitive or emotional goals, such as decreasing anxiety or improving attention, confidence, self-esteem, and motor skills. Music lessons teach musical skills such as singing or playing instruments, and lessons may need to be adapted to meet the special needs of students with Williams syndrome (Coleman, 1998). Learning by ear as opposed to notation seems to work best, as does a positive, supportive teacher (Lenhoff, 1998). Although musical interests or talents may vary widely among individuals with Williams syndrome, musical interventions may nonetheless be of value in promoting self-esteem and developing new avenues of fun.

FAMILY CONSIDERATIONS

Family stress and support have yet to be widely studied in Williams syndrome, and research is greatly needed on how family issues change over the course of development. Infants and toddlers with Williams syndrome, for example, are often irritable and fussy, with hypotonia, feeding problems, and discomfort related to hypercalcemia (Morris et al., 1988). The early years may also be marked by corrective surgeries for cardiac problems. All of these set the stage for high levels of family stress.

> *Family stress and support have yet to be widely studied in Williams syndrome, and research is sorely needed on how family issues change over the course of development.*

Family stress may lessen or shift as the child with Williams syndrome becomes more medically stable and shows increasing cognitive and linguistic competencies as well as a social personality. Yet another shift may occur as families learn to cope with their child's anxieties, fears, learning problems, and hyperactivity. How families function day to day may thus be a by-product of family resources and supports, and of both the positive and negative characteristics of their offspring with Williams syndrome. Indeed, examining 31 families of children and adolescents ages 2–21 years, researchers found that inattention and acting out problems predicted family stress, but that such risks were offset or buffered by the positive effects of these children's social, empathic, and kind-spirited personalities (Fidler, Most, Hodapp, & Dykens, 1999).

Many families continue to care for their offspring with Williams syndrome well into the adult years (Udwin, Howlin, Davies, & Mannion, 1998). Although adults may show diminished problems with hyperacusis, anxiety, and impulsivity (Gosch & Pankau, 1997; Udwin et al., 1998), this is not always the case. Further, many adults continue to struggle with fears and social disinhibition, and they require high needs for supervision for everyday safety and adaptive skills such as dressing and cooking (Udwin, 1990). The level of support these adults receive may differ by the country in which they live: Udwin et al. (1998) found that many families residing in the United Kingdom do not receive appropriate support or respite services, despite the persistent medical and psychological needs of their adult family member with Williams syndrome. The outlook for families may improve in the years ahead due to the outreach and support provided by Williams syndrome parent and family support groups both in this country and abroad (see Resources for information on the National Williams Syndrome Association).

NEXT STEPS

Despite a groundswell of studies on cognition and language, many other aspects of behavior in those who have Williams syndrome remain largely unexplored:

- Adaptive and social competencies and personality strengths such as empathy, and how all these relate to educational, vocational, and personal adjustment
- Optimal treatments and interventions for anxiety, fears, and phobias, as well as for attentional impairments
- The efficacy of social skills training programs in increasing friendships and curbing social disinhibition, indiscriminate relating, and risks of abuse or exploitation
- Gene–brain behavior relationships that cast a wider net of behavioral correlates, including anxiety
- The efficacy of specific educational curricula that capitalize on cognitive-linguistic strengths and minimize weaknesses

Future work needs to better describe these and other aspects of Williams syndrome.

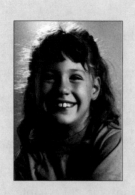

5

Fragile X Syndrome

Fragile X syndrome was first identified just decades ago in the 1970s, yet it has already had a profound impact on the study of mental retardation. The discovery of fragile X syndrome underscored the importance of X-linked disorders as a major cause of developmental disabilities. Furthermore, with unexpected research interest in the cognitive and behavioral features of fragile X, this disorder helped legitimize and solidify the study of behavioral phenotypes in general. Indeed, relative to several of the other syndromes summarized in this book, fragile X syndrome leads the way as a model neurodevelopmental disorder for making novel gene–brain behavior associations.

Fragile X features many intriguing genetic and clinical features. To highlight just a few, fragile X syndrome

- Is the most common known inherited cause of mental retardation
- Is the first known human disease attributed to a trinucleotide repeat; a genetic breakthrough that has led

the way to discoveries of repeats in Huntington disease, myotonic dystrophy, and other diseases

- Results in a wide range of cognitive involvement, from mild learning disabilities to moderate mental retardation

- Results in problems relating to others, which range in severity from shyness to autism

- Has generated considerable controversy regarding who to test and screen for this disorder

After providing a brief history of fragile X syndrome, this chapter examines these and other features of this complex developmental disorder.

HISTORY

The fact that many more males are affected by mental retardation than females has long been acknowledged. It was only in the early 1970s, however, that social theories explaining this discrepancy finally gave way to genetic explanations and X-linked mental retardation was accepted as a distinct diagnostic category. As reviewed in Chapter 2, males have only one X (or sex) chromosome and are vulnerable to a wide range of disabling conditions from which their female counterparts, by virtue of a second X, are protected.

In 1943, Martin and Bell described a large family in which multiple males were affected by mental retardation, apparently inherited through minimally or unaffected females. No laboratory test existed for this X-linked condition, but affected males had a recognizable pattern of clinical characteristics that included large ears, a long and narrow face, and enlarged testicles. This last feature, technically referred to as *macroorchidism,* became the hallmark characteristic of the so-called Martin-Bell syndrome. Only a handful of families were ever clinically diagnosed as having Martin-Bell syndrome, and it took almost four decades before a direct connection could be made between this disorder and the one we now know as fragile X syndrome.

In 1969, Herbert Lubs reported the presence of an abnormal "marker X" chromosome in a family of males with X-linked mental retardation. The marker was an X chromosome with a small, pinched-off piece of genetic material at the bottom of its "q" (or long) arm (see Figure 5.1). Few labs could reproduce Lubs' finding, and its significance remained unrecognized for almost a decade, until 1977. At that time, Grant Sutherland first identified the specific laboratory techniques necessary for the marker X to show itself. Soon after, the marker X became known as the "fragile X" because of its thread-like appearance, and laboratories throughout the world began to offer fragile X chromosome analysis as a diagnostic test for males with mental retardation. Blood samples from the original family identified by Martin and Bell were studied in 1981 (Proops & Webb, 1981), and it was confirmed that members had the fragile X. Thus, the clinical descriptions of the Martin-Bell males were linked to an objective laboratory marker, and a distinct form of X-linked mental retardation, called fragile X syndrome, was confirmed.

GENETICS

Diagnosis

Until 1991, when the exact genetic mutation underlying fragile X syndrome was first identified, the diagnosis was made by visualizing the fragile X chromosome in cytogenetic preparations. This technique was highly accurate for diagnosing affected males, and could also identify more than 90% of fragile X females with mental retardation. Fragile X chromosome testing could not, however, detect most unaffected female and male carriers, nor could it be used reliably for prenatal diagnosis.

In 1991, the gene responsible for fragile X syndrome was discovered (Verkerk et al., 1991). Dubbed with the acronym FMR1 (fragile X mental retardation 1), the gene in its normal state produces a protein product thought to play a key role in both pre- and postnatal brain development. The FMR1 gene contains a repetitive sequence of the trin-

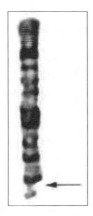

Figure 5.1. Cytogenetic view of the fragile X marker.

ucleotide CGG, which in most people is repeated anywhere from 6 to 50 times. Most intellectually typical fragile X carriers have an expanded FMR1 gene sequence, ranging from 50 to 200 CGG repeats in size. Repeat sizes within this range are called *fragile X premutations* and do not appear to affect the production of FMR1 protein.

Male and female premutation carriers show no outward signs of fragile X syndrome; their cognitive or behavior functioning is not affected (Mazzocco & Holden, 1996; Reiss, Freund, Abrams, Boehm, & Kazazian, 1993). Individuals who carry the premutation, however, can pass the mutation to their children. In females, fragile X premutations are unstable and can expand further when passed down to the next generation. If the CGG sequence expands to larger than 200 repeats in size it is called a *full mutation*. An FMR1 gene with a full mutation becomes inactive, or *methylated,* and does not make its protein product, resulting in symptoms of fragile X syndrome. Virtually all males with a methylated full mutation show clinical characteristics of fragile X syndrome. More than half of females with a full mutation have fragile X symptoms, the others being protected from symptoms by the normal FMR1 gene on their second X chromosome.

Direct deoxyribonucleic acid (DNA) testing of the FMR1 gene has now replaced the earlier chromosome test in most instances. The testing can distinguish among normal, premutation, and full mutation size gene sequences, meaning that unaffected male and female family members can find out whether they are fragile X carriers. DNA studies can also tell the extent to which the FMR1 gene is inactivated, which is sometimes helpful for determining a child's prognosis. DNA for fragile X testing is usually extracted from blood samples, or from fetal cells in amniotic fluid or other tissues for prenatal diagnosis.

Hereditary Implications for Families

Because of the existence of both pre- and full mutations, as well as the sex chromosomal differences among males and females, fragile X syndrome has a particularly complex inheritance pattern. Carrier females can pass their fragile X mutation to children of either sex. Carrier males can only transmit the fragile X mutation to their daughters, never to their sons; as in all X-linked disorders, there is no male-to-male inheritance. The fragile X premutation does not expand in size when passed from an unaffected father to his daughters, and they too are unaffected. As females though, they are at risk for having children with an expanded full mutation. Whenever one person in a family is found to have fragile X syndrome, the gene mutation can almost always be traced back to previous generations, even though many of the gene carriers in a family may be unaffected.

Whenever one person in a family is found to have fragile X syndrome, the gene mutation can almost always be traced back to previous generations, even though many of the gene carriers in a family may be unaffected.

For example, a boy with fragile X syndrome may be the only person in his family with significant mental retardation. Because of its inheritance pattern, however, we know that he received the fragile X from his mother, who must have inherited either a pre- or full mutation from one of her parents. Although unaffected, the boy's mother is at high risk for having other children with fragile X syndrome. Likewise, the mother's siblings and cousins could also be carriers. The boy's unaffected sister has a strong chance of carrying a fragile X pre- or full mutation, which might then result in fragile X syndrome in her future children. The boy's unaffected brother could carry a fragile X premutation, which all of his daughters would inherit, putting his future grandchildren at high risk for having fragile X syndrome. This common condition clearly has far-reaching genetic implications for the extended family, once again illustrating the importance of identifying the diagnosis in people with mental retardation and other developmental disabilities.

Prevalence

The fragile X chromosome test did not become widely available until the mid-1980s, and until then, few researchers anticipated the high prevalence of the syndrome or its wide-ranging effects in both males and females. Although initial prevalence estimates have recently been revised downward, fragile X syndrome continues to rank as the most common known inherited cause of mental retardation, occurring in 1 in 4,000 males and at least half as many females (Turner, Webb, Wake, & Robinson, 1996). Furthermore, as many as 1 in 259 women in the general population may be a fragile X premutation carrier and at risk for having affected children (Rousseau, Rouillard, Morel, Khandjian, & Morgan, 1995). Fragile X syndrome appears in all racial and ethnic groups and has been found to account for up to 14% of unexplained mental retardation in males. Approximately one third of all X-linked mental retardation is due to fragile X syndrome.

PHYSICAL FEATURES

The physical characteristics associated with fragile X syndrome are non-specific and may be found in people without this disorder. Macro-orchidism, the much-publicized hallmark of Martin-Bell syndrome, is uncommon among prepubertal boys with fragile X syndrome, although it may be seen in as many as 80% of postpubertal boys and men with this disorder. Indeed, mean testicular volumes of adult men with fragile X syndrome may be twice that seen in typical men without this syndrome (Hagerman, 1996). Other physical features are subtle in childhood and become more pronounced with advancing age, including a long, narrow face and prominent ears. Figures 5.2 and 5.3 depict the faces of a child and two adults with fragile X syndrome, respectively. More variable physical features seen in childhood include those related to loose connective tissue, including hyperextensible finger joints, flat feet, and soft skin. Many of these physical features are so common in the general population that they are only marginally useful for identifying individuals with fragile X syndrome, many of whom do not look particularly distinct from other people with similar disabilities.

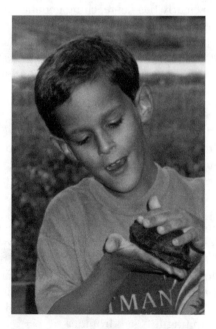

Figure 5.2. Young, fully affected boy with typical fragile X facial features.

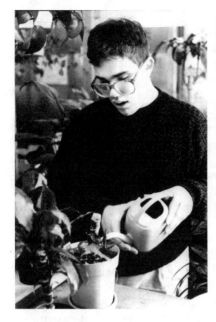 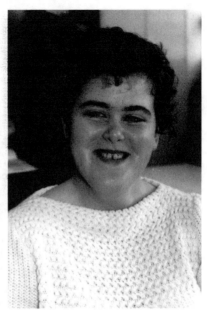

Figure 5.3. Adults with fragile X syndrome.

Few significant medical problems are associated with fragile X syndrome, and most affected males and females are physically healthy. Chronic ear infections are common in childhood, and there is a high frequency of mitral valve prolapse, a minor heart problem that usually requires no treatment. Seizures are seen in about 20% of children with fragile X syndrome, and typically these are easily controlled (Hecht, 1991). Some children also show strabismus and scoliosis. Fortunately, there is no evidence to suggest a reduced life span among people with fragile X syndrome. Similarly, the syndrome has not been associated with any increased incidence of dementia or other signs of abnormal aging.

COGNITIVE FUNCTIONING

As suggested previously, the level of cognitive functioning in people with fragile X syndrome depends on their genetic status and gender. As we show later in the chapter, cognitive level also depends on age. The next section examines these and other factors and how they affect cognitive functioning in individuals with fragile X syndrome.

Cognitive Levels

Males   At present, three types of genetically distinct males have been identified; each seems to be associated with different IQ levels. The largest group of males are fully affected, with fully methylated CGG repeats that effectively shut down the production of FMR1 protein. These males invariably have mental retardation, with IQ scores that fall in the mild to moderate range, depending on when they are tested.

A second, smaller group of males are mosaic for fragile X syndrome, meaning that some of their cells have an unmethylated FMR1 gene, although other cells have a nonfunctional, fully mutated gene. These males produce some FMR1 protein and have higher IQ scores than their fully affected counterparts, often with IQ scores that fall in the borderline to low average range.

A small number of males have been identified who show an unusual pattern. These males show full CGG expansions (in excess of 200 repeats), but, for unknown reasons, they have partial methylation. These males thus produce some FMR1 protein, though at less than normal levels (Hagerman et al., 1994; Merenstein et al., 1996). These males have the highest IQ scores of all, showing average to low-average cognitive performance. Although only about a dozen of these males have been identified, they further demonstrate that the degree of cognitive delay in males with fragile X syndrome depends on the amount of FMR1 protein produced.

Recently, Tassone et al. (1999) refined these observations even more by correlating IQ domains, behavior problems, and physical characteristics to FMR1 protein status in three groups of males: those with 1) mosaicism, 2) partially methylated full mutations, and 3) full mutations. FRM1 protein status was strongly correlated with both performance and verbal IQ in males with partial methylation; these correlations were less strong among mosaic males. FMR1 protein accounted for 68% of the IQ variance in males with partial methylation, and 38% in mosaic males. As expected, no relationship was found among FMR1 protein and IQ in fully methylated males, as they produce little to no protein. For all groups, correlations were nonsignificant among FMR1 protein and measures of physical or behavioral involvement.

Females   The level of cognitive functioning in affected females also depends on the amount of FMR1 protein produced, yet with an additional twist. All females (with or without fragile X syndrome) have two X chromosomes, and one of these is randomly inactivated in all cells. The degree of involvement in fragile X females thus depends on the proportion of activated cells with normal X chromosomes relative to activated cells with the fragile X gene. If the normal X is inactivated in the majority of cells, the female will be more cognitively and clinically affected with fragile X syndrome, and vice versa. Although data are equivocal, it appears that IQ and other features of females with fragile X syndrome are related to the so-called "activation ratio," or the proportion of normal active X chromosomes to the total active plus the inactive normal X chromosomes. In general, then, females with full mutations are less cognitively affected than are males because they produce some FMR1 protein from their normal X chromosome.

Among girls with fragile X syndrome, FMR1 protein status is a powerful predictor of IQ, more so than mean level of parental IQ (Reiss, Freund, Baumgardner, Abrams, & Denckla, 1995). Although parental IQ predicts close to half of the variance of IQ in girls without fragile X syndrome, in girls with fragile X, it predicts just 26% of the variance, while FMR1 protein status predicts 33% of the variance (Reiss et al., 1995).

It may be, then, that deficient FMR1 protein in females is more strongly associated with physical features than with cognitive ability, whereas impairments in protein in males are conversely more predictive of cognitive abilities than of physical involvement.

These findings are consistent with Tassone et al. (1999), who correlated FMR1 protein status in females with a full mutation to IQ, as well as to physical and behavioral indices of fragile X syndrome. Protein status accounted for 31% of the IQ variance in these females, yet only the performance IQ was correlated with protein status. Among females, verbal skills may be somewhat spared relative to performance-based abilities (see also de Vries, 1996). Furthermore, unlike males, FMR1 protein status in these females was strongly and negatively correlated with their indices of physical involvement (Tassone et al., 1999).

It may be, then, that deficient FMR1 protein in females is more strongly associated with physical features than with cognitive ability, whereas impairments in protein in males are conversely more predictive of cognitive abilities than of physical involvement. This hypothesis gains support from studies of women with premutations. Although women with premutations did not show cognitive or behavioral differences, Riddle et al. (1998) found that these women were more apt than were unaffected women to show some of the syndrome's physical features, such as prominent ears; jaw; and, to a some extent, a high, arched palate.

Future studies are necessary to show how FMR1 protein levels in females with fragile X syndrome interact with other correlates of IQ,

　　　　　　　　　　　　　　　　　　　　　　　　　　　Genetic Disorders

such as stress, sociocultural adversity, and intensity of special and early intervention services.

No correlations have as yet been found among protein status in males or females and overall indices of behavioral problems or symptoms of attention-deficit/hyperactivity disorder (ADHD). Yet more refined measures of behavioral or emotional difficulties may be needed to uncover such relationships.

Cognitive Profiles

Males Many fully affected males with fragile X syndrome show particular patterns of cognitive strength and weakness (see Table 5.1). As found across many studies, these males show difficulties with short-term memory tasks, including auditory-verbal and visual-perceptual short-term memory (Dykens, Hodapp, & Leckman, 1987; Freund, Peebles, Aylward, & Reiss, 1995; Kemper, Hagerman, & Altshul-Stark, 1988; Maes, Fryns, Van Walleghem, & Van den Berghe, 1994b). These difficulties may impede performance in sequentially based tasks, in which stimuli need to be retained in the working memory long enough to be placed in serial or temporal order. Indeed, difficulties in sequential processing seem more pronounced in fragile X males than in typical males (Crowe & Hay, 1990; Hodapp et al., 1992), though this may not be as apparent among older, institutionalized, or low-functioning men (Maes et al., 1994a; Simon, Rappaport, Papka, & Woodruff-Pak, 1995). Although many males also show relative weaknesses in visual-spatial and visual-motor tasks (Crowe & Hay, 1990), they may perform better when these visual-spatial tasks do not require short-term memory,

Table 5.1. Cognitive and adaptive strengths and weaknesses in males and females with fragile X syndrome

Strengths	Weaknesses
Verbal skills	Auditory-verbal short-term memory
Repertoire of acquired knowledge	Visual-perceptual short-term memory
Long-term memory for learned information	Sustaining attention, effort
Verbal long-term memory	Sequential processing
Expressive and receptive vocabularies	Certain visual-spatial and perceptual organization tasks
Adaptive daily living skills, especially domestic and personal grooming tasks (males)	Shifting problem-solving strategies
	Integrating information (more readily measured in females)
	Adaptive socialization skills (females and males with autism)

and are instead embedded in a familiar context (Freund & Reiss, 1991; Maes et al., 1994b). Some studies find that males show impairments in quantitative reasoning (Freund et al., 1995), yet other work finds no particular weaknesses in arithmetic skills (Maes et al., 1994a).

In contrast to experiencing these difficulties, males with fragile X syndrome often excel in verbal skills, especially with tasks that tap their repertoire of acquired knowledge and their expressive and receptive vocabularies (Dykens et al., 1987; Freund & Reiss, 1991; Maes et al., 1994b). Long-term memory for so-called "crystallized" knowledge, or information acquired through environmental learning, is typically much better developed than is the ability to solve problems with novel stimuli or with short-term memory. Indeed, many boys show steady increments in acquired knowledge and vocabulary over the course of development, whereas no such age-related improvements are seen in sequentially based, short-term memory (Hodapp, Dykens, Ort, Zelinsky, & Leckman, 1991). In general, then, males often do well when tasks or lessons to be learned are embedded in a familiar context that draws on information stored in long-term memory. These and other implications for intervention are discussed later in the chapter.

Females A recent flurry of research points to similar profiles of strength and weakness in females with fragile X syndrome (see Table 5.1). In general, verbal skills are relatively spared, with women instead showing difficulties in visual-perceptual and spatial construction, or more right hemisphere functioning (Abrams et al., 1994; Mazzocco, Hagerman, & Pennington, 1992; Mazzocco, Pennington, & Hagerman, 1993; Thompson, Rogeness, McClure, Clayton, & Johnson, 1996). Strikingly, the activation ratio (variations in X inactivation patterns and levels of subsequent FMR1 protein) correlates best with specific IQ subtests that assess these areas of relative weaknesses, such as the Wechsler-based Block Design, Coding, and Picture Arrangement (Wechsler, 1991), and the Performance IQ (Abrams et al., 1994; Reiss, Abrams, Greenlaw, Freund, & Denckla, 1995). As verbal skills are relatively spared, correlations are nonsignificant among the activation ratio and verbal IQ subtests.

Many women with fragile X syndrome also show difficulties with cognitive skills that reflect frontal lobe function. These women may have problems sustaining attention, shifting their problem-solving strategies, and integrating information (Mazzocco et al., 1992; Mazzocco et al., 1993; Sobesky et al., 1996). Some researchers hypothesize that these difficulties may lead to a set of emotional or psychiatric vulnerabilities in affected females, including lability; perseverative and tangential speech; and strained, unusual, or odd thinking (Mazzocco et al., 1993). Others, however, do not find that frontal lobe impairments cause emotional difficulties, though they may serve to worsen them (Sobesky et al., 1996).

Some of these IQ and cognitive profile findings may also be related to certain anomalies in brain functioning. Mostofsky et al. (1998) found that, relative to controls, females with fragile X syndrome showed decreased posterior vermis sizes, though these decreases were not as pronounced as those found in males with fragile X syndrome. Posterior vermis size predicted a significant proportion of the variance on visual-spatial IQ measures, as well as a proportion of the activation ratio. Intriguingly, injuries to the cerebellum and neocerebellum, which include parts of the posterior vermis, often lead to problems with cognitive and motor planning, detecting errors, and shifting strategies to solve problems; all are issues commonly seen in females with fragile X syndrome. Findings encourage further studies that link FMR1 status to neuroanatomical and cognitive-behavioral functioning.

IQ Trajectories

Several well-designed studies find that many fully affected males with fragile X syndrome show declines in their IQ scores over time (Dykens et al., 1989; Fisch et al., 1996; Hodapp et al., 1990; Lachiewicz, Gullion, Spiridigliozzi, & Aylsworth, 1987; Wright-Talamante et al., 1996). Both cross-sectional and longitudinal studies point to a downward trajectory of IQ over the course of an individual's development, especially in late childhood and adolescence. Although these IQ trajectory studies differ in sample sizes, types of IQ tests used, ages of IQ testing, and prospective versus retrospective approaches, all report significant age-related declines in IQ test standard scores.

An example of this decline is presented in Figure 5.4, which depicts a cross-sectional analysis of IQ scores from 130 boys (Dykens, Ort, et al., 1996). In this cohort of fully affected males, IQ declined from a mean of 55 in the group of children ranging from 1 to 5 years old to a mean IQ of 39 among the 16- to 20-year-old participants. Longitudinal data likewise show IQ declines (see Dykens, Hodapp, & Leckman, 1994, for a review). Four aspects of these robust findings are particularly intriguing:

1. *IQ declines do not represent a regression or loss in cognitive skills per se but instead suggest a slowing in the rate of acquisition of these skills.* As IQ scores decline, mental-age (MA) scores and success with specific cognitive tasks may be stable in some individuals, although others may even show modest increases in age scores or new successes with items on IQ tests (Hodapp et al., 1991). Yet such stability or gains in age scores are not in keeping with the rate of learning predicted by early IQ scores, contributing to the decline in IQ standard scores.

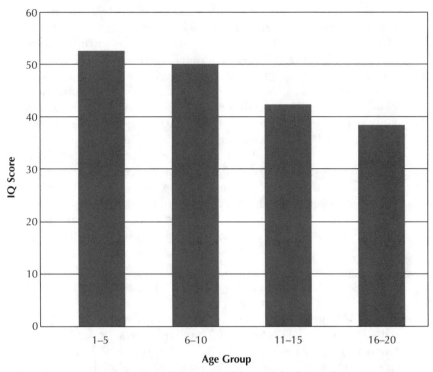

Figure 5.4. Cross-sectional analysis of IQ scores in 130 boys with fragile X syndrome. Mean IQ score in the 1- to 5-year-old group = 55; 6- to 10-year-old group = 50; 11- to 15-year-old group = 43; 16- to 20-year-old group = 39.

2. *Reasons for this slowed rate of cognitive development are unclear.* Early hypotheses suggested that boys with fragile X slowed in their rate of development because of their difficulties with certain items on IQ tests; however, which items made them appear to have slowed in their learning were never specified. Recent neuroanatomical and genetic findings hold more promise for understanding the IQ decline phenomenon. Reiss, Lee, and Freund (1994) found age-related changes in the size of the superior temporal gyrus, hippocampus, and lateral ventricles, structures that are important in learning, memory, attention, and language (see Abrams & Reiss, 1995, for a review). These data suggest a deleterious effect of the lack of FMR1 protein that extends beyond early brain development to include the childhood and adolescent years. To build on these findings, studies are now needed to longitudinally examine brain and IQ changes in the same group of boys with fragile X syndrome.

Recent findings fine-tune these observations by showing that males who produce some amount of FMR1 protein seem protected against the IQ decline. Specifically, the few cases of fully affected males with less than 50% methylation have not shown IQ declines, and these males maintain their average IQs into the adult years (Hagerman et al., 1994; Merenstein et al., 1996; Wright-Talamante et al., 1996). Similarly, IQ declines are not observed among the majority of females with fragile X syndrome who produce some FMR1 protein as related to their activation ratio (Abrams et al., 1994; Wright-Talamante et al., 1996). Only a small percentage of fully affected females show IQ declines, and these declines are generally less steep or less severe as those seen in males (Brun et al., 1995; Fisch, Simensen, Arinami, Borgfgraef, & Fryns, 1994). Presumably, however, those few women with limited to no FMR1 protein production may show IQ declines more in keeping with their male counterparts.

3. *It is unclear when males are most vulnerable to a slowing of development and subsequent IQ decline.* Cross-sectional analyses of young boys up to age 5 years do not show evidence of IQ score decline (Freund, Rice, & Abrams 1995), whereas young boys followed longitudinally showed some declines in IQ standard scores (Bailey, Hatton, & Skinner, 1998). Moreover, a variable developmental course was found among 46 young boys followed longitudinally, with some boys showing relative stability in age-equivalent scores, and others showing modest to striking gains in developmental age-scores over time (Bailey et al., 1998). Stability in age scores and a downward trend in IQ scores have been observed among older males ranging from 8 to 15 years (Hagerman et al., 1989; Hodapp et al., 1990; Lachiewicz et al., 1987), and into the adult years (Dykens et al., 1989; Fisch et al., 1991). Although the exact age of plateauing thus remains unclear, it appears that boys may be vulnerable to slowed development anywhere from late childhood into adolescence and adulthood.

4. *Finally, the trajectory of IQ in fragile X syndrome differs from rates of development found in people with mental retardation in general, as well as from people with other genetic syndromes.* Stability in IQ scores over time is observed in longitudinal studies of people with mixed or nonspecific mental retardation (e.g., Silverstein, Legutkin, Friedman, & Takayama, 1982), with increased variability among those with mild to borderline levels of delay (e.g., Keogh, Bernheimer, & Gutherie, 1997). Relative stability is seen as well in IQs of people with Prader-Willi syndrome (Dykens, Hodapp, Walsh, & Nash, 1992a),

although children who have Down syndrome may alternate among periods of cognitive-adaptive gains and plateaus (see Hodapp, 1996, for a review). Although comparative studies are needed, the distinctiveness of the IQ trajectory in fragile X syndrome underscores the possibility that the lack of FMR1 protein is deleterious to functioning over the course of development.

ADAPTIVE PROFILES AND TRAJECTORIES

Many researchers and parents contend that the adaptive behavior of people with fragile X syndrome is a more accurate estimate of their level of functioning than IQ. This is because measures of adaptive behavior, such as the widely used Vineland Adaptive Behavior Scales (VABS, Sparrow, Balla, & Cicchetti, 1984), rely on parental or caregiver reports, and circumvent certain challenges in directly testing people with fragile X syndrome. Indeed, many individuals with fragile X syndrome may be uncomfortable with the social-interpersonal demands of the testing situation, showing gaze avoidance and social anxiety, as well as hyperactivity and distractibility. All of these behaviors may detract from optimal IQ test performance (Cohen et al., 1996).

Many researchers and parents contend that the adaptive behavior of people with fragile X syndrome is a more accurate estimate of their level of functioning than IQ.

Despite these possible testing difficulties, impressively high correlations are typically found among IQ and adaptive behavior scores in males with fragile X syndrome (Dykens, Ort et al., 1996; Dykens, Ort, et al., 1993). For many, adaptive levels are either commensurate with or exceed IQ expectations (Dykens, 1995a; Fisch et al., 1996, Wiegers, Curfs, Vermeer, & Fryns, 1993), and males with some FMR1 protein production, such as those with mosaicism, may show better-developed adaptive skills than fully affected males show(Cohen et al., 1996).

Profiles

Many males with fragile X syndrome show significant strengths in daily living or self-help skills relative to other adaptive domains such as communication or socialization (Dykens et al., 1993; Dykens, Ort, et al., 1996; Maes et al., 1994a; Wiegers et al., 1993). Such strengths are seen in males who are both institutionalized and home-reared, and these strengths are also apparent relative to others with mental retardation (Dykens, Leckman, Paul, & Watson, 1988; Maes et al., 1994a). Many males seem to perform particularly well with domestic or household chores and duties, as well as with personal grooming tasks; these strengths seem especially apparent in males from late childhood through adulthood (Dykens, Ort, et al., 1996). Although reasons for these strengths are unknown, they may relate to the cumulative prac- tice effects of tasks that are inherently repetitive, rote, and "hands-on," as well as embedded in a meaningful context.

In contrast, females with fragile X syndrome do not share these particular strengths in daily living skills and instead show relative weaknesses in socialization skills, especially in interpersonal skills (Freund et al., 1993). Although preliminary, such observations seem directly related to a host of emotional and psychiatric vulnerabilities shown by these girls and women, including shyness, avoidance, and other oddities in relating. Of note is that socialization skills do not emerge as a salient weakness in most males with fragile X syndrome, except for the minority of males with a co-morbid autistic disorder (Cohen, 1995a).

Trajectories

Although adaptive skills may be better developed than cognition in some males, both domains show a downward trajectory or slowed rate of development over time. Declines in VABS standard scores were seen in large, cross-sectional studies of more than 130 males with fragile X, as well as in longitudinal studies of males tested at least twice with the VABS (see Dykens, 1995a, for a review). Declines in adaptive behavior standard scores may be more steep or pronounced than declines in cog- nition (Fisch et al., 1996), and age-related declines in Vineland commu- nication and socialization standard scores were observed even in a small sample of preschool boys (Freund et al., 1995).

In general, however, boys with fragile X syndrome appear to show slow, steady gains in adaptive behavior age-equivalent scores across various domains of functioning (Bailey et al., 1998; Dykens, Ort, et al., 1996). Figure 5.5, for example, shows gains in VABS age-equivalent scores in 18 boys tested twice in the 1- to 10-year-old period, and relative stability in 11 males tested twice in the 11- to 20-year-old period. Further- more, cross-sectional analyses of VABS data from 130 boys suggest that adaptive gains are most striking in the 1- to 5-year-old period, and less striking—though still apparent—in 6- to 10-year-olds. After individuals reach 10 years of age, increased variability is suggested in their adaptive

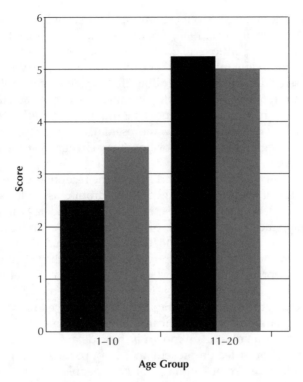

Figure 5.5. Longitudinal analyses of Vineland age-equivalent scores. Significant gains were seen from first to second testing in the 1- to 10-year-old group (from a mean of 2.53 to 3.37). No significant gains were seen from first to second testing in the 11- to 20-year-old group (means = 5.16 and 5.04, respectively). (Key: ■ = first testing, ■ = second testing)

skills acquisition. Although some males show gains in age-equivalent scores into adulthood, especially in domestic and personal grooming skills (Cohen, 1995a; Wiegers et al., 1993), on average these older males show relative stability in age-equivalent scores at least through age 40 years (Dykens, Ort, et al., 1996). As with IQ, further work is needed that relates adaptive skills to FMR1 protein status and neuroanatomical functioning in both boys and men with fragile X syndrome.

LINGUISTIC FUNCTIONING

Relative to other behavioral domains, little work has yet been accomplished on the speech and language characteristics of people with fragile X syndrome, especially females (see Dykens, Hodapp, & Leckman, 1994, for a review). Many males show uneven and unpredictable rates of speech, alternating between short, rapid bursts of speech and longer pauses (Wolf-Schein et al., 1987). Speech is also characterized by whole- and part-word repetitions (e.g., repeating sounds or words), substitutions or omissions of sounds, and cluttering (i.e., a type of verbal clumsiness or difficulty in controlling the sequence of complex motor movements required in speaking) (Hanson, Jackson, & Hagerman, 1986; Paul, Cohen, Breg, Watson, & Herman, 1984; Paul et al., 1987). Studies have yet to assess how representative are these features of males with fragile X syndrome or how they change over the course of development.

Delays are consistently found in both the receptive and expressive vocabularies of males with fragile X syndrome, as well as in their syntactic development. Indeed, expressive language delays are often the precipitating factors that initially bring young boys with fragile X syndrome to professional attention. It is unclear if males show uneven development across their receptive versus expressive vocabularies (Madison, George, & Moeschler, 1986; Paul et al., 1987), yet the repertoire of both receptive and expressive vocabulary words is a cognitive-adaptive strength among older fragile X males relative to controls (Maes et al., 1994a). Although males typically show delays in syntactic or grammatical development, it is unknown if these delays are commensurate with their MA or instead represent an area of particular impairment.

The adaptive use of language, or how people with fragile X syndrome converse and communicate with others, has perhaps been more captivating to researchers than have other speech-language domains. Referred to as *pragmatics*, findings from this body of work suggest that many males with fragile X syndrome are tangential in their conversations and that they overuse highly routinized phrases and jargon (see Abbeduto & Hagerman, 1997, for a review). Furthermore, both linguistic and behavioral studies find that males with fragile X syndrome tend to perseverate, or excessively repeat a word, a phrase, or a topic. Perseveration is elevated even compared with others with mental retardation (Ferrier, Bashir, Meryash, Johnston, & Wolff, 1991; Reiss & Freund, 1992; Sudhalter, Cohen, Silverman, & Wolf-Schein, 1990). Similarly, females with fragile X syndrome may show perseverative, tangential, loosely organized, and run-on language as well as an overreliance on routinized or automatic phrases (Madison et al., 1986; Mazzocco et al., 1993). Some of these difficulties likely relate to these females' relative weaknesses in certain neurocognitive tasks, including the ability to anticipate or plan, to use feedback to shift response sets, and to integrate information.

Reasons for the high rates of perseveration in people with fragile X syndrome are unknown. Some researchers frame perseveration as a response to problems with word-retrieval or expressive syntax, others to being overaroused and stimulated (see Abbeduto & Hagerman, 1997, for a review). MRI studies suggest that perseverative language may have distinctive neurological correlates. Specifically, many males and females show increased volume of the caudate nucleus, which stems from inadequate pruning of neural connections (Reiss et al., 1995). The caudate nucleus is involved in frontal lobe circuits regulating cognitive and emotional functioning, including the ability to inhibit responses (Reiss, Abrams, et al., 1994). Perseveration, then, may be related to increased neural connections and arousal (due to inadequate pruning) coupled with a failure to properly inhibit these responses.

Even though speech and language findings to date are intriguing, these domains remain largely unexplored. Studies have yet to relate variability in speech-language profiles to molecular genetic status or FMR1 protein production, especially in girls and women with pre- and full mutations. Work also needs to link language to cognition and assess if the developmental trajectories in cognitive and adaptive functioning are seen as well in the speech and language arena. As suggested by Abbeduto and Hagerman (1997), studies are also needed that assess more unusual language features, including selective mutism in girls (not speaking in certain contexts) and self-talk in boys, which includes mumbling to oneself, sometimes with shifts in register and voice, and mimicry of cartoon or other characters. All of these research efforts need to be made with an eye toward improving speech-language services, including outcome studies of various speech-language therapies (Abbeduto & Hagerman, 1997).

All of these research efforts need to be made with an eye toward improving speech-language services, including outcome studies of various speech-language therapies.

MALADAPTIVE BEHAVIOR—PSYCHOPATHOLOGY

Males

Fragile X Syndrome and Autism Early work on psychopathology focused almost exclusively on possible ties between autism and fully affected boys with fragile X syndrome. Much of this work was sparked by the hope that fragile X syndrome would emerge as a reasonably common genetic cause of autism. Yet, this flurry of research

faded as researchers developed a better sense of the autistism-like behaviors shown by these males, as well as a new appreciation for the
wide range of genetic and phenotypic expressions of fragile X syndrome. More recent work, then, moves away from autism per se and instead describes a host of behavioral vulnerabilities in males and females with both pre- and full mutations (see Table 5.2).

Before this broadened perspective, however, researchers spent
considerable time probing the autism–fragile X link, especially during
the 1980s and early 1990s. This work was based on early research and
case reports of autistism-like features in fully affected males, including
poor eye contact, language delay, perseveration, echolalia, self-injury
(e.g., hand and arm biting), stereotypies (e.g., hand flapping and body
rocking), hypersensitivity to auditory stimuli or environmental change,
tactile defensiveness, preoccupations with a narrow range of stimuli,
and poor peer and social relating (e.g., Gillberg, Persson, & Whalstrom,
1986; Meryash, Szymanski, & Gerald, 1982).

Following up on these observations, some researchers screened
groups of males with autism for the fragile X marker. As summarized
in Table 5.3, rates of fragile X among autistic males ranged from 0% to

Table 5.2.   Characteristic maladaptive vulnerabilities in individuals with fragile X syndrome

Gaze avoidance
Attention deficits
Hyperactivity
Shyness
Social isolation
Social anxiety
Perseveration
Hyperarousal
Tactile defensiveness[a]
Self-injury[a]
Stereotypies[a]
Low self-esteem[b]
Depressive features[b]
Oddities in thinking and affect[b]
Tangential thinking[b]
Unrealistic or distorted view of self, denial of difficulties [b]

[a]More likely to be seen in fully affected individuals.
[b]More likely to be seen in higher-functioning individuals.

Table 5.3. A sampling of studies assessing fragile X syndrome in autism

Study	Number of individuals with autism	Percentage with fragile X syndrome
Watson et al., 1984	76	5.3
Venter et al., 1984	40	0
Jorgensen et al., 1984	23	4
Goldfine et al., 1985	37	0
Blomquist et al., 1985	102	16
Pueschel et al., 1985	18	0
McGillivray et al., 1986	33	9
Wright et al., 1986	40	2.5
Wahlstrom et al., 1986	143	13
Fisch et al., 1986	144	12.5
Brown et al., 1986	183	13.1
Payton et al., 1989	85	2.4
Wahlstrom et al., 1989	52	9
Ho & Kalousek 1989	45	2
Cantu et al., 1990	67	1
Tranebjaerg & Kure,1991	32	6
Bailey et al., 1993	123	1.6

From Dykens, E.M. & Volkmar, F.R. (1997). Studies of autism in fragile X syndrome In D.J. Cohen & F.R. Volkmar (Eds.), *Handbook of autism and pervasive developmental disorders* (2nd ed, p. 392). Copyright 1997 John Wiley & Sons. Reprinted by permission of [Wiley-Liss, Inc., a subsidiary of] John Wiley & Sons, Inc.

16% (see Dykens & Volkmar, 1997, for a review). Variability in rates across studies is likely attributed to different sample sizes and ascertainment biases. Also, at the time of these studies, fragile X was still identified cytogenetically, and laboratories often used different criteria for making the fragile X diagnosis (e.g., percentages of cells showing the fragile site).

Other studies assessed to what extent groups of boys with fragile X syndrome could be diagnosed with autism. As depicted in Table 5.4, overlap among the two disorders was even more disparate, with rates of autism in individuals with fragile X ranging from 5% to 60%. In addition to variable sample sizes, major methodologic problems in these studies included inconsistent or poorly defined diagnostic criteria for autism and a lack of inter-rater reliability in making autism diagnoses (Dykens & Volkmar, 1997).

A decade and more than 40 studies later, most researchers concluded that rates of full-blown autism among males with fragile X may

Table 5.4. A sampling of studies assessing autism in fragile X syndrome

Study	Number of participants with fragile X syndrome	Percentage of participants with autism	Autism diagnostic criteria
Brown et al., 1982	22	23	Rutter
Fryns & Van den Berghe, 1983	30	16	Not stated
Jacobs et al., 1983	9	22	Not stated
Levitas et al., 1983	10	60	DSM-III
Nielsen 1983	27	33	Four behaviors
Fryns et al., 1984	21	14	Two behaviors
Partington, 1984	61	5	Three behaviors
Rhoads, 1984	17	18	Not stated
Benezech & Noel, 1985	28	53	DSM-III
Brown et al., 1986	150	17	DSM-III
Hagerman et al., 1986	50	46	DSM-III
Borghgraef et al., 1987	23	39	Autiscale
Bregman et al., 1988	14	7	DSM-III
Reiss & Freund, 1990	17	18	DSM-III-R
Bailey et al., 1998	57	15	CARS

From Dykens, E.M. & Volkmar, F.R. (1997). Medical conditions associated with autism in fragile X syndrome. In D.J. Cohen & F.R. Volkmar (Eds.), *Handbook of autism and pervasive developmental disorders* (2nd ed, p. 392). Copyright 1997 John Wiley & Sons. Reprinted by permission of [Wiley-Liss, Inc., a subsidiary of] John Wiley & Sons, Inc.

be no higher than are rates found in the general population of males with mental retardation (Einfeld, Molony, & Hall, 1989; Einfeld, Tonge, & Florio, 1994). In some studies the overlap among these two disorders was shown to be about 5%–7% (Bailey et al., 1993; Bailey et al., 1998; Fisch, 1992). More recent estimates, however, are higher (15%–25%), as they take into account those males with high-functioning or milder forms of autism (Bailey et al., 1998; McCabe, de la Cruz, & Clapp, 1999). Furthermore, rates may be slightly higher among young boys, as some children "outgrow" their autism, and others may be diagnosed as having autism so that they may receive certain school-based services (Bailey et al., 1998).

Autistism-Like Behavior Instead of autism per se, most males can be placed along a spectrum of problems involving gaze avoidance, social relating, anxiety, and hyperarousal. Many males with fragile X syndrome show a unique pattern of gaze, whereby they initially avert gaze, wait for the other person to look elsewhere, and then return the gaze (Cohen et al., 1988; Cohen, Vietze, Sudhalter, Jenkins, & Brown, 1991). Although direct gaze is aversive to them, most males with fragile X syndrome seem interested in others and are much more socially attuned to people than are their counterparts with autism.

This seemingly contradictory behavior (a willingness to interact coupled with gaze aversion) is aptly demonstrated in the so-called "fragile X handshake." In a clever set of experiments, Wolff, Gardner, Paccia, and Lappen (1989) compared the greeting behavior of 18 males with fragile X syndrome with that of IQ-matched males without fragile X syndrome. Unlike their counterparts with mental retardation, males with fragile X syndrome displayed a distinctive sequence of greeting behaviors. As depicted in Figure 5.6, they routinely took the hand of others but turned their head as they did so, mumbled a conventional social greeting, and then later returned the gaze (Wolff et al., 1989).

Furthermore, unlike males with autism, fragile X males are sensitive to the facial emotional cues of others (Simon & Finucane, 1996; Turk & Cornish, 1998), and most relate well and are warmly attached to their parents and other care providers. Some may be initially wary or avoidant of others, and then become increasingly comfortable with them over time, as seen in a "slow-to-warm" stance or temperamental style (e.g., Kerby & Dawson, 1994). Many males are thus shy and socially anxious or withdrawn and upset by novel people or environments, even as compared with others with developmental delay (Einfeld et al., 1994; Freund et al., 1995; Reiss & Freund, 1992). Some

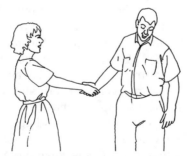

Figure 5.6. The "classic" fragile X syndrome handshake (turn trunk, extend hand, avert gaze, mumble a greeting, and return gaze after the other person looks away). (From Wolff, P.H., Gardner, J., Paccia, J., & Lappen, J. [1989]. The greeting behavior of fragile X males. *American Journal on Mental Retardation, 93,* 408; reprinted by permission.)

may even meet *Diagnostic and Statistical Manual of Mental Disorders, Fourth Edition* (American Psychiatric Association, 1994) criteria for generalized or social anxiety disorders, or for pervasive developmental disorder (e.g., Bregman, Leckman, & Ort, 1988; Reiss & Freund, 1990).

Other autism-like behaviors such as stereotyped motor movements (e.g., hand-flapping, rocking) also seem more common among boys with fragile X syndrome than among other boys with mental retardation (Baumgardner, Reiss, Freund, & Abrams, 1995; Einfeld et al., 1989; Reiss & Freund, 1992). Along with tactile defensiveness, perseveration, hand-biting, social anxiety, and shyness, stereotypies may relate to a generalized hyperarousal of the autonomic nervous system (Cohen, 1995b). Hyperarousal and subsequent behavioral responses are most likely seen in social situations, with demands to perform, and with changes in routine. In these ways, then, autism features in fragile X syndrome may be best associated with anxiety and hyperarousal and less so to the profound social indifference that is the hallmark of autism (Fisch, 1992; Hagerman, 1996).

In addition, the vast majority of clinically referred boys with fragile X syndrome present with hyperactivity and inattention (Bregman et al., 1988; Hagerman, 1996). Relative to others with mental retardation, rates of restlessness, overactivity, and impulsivity may be high even among nonclinical samples of males with fragile X syndrome (Baumgardner et al., 1995). Other researchers, however, have found that hyperactivity is no more common among children with fragile X syndrome than IQ-matched control participants (Einfeld et al., 1994). Interestingly, overactivity is observed in animal models of fragile X syndrome (Willems, Reyniers, & Oostra, 1995), suggesting some vulnerability toward overactivity in the fragile X behavioral phenotype.

Neuroanatomical findings clarify many of these behavioral observations. In a series of neuroimaging studies, Mostofsky et al. (1998) and Reiss and colleagues (1991, 1995) found smaller posterior cerebellar vermis sizes in males with fragile X syndrome. The posterior cerebellar vermis is involved with processing sensory stimuli and modulating motor activity, and anomalies in its size may be associated with the hyperactivity and hypersensitivity to tactile and auditory stimuli seen in males with fragile X syndrome.

In addition, the caudate nucleus is enlarged in males with fragile X syndrome (Reiss et al., 1995), and caudate nucleus volume appears inversely correlated with IQ. The caudate nucleus is involved with several frontal subcortical circuits, and interruptions or lesions to these circuits are known to produce problems in executive function, in regulating affect and motor functioning, and in the ability to inhibit responses and to respond flexibly to environmental cues. Anomalies in the caudate nucleus, then, may be related to many salient features of fragile X syndrome, including verbal perseveration; stereotypies; hyperactivity and attention impairments; impulsivity; emotional lability; inflexibility; and difficulties with organization, planning, and sequencing information. Findings from these neuroanatomical studies encourage further research relating cognitive, emotional, and behavioral features of fragile X syndrome to specific regions of the brain.

Females

In contrast to the early years of study on fragile X syndrome, considerable work has now been devoted to the emotional and behavioral vulnerabilities of women and girls with both pre- and full fragile X mutations. In general, females with full mutations show similar—albeit less severe—emotional and maladaptive behavioral concerns to their male counterparts. The extent to which cognitively unaffected women with premutations also show certain emotional or psychiatric vulnerabilities, however, is less clear.

Problems relating to others have now been noted in women with fragile X syndrome, even as compared with women in a variety of contrast groups. Early work, for example, identified increased risks of schizoptypal features in women with full mutations (Freund, et al., 1993; Freund, Reiss, Hagerman, & Vinogradov, 1992; Reiss, Hagerman, Vinogradov, Abrams, & King, 1988; Reiss, Freund, Vinogradov, Hagerman, & Cronister, 1989). Common symptoms included shyness, social withdrawal, avoidance, isolation, awkwardness, gaze avoidance, and oddities in thinking. More recent work, based on Minnesota Multiphasic Personality Inventory (MMPI-2; Hathaway & McKinely, 1989) scores and interviews, suggested that women with full mutations also have unrealistic or distorted views of themselves, which may include denying their problems and having difficulty integrating historical information into their current lives (Sobesky, Hull, & Hagerman, 1994; Sobesky, Pennington, Porter, Hull, & Hagerman, 1994; Steyaert, Decruyevaere, Bohrgraef, & Fryns, 1994). Some of these challenges seem related to the neurocognitive frontal lobe impairments often seen in these women (Mazzocco et al, 1992; 1993).

Expanding these findings, Sobesky and colleagues (1995; 1996) assessed several groups: women with premutations; women with full mutations; and as control groups, women without fragile X syndrome who grew up in homes with family members with fragile X, and women without fragile X syndrome or without fragile X in the family. Women with full mutations showed more social discomfort than did other participants, exhibiting behaviors that included social isolation, poor eye contact, and difficulties establishing rapport with others (Sobesky et al., 1995). Although interested in social relationships and exchanges, many of these women lacked the requisite skills to interact successfully or comfortably with others.

Similar vulnerabilities have also been hinted at in women with premutations, however. Women with both pre- and full mutations show increased risks of emotional lability, and those with premutations may actually be more socially sensitive or anxious than are those with full mutations (Sobesky et al., 1994). Although women with both pre- and full mutations may exhibit certain schizotypal personality traits, those with full mutations are more apt to show oddities in language and interaction, as well as problems with goal-directed thinking and appropriate displays of affect (Sobesky, Hull, et al., 1994). More recent findings, however, do not find widespread support for emotional vulnerabilities occurring in women with premutations (Riddle et al., 1998).

Depressive affect and disorders have also been described in women and mothers with fragile X syndrome, even as compared with mothers of children who have other types of developmental disabilities.

Depressive affect and disorders have also been described in women and mothers with fragile X syndrome, even as compared with mothers of children who have other types of developmental disabilities (Reiss et al., 1988; 1989). In general, rates of depression and dysthymia (persistent, mild depression) seem comparable across women with both pre- and full mutations (Reiss et al., 1989; Thompson et al., 1994). Similarities in rates across individuals in these two groups may be associated with the stress of raising a child with developmental disabilities, as well as with lingering guilt or self-blame for having transmitted a genetic disorder to their children.

Furthermore, rates of depression among these women may be higher than previously thought. Compared with women in the general population and with mothers of children with other types of disabilities, Thompson et al. (1994) and Thompson, Rogeness, McClure, Clayton, and Johnson (1996) identified high rates of lifetime depression, up to 80%, in women with fragile X who have average IQs and pre- or full mutations. Such rates may indicate a three-fold increase in affective disorders among women with fragile X syndrome relative to women in the general population (Franke et al., 1996). At the same time, however, women in this study showed similar rates of affective disorder as did mothers of children with autism, suggesting that the demands of raising a child with disabilities may also relate to these high rates of depressive disorders.

Similar to women with fragile X syndrome, young girls with this syndrome are prone to shyness and social withdrawal. Relative to other girls, parents and teachers rate girls with fragile X syndrome as more socially withdrawn, sad, and anxious and as showing more salient weaknesses in interpersonal social skills (Freund et al., 1993; Hagerman et al., 1986; Lachiewicz 1992; Lachiewicz & Dawson, 1994). Withdrawal and social problems were also elevated in eight girls with fragile X relative to their unaffected sisters, suggesting that family environment is not solely responsible for the social difficulties seen in affected girls (Mazzocco, Baumgardner, Freund, & Reiss, 1998).

Increased rates of hyperactivity, impulsivity, and inattention have also been observed among girls with fragile X (e.g., Lachiewicz, 1992; Lachiewicz & Dawson, 1994). Indeed, these girls are at risk for ADHD, showing higher rates of ADHD than do girls in the general population, but lower rates than were commonly seen in boys with fragile X syndrome. Symptoms of ADHD exhibited by girls with fragile X may not be as severe as those seen in boys with fragile X, and many girls present primarily with inattention and impulsivity, only secondarily with motoric hyperactivity.

INTERVENTION IMPLICATIONS

The cognitive, adaptive, and behavioral/psychiatric profiles of males and females with fragile X syndrome suggest specific treatment and intervention guidelines. As with other etiology-specific recommendations, these guidelines have yet to be formally evaluated. Although they make sound clinical sense and are congruent with an extensive data base, it is unclear if they are any more effective in terms of long-term outcome and success than more generic ways of educating or supporting people with mental retardation in general.

Educational-Vocational Considerations

In light of the cognitive and adaptive profiles summarized in Table 5.1, many children and adults with fragile X syndrome do well with teaching approaches that emphasize simultaneous processing and verbal long-term memory and that are embedded in a familiar context. As opposed to sequential processing tasks in which students are required to place stimuli in serial or temporal order, many students with fragile X syndrome perform better with integrative tasks that stress the overall meaning of the concept to be learned. Particularly helpful are integrative tasks that draw on acquired words, have a visual or hands-on component (e.g., pictures, diagrams), or use a familiar context (e.g., snapshots of the child's classroom, favorite toys, family members, objects of special interest). Practical strategies might involve teaching number concepts with license plates, clocks, cooking, and other real-life activities (see Braden, 1992, and Scharfenaker, Hickman, & Braden, 1991, for more details).

Given the behavioral vulnerabilities outlined in Table 5.2, many students with fragile X syndrome need help staying attentive and focused on the task at hand. Classroom techniques for reducing visual and auditory distractors often work well, such as using study cubicles, placing the desk at the front of the room, or having periods of quiet time. In addition, many teachers and parents find it helpful to avoid or de-emphasize short-term memory tasks in which the children are expected to act on a set of verbal instructions, without the benefit of visual cues. Finally, many boys and girls respond well to stimulants or other medications commonly used to treat children with ADHD (Hagerman, Murphy, & Wittenberger, 1988).

> Given the behavioral vulnerabilities... many students with fragile X syndrome need help staying attentive and focused on the task at hand.

Although children with fragile X syndrome are interested in others, their overactivity, hyperarousal, and difficulties with change all suggest that they may respond well to certain changes in their environments. Specifically, these children benefit from a reduced flow of people through the classroom, a predictable daily routine, and other calm-ing strategies such as sensory stimulation, music, and relaxation techniques (see Scharfenaker et al., 1991). Furthermore, many socially anxious or shy boys and girls may benefit from social skills training programs. Unlike other participants in such programs, however, increasing direct gaze or eye contact should not be a goal for children with fragile X syndrome, as doing so may increase their anxiety and distress. Instead, their distinctive patterns of gaze need to be respected as does their variability in approaching and interacting with others.

The vocational and residential outcomes of fully affected men and women have yet to be carefully documented. Though adults live and work in a variety of settings, they may perform best in slower paced work programs, in which each day they interact with a few people in a predictable and set routine. Depending on their tolerance for others, more individualized work tasks accomplished in a parallel manner with others may be in order, as opposed to jobs that depend on successfully interacting with others. People with fragile X syndrome may excel in tasks that tap domestic daily living skills or that are predictable and routine. Similar to their younger counterparts, adults may also respond well to visual cues or tasks that touch on verbal long-term memory.

Therapy and Family Support

Supportive psychotherapy and counseling may be beneficial for many higher functioning males and affected or unaffected females (Hagerman & Sobesky, 1989). Specific concerns of these individuals often include shyness, low self-esteem, depression, learning disabilities, guilt associated with having a transmittable genetic disorder, feelings toward their child or children with disabilities, and worries regarding the reproductive decisions faced by their carrier daughters. If depression or dysthymia are salient, many people benefit as well from standard psychotropic interventions. Social skills training and therapy groups may also prove beneficial to some men and women with fragile X syndrome.

Although individual approaches are helpful, family support models are increasingly used in the developmental disability field. Such approaches are particularly relevant to fragile X syndrome. As a transmittable condition, more than one member of the immediate or extended family is invariably touched by fragile X syndrome. Some family members may readily seek services for themselves or their relatives. In contrast, others may not seek services, especially affected women who are shy or avoidant or who deny or minimize their difficulties. Such families are especially challenging for clinicians, as are families with more than one affected child and families with mothers who have cognitive impairments or who are less educated (Meryash, 1989). These families may require more intensive, long-term, or flexible supports, including at-home interventions, parent aides, respite care providers, and advocates who help parents negotiate educational and social services delivery systems (Dykens & Leckman, 1990).

Testing and Screening for Fragile X Syndrome

A final intervention implication moves away from behavior per se and takes up concerns that stem from the genetics of fragile X syndrome. As fragile X syndrome is characterized by complicated inheritance patterns, professionals who work with these families should ensure that family members have appropriate genetic counseling regarding their genetic status and inheritance risks. Feedback from families suggests that women want this counseling information, and that they want their daughters to grow up knowing their own carrier status, from early adolescence on (McConkie-Rosell, Spiridigliozzi, Iafolla, Tarleton, & Lachiewicz, 1997). With counseling, families make more informed family planning choices (Robinson, Wake, Wright, Laing, & Turner, 1996), suggesting that genetic counseling is both effective and in high demand.

Furthermore, as recommended in the policy statement of the American College of Medical Genetics (Park, Howard-Peebles, Sherman, Taylor, & Wulfsberg, 1994), certain individuals should be routinely referred for fragile X testing. These include

- Individuals of either sex with mental retardation, developmental delay, or autism, especially if they have 1) any physical or behavioral characteristics of fragile X syndrome, 2) a family history of fragile X syndrome, or 3) male or female relatives with undiagnosed mental retardation
- Individuals seeking reproductive counseling who have 1) a family history of fragile X syndrome or 2) a family history of undiagnosed mental retardation
- Fetuses of known carrier females
- People with unclear, inconsistent, or ambiguous previous fragile X testing

Fragile X testing should thus be considered in any person with (or related to someone with) mental retardation of unknown etiology, regardless of gender and even in the absence of "typical" fragile X physical or behavioral features.

More controversial, however, is the issue of widespread, population-based screening for fragile X syndrome. The American College of Medical Genetics policy statement (Park et al., 1994) does not recommend population-based screening at this time. The statement cites concerns with the significant lag in educating both professionals and the general public about fragile X syndrome, and with the logistical challenges in providing follow-up genetic counseling for a complex disorder on a large-scale basis (see also McCabe et al., 1999).

Yet, others argue that obstacles to population-based testing are surmountable, including "thoughtful and sound strategies for cost-containment, appropriate patient education, and quality genetic counseling" (Finucane, 1996, p. 781). Finucane, in particular, make persuasive arguments for offering fragile X testing to all pregnant women. She predicts that some form of population testing, such as in pregnant or preconceptual women, is on the horizon. In light of these predictions, professionals from many disciplines have a growing obligation to be knowledgeable about fragile X syndrome, including its genetic, behavioral, and developmental characteristics. This chapter is one small step in that direction.

NEXT STEPS

Rapid advances are being made in the genetics of fragile X syndrome and even in the connections of genetics, brain, and behavior. Yet, many issues remain unresolved in this syndrome:

- To what extent do FMR1 protein levels in girls and women relate to behavioral characteristics other than IQ, particularly to shyness, social withdrawal, or behavior problems?

- How are females with fragile X syndrome and people who have brain injuries to their cerebellum similar and different, given that both show changes (are either smaller sized or damaged) to the brain's posterior vermis region?

- To what extent do males with fragile X syndrome show slower rates of development across cognition, language, and adaptive skills? To what extent are these skills separate or related?

- What domains of language constitute relative weaknesses for males and females with fragile X syndrome? Are difficulties in, say, grammar similar to those shown in overall MA, or is this an area of relative weakness?

- For individuals with fragile X syndrome, how effective are interventions that focus on simultaneous processing or that capitalize on routines and repetition?

- What are the relative effects of a child (or children) with fragile X on family functioning, and how do these effects relate to the genetic status of mothers?

6

Prader-Willi Syndrome

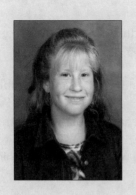

"We are amazed by discoveries in Prader-Willi and Angelman syndromes ... imprinting changes the rules of mammalian genetics ... we now have a mechanism to explain things that we have not understood for years."

—Dr. Judith Hall, The New York Times, July 16, 1991

Prader-Willi syndrome, first identified in the mid-1950s, continues to fascinate both researchers and interventionists. Part of the disorder's intrigue arises from its hallmark symptoms of hyperphagia, or overeating, and marked propensity to obesity—unique features of the syndrome. But as Judith Hall (1991) highlighted in *The New York Times*, Prader-Willi syndrome is also noteworthy for its pivotal role in recent molecular genetic history. To this day, Prader-Willi syndrome captivates genetic and behavioral researchers alike, and as a result the past decades have witnessed a ground swell of new knowledge about this disorder. As summarized in this chapter, we now know that Prader-Willi syndrome

- Is the first known human disorder to show the effects of genomic imprinting, leading to revolutionary changes in the field of molecular genetics
- Is the leading known genetic cause of obesity

- Shows two distinctive stages in early childhood—difficulty sucking and failure to thrive in infancy followed by hyperphagia, or eating too much and thriving too well
- Includes many individuals who have a fondness for (and, possibly, strengths in) solving jigsaw puzzles
- Involves increased risks of compulsive behaviors, as well as other maladaptive features
- Presents unique challenges related to food management and choice and self-determination

HISTORICAL BACKGROUND

In 1956, Prader, Labhart, and Willi published in a German journal a short paper entitled "A Syndrome of Obesity, Short Stature, Hypogonadism, and Learning Disability, with Hypotonia During the Neonatal Period" (see Clarke, Boer, & Webb, 1995). Similar to Langdon Down's short paper on Down syndrome, the article introducing Prader-Willi syndrome is noteworthy for its brief but careful description of the syndrome. Reporting on nine individuals, Prader et al. described their patients' obesity, short stature, hypotonia, and failure to thrive during infancy. The authors even speculated that Prader-Willi syndrome "appears, therefore, to be a hypothalamic disorder" (1956, p. 39). Although researchers have made many advances in this syndrome, hypothalamic anomalies remain the leading—and still unresolved—culprit of at least some of the disorder's cardinal clinical features (Swaab, 1997).

We now know that the disorder generally results from one of two causes—paternal deletion or maternal uniparental disomy (to be discussed in the next section on genetics)—and that the prevalence rate of Prader-Willi syndrome ranges from 1 in 10,000 to 1 in 15,000 individuals. In recent years, researchers have also come to appreciate the "multisystem" nature of this disorder, or the many physical, diagnostic, and behavioral issues that, along with the food issues, deserve attention.

GENETIC, MEDICAL, AND PHYSICAL ISSUES

Although the exact hypothalamic impairment has yet to be identified, considerable progress has been made in identifying the genetic basis of Prader-Willi syndrome. From the early 1980s on, it was understood that most individuals with the syndrome have a small deletion at a certain area (q11-13) on the long arm of chromosome 15 (Ledbetter et al., 1981). With a few exceptions, the remainder of individuals with Prader-Willi syndrome have typical-appearing chromosomes under the microscope.

But what causes Prader-Willi syndrome in the remaining individuals? As molecular genetic technology improved in the late 1980s, researchers discovered two things. First, the deletions causing Prader-Will syndrome always occurred solely in the chromosome 15 inherited from the father (Butler, 1990; Nicholls, Knoll, Butler, Karam, & Lalande, 1989). Second, those individuals without a deletion had two chromosome 15s inherited from the mother, and no chromosome 15 from the father—a situation called *maternal uniparental disomy*, or *UPD* (Nicholls et al., 1989). In individuals with UPD, the chromosomes themselves are typical in number and structure, but the inheritance pattern is wrong. In effect, all individuals with Prader-Willi syndrome have it because they lack the father's contribution to the specific region of the long arm of chromosome 15 associated with this disorder.

In effect, all individuals with Prader-Willi syndrome have it because they lack the father's contribution to the specific region of the long arm of chromosome 15 associated with this disorder.

The genetic findings in Prader-Willi syndrome can be explained by a phenomenon called genetic (or genomic) imprinting (see Chapter 2). In imprinting, genes or groups of neighboring genes are expressed differently depending on the sex of the parent from whom they were inherited. The genes themselves are not altered, but instead some genes are inactivated or switched off. In the typical situation, the maternally derived copies of chromosome 15 in the critical region for Prader-Willi syndrome are inactivated, and only the paternally derived region is expressed in cells. But when the paternal copy of this region is missing—by deletion or by complete absence as in maternal disomy—there is no active copy of the genetic information, and an abnormality in development results in Prader-Willi syndrome (Nicholls, 1993). Although several paternally expressed genes have been identified in the Prader-Willi critical region, only the disruption of one of these genes (called *SNRPN* and perhaps another gene called *NDN*) is significant to the Prader-Willi phenotype (Khan & Wood, 1999).

Prader-Willi syndrome is caused, then, by the absence of the typically active, paternally inherited genes at a particular location on the long arm of chromosome 15. In about 70% of cases, this absence is due to a deletion on the chromosome 15 inherited from the father; most remaining individuals have UPD, or two copies of chromosome 15 from the mother (Mascari et al., 1992; Nicholls et al., 1989; Robinson et al., 1991). An additional 5% of individuals have a translocation or other structural abnormality involving chromosome 15. Finally, a very small percentage (1%–5%) have neither deletion nor UPD, but rather a micro-deletion in the center controlling the imprinting process within 15q11-q13 (Buiting et al., 1995; Saitoh et al., 1997). Though small, this last group includes virtually all cases in which there has been a recurrence of Prader-Willi syndrome within a family.

More refined understandings of the genetics of Prader-Willi syndrome have led researchers to examine possible phenotypic differences across the various genetic subtypes of this disorder. Physically, those with paternal deletions seem more apt to show the syndrome's typical facial features, as well as hypopigmentation (Butler, 1989; Cassidy et al., 1997; Gillessen-Kaesbach, Robinson, et al., 1995; Mitchell et al., 1996). Hypopigmentation, or fair complexion or coloring, is attributed to the deletion of a gene for tyrosinase positive albinoidism in the Prader-Willi critical region. Relative to those with deletions, people with UPD may have increased birth weight, a shorter course of gavage feeding (feeding through a tube) in infancy, and a later onset of hyper-phagia (Gillessen-Kaesbach, Robinson, et al., 1995; Mitchell et al., 1996); some of these features, however, are not observed as being consistent. (Gunay-Aygun, Heeger, Schwartz, & Cassidy, 1997). Advanced mater-nal age is also seen among mothers who bear children with UPD. More subtle physical features in offspring with maternal UPD may lead to a later age of diagnosis in these individuals (Gunay-Aygun et al., 1997). The relatively few individuals with Prader-Willi syndrome who have microdeletions in the imprinting center seem phenotypically similar to others, except that they do not have hypopigmentation (Saitoh et al., 1997). Observations regarding physical features have provoked a new series of studies on possible behavioral differences across deleted ver-sus UPD cases; preliminary findings are presented later in this chapter.

Diagnosis

Given the recent and fast-paced developments in the genetics of Prader-Willi syndrome, many people were first diagnosed clinically—that is, from their physical and behavioral features. And, as the disor-der is relatively rare (making the costs of widespread genetic testing prohibitive), in 1993 professionals working in this syndrome published a list of "consensus clinical criteria" for the disorder (Holm et al., 1993). Although genetic testing has evolved to the point of being both highly accurate and readily available, these clinical criteria, listed in Table 6.1, are still extremely valuable in suggesting the diagnosis and indicating the need for diagnostic testing. No one individual will have all of the manifestations of the disorder listed in Table 6.1, and considerable variability exists in the severity of each of the clinical criteria.

Table 6.1. Summary of the clinical diagnostic criteria for Prader-Willi syndrome

Major criteria (1 point each)	Minor criteria ($^1/_2$ point each)	Supportive criteria (no points)
Infantile central hypotonia	Decreased fetal movement and infantile lethargy	High pain threshold
Infantile feeding problems/failure to thrive	Typical behavior problems	Infrequent vomiting
Rapid weight gain between 1 and 6 years old	Sleep disturbance/sleep apnea	Temperature control problems
Characteristic facial features	Short stature relative to the family by age 15 years	Scoliosis and/or kyphosis
Hypogonadism: genital hypoplasia, pubertal deficiency	Hypopigmentation	Early adrenarche
Developmental delay/mental retardation	Small hands and feet for height age	Osteoporosis
	Narrow hands with straight ulnar border	Unusual skill with jigsaw puzzles
	Esotropia, myopia	Normal neuromuscular studies
	Thick, viscous saliva	
	Speech articulation difficulties	
	Skin picking	

From Holm et al. (1993). Diagnostic criteria for Prader-Willi syndrome. Prader-Willi syndrome: Consensus diagnostic criteria. *Pediatrics, 91,* 399. Elk Grove Village, IL: American Association of Pediatrics; reproduced by permission of *Pediatrics.*

The diagnosis of Prader-Willi syndrome should be strongly suspected in children younger than 3 years of age with a score of 5 points—three from major criteria—or in those older than 3 years with 8 points—four from major criteria. The original diagnostic criteria included a major criterion of chromosome 15 deletion or other chromosome 15 anomaly.

Several genetic tests can now be used to detect Prader-Willi syndrome. Although high resolution cytogenetic analysis can often detect the 15q11-q13 deletion, this technique gives unacceptably high false-negative and false-positive rates. For these reasons, cytogenetic tests are no longer considered sufficient for diagnostic purposes. Instead, the definitive diagnostic test for the common size deletion causing Prader-Willi syndrome is FISH (see Chapter 2). The American Society of Human Genetics/American College of Medical Genetics Test and Technology Transfer Committee has recently published a statement regarding the status of genetic testing for Prader-Willi syndrome (ASHG/ACMG Statement, 1996). Prenatal detection of Prader-Willi syndrome is also now possible.

Although to date there have been no reports of recurrence of Prader-Willi syndrome in families in which one child has Prader-Willi syndrome from either a deletion or from UPD, theoretically the syndrome can recur in a family. Because UPD, in particular, is caused by a chromosomal nondisjunction (which can recur and is related to advanced maternal age), there is some risk of families having a second child with UPD. In both deletion and UPD, a 1% or less recurrence risk has been deemed appropriate for genetic counseling purposes. In contrast, in the small number of families with an imprinting mutation, a recurrence risk of up to 50% pertains, as the imprinting mutation likely involves a dominant mutation in the paternal grandmother's germline.

Two Stages

Individuals with Prader-Willi syndrome are often described as going through two distinct developmental phases. Even before birth, infants with Prader-Willi syndrome are hypotonic, with decreased fetal movement, frequent abnormal fetal position, and difficulty at the time of delivery (often necessitating cesarean section; Cassidy, 1984; Holm et al., 1993). During infancy, hypotonia is usually associated with a poor suck, and many infants are diagnosed as having "failure to thrive." Many infants require gavage or other special feeding techniques. Infantile lethargy, with decreased arousal and weak cry, are also prominent symptoms, often leading to the need to awaken the child to feed. Reflexes may be decreased or absent. Delayed motor milestones are evident; for example, the average age of sitting is 12 months and for walking, the average age is 24 months. The "first stage" of Prader-Willi syndrome therefore involves central infantile hypotonia as well as concomitant difficulties in gaining weight and achieving motor milestones. In striking juxtaposition to these early months, a dramatic shift occurs in this failure-to-thrive pattern sometime during the 1- to 6-year-old period.

At this point, typically from around 3–4 years of age, toddlers and preschoolers begin a lifelong pattern of hyperphagia. Food preoccupations become common; children tend to ask about food or meals, and older individuals may also food-seek, hoard or forage for food, or eat unappealing substances. Low muscle tone and a disinclination to exercise add to the deleterious effects of

In striking juxtaposition to these early months, a dramatic shift occurs in this failure-to-thrive pattern sometime during the 1- to 6-year-old period.

the drive to eat excessively. A high threshold for vomiting may complicate bingeing—no matter how much food these individuals eat, they rarely vomit. It is also from this point on that, without sustained dietary interventions, large weight gains can occur; in some they assume life-threatening proportions.

Figure 6.1 shows a child and an adolescent with Prader-Willi syndrome. As is common in this disorder, the weight on these individuals is centrally located, not in the hands, feet, arms or lower legs. Even individuals with Prader-Willi syndrome who are not obese tend to store

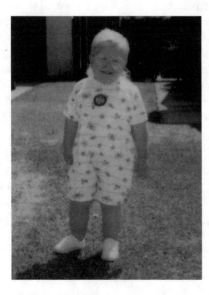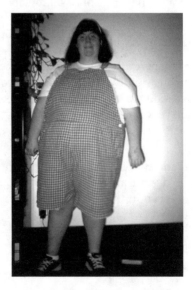

Figure 6.1.   A child and a young adult with the typical facial and body features of Prader-Willi syndrome.

fat on the abdomen, buttocks, and thighs. Typical of most people with the disorder, the individuals in Figure 6.1 have sloping shoulders and a heavy mid-section, and short stature. Indeed, average adult height is 5'1" for males and 4'10" for females (Cassidy, 1984; Hudgins, McKillop, & Cassidy, 1991). People with Prader-Willi syndrome generally have small, narrow hands and short, broad feet, with an average adult shoe size of 3 for females and 5 for males.

Figure 6.1 also depicts the characteristic facial features associated with Prader-Willi syndrome. These include a narrow face with almond-shaped eyes, narrow nasal bridge, and a down-turned mouth with a thin upper lip. Many of these are subtle at birth, and evolve over the course of development.

Other Medical Issues

Since first described in 1956, it has been apparent that many of the features of Prader-Willi syndrome arise from insufficient function of the hypothalamus. In addition to controlling hunger and thirst, the hypothalamus regulates sleep–wake cycles, and temperature regulation. The hypothalamus also releases hormones that travel to the pituitary gland, controlling the release of other hormones such as growth hormone, the sex hormones (gonadotropins), and thyroid-stimulating hormones that control basal metabolic rate.

As indicated in the list of medical concerns below, many of the typical homeostatic functions of the hypothalamus are disrupted in Prader-Willi syndrome, and hypothalamic anomalies likely contribute to many of the syndrome's medical issues. Many of these problems are inconsistently manifest across people with the syndrome; even the drive for food varies across individuals. Although details of medical problems are beyond the scope of this chapter (see Greenswag & Alexander, 1995), major issues include

- Sleep disturbances, especially excessive daytime sleepiness, oxygen desaturation in REM sleep, and sleep apnea. These seem common even in the absence of obesity
- Hypogonadism (i.e., insufficiently developed reproductive organs) in both males and females
- Growth hormone deficiency and characteristic short stature
- Hyperphagia and overeating, most likely due to impaired satiety
- Heart and circulation problems resulting from excessive obesity (e.g., hypertension, thrombophlebitis, chronic leg edema)

- Hypopigmentation (due to deletion of gene for albinoidism in the Prader-Willi critical region)
- A high pain threshold
- Temperature regulation problems
- Thick, viscous saliva that may predispose individuals to cavities and contribute to articulation abnormalities
- Diabetes mellitus (Type II), especially with increased obesity
- Joint problems, including osteoporosis, scoliosis (i.e., curvature of the spine), and kyphosis (i.e., backward curvature of spine; this begins mainly during early adulthood)

Despite this long list of associated health issues, if people with Prader-Willi syndrome can avoid obesity, they generally enjoy good health. Indeed, parents often report that their child with Prader-Willi syndrome is healthier than are his or her unaffected siblings. Yet, to this day, complications of obesity are the major cause of morbidity and mortality in people with Prader-Willi syndrome; if morbid obesity can be controlled in these individuals, life spans may be nearly typical (Cassidy, Devi, & Mukaida, 1994; Greenswag, 1987). Other behavioral aspects of the drive for food are discussed later in the chapter.

COGNITIVE AND LINGUISTIC FUNCTIONING

Although the range of IQ scores in Prader-Willi syndrome has been well-described over the years, researchers have only recently begun to examine other aspects of cognition, language, and adaptive behavior in this syndrome.

Range of Intellectual Abilities

Compared with people with genetic mental retardation syndromes such as fragile X syndrome or Down syndrome, most people with Prader-Willi syndrome have high levels of intelligence. In many studies, the average IQ score is about 70 (e.g., Dykens, Hodapp, Walsh, & Nash, 1992a). Aggregating IQ data from 575 participants in 57 published studies, Curfs (1992) found that 32% of individuals had IQ scores above 70, 34% showed mild mental retardation, 27% had moderate delays, and only 6% showed severe to profound levels of impairment. Of the 32% of people with IQ scores above 70, 27% showed borderline (IQ 70–84) levels of intelligence and 5% showed average IQ scores (IQ 85 and above). Adaptively, however, even high-functioning individuals rarely function at a level commensurate with their IQ scores because of interference from food-related and other behavior problems.

Cognitive Profiles

Early clinical observations suggested that many children with Prader-Willi syndrome showed significant relative strengths in reading and weaknesses in arithmetic (e.g., Holm, 1981; Sulzbacher, Crnic, & Snow, 1981). Yet, studies of achievement do not provide overwhelming support for such a profile. Administering the Kaufman Assessment Battery for Children (K-ABC; Kaufman & Kaufman, 1983) to 21 adolescents and adults with Prader-Willi syndrome, Dykens et al. (1992a) found a nonsignificant discrepancy in age-equivalent scores in arithmetic versus reading (7.68 years versus 8.55 years, respectively). Similarly, Taylor (1988) reported a mean standard achievement test score of 70 in math and 73 in reading, again providing only modest support for a "reading over math" profile of academic abilities.

Only a handful of studies have moved beyond academic achievement to identify other aspects of cognitive processing in Prader-Willi syndrome. Examining global cognitive patterns with Wechsler-based tests, Borghgraef, Fryns, and Van den Berghe reported "great differences" (1990, p. 148) in Verbal versus Performance IQ scores in 8 of their 12 participants with Prader-Willi syndrome. Three of these individuals showed at least a 15-point discrepancy in favor of the Verbal IQ. Significant Verbal versus Performance IQ differences were also found in a study of 26 children with Prader-Willi syndrome, ages 7–15 years, but 10 participants showed elevations in the Performance IQ, and only 3 in the Verbal IQ (Curfs, Wiegers, Sommers, Borghgraef, & Fryns, 1991). Findings are thus inconsistent, with perhaps a slight favoring of Performance IQ.

More fine-tuned studies of specific cognitive processes shed some light on these inconsistent findings. Table 6.2 summarizes these studies. Taylor (1988) compared with Wechsler Intelligence scale for Children–Revised (Wechsler, 1991) subtests in an unspecified number of participants with Prader-Willi syndrome with a sample of obese individuals with mental retardation (but not Prader-Willi syndrome). The two groups showed comparable subtest scores, with just one exception: Relative to the obese individuals, participants with Prader-Willi syndrome showed significantly higher scores on Block Design, a task tapping visual-motor functioning. Similarly, Curfs et al. (1991) found that one half of their sample showed significant WISC–R subtest scatter, and 9 of these 13 children had relative strengths in Block Design.

Visual processing strengths are also suggested by Gabel et al. (1986), who administered a battery of attentional, visual-spatial and psychomotor tasks to 15 children with Prader-Willi syndrome and 15 age- and sex-matched typical children. Not surprisingly, the Prader-Willi group scored consistently lower than the typical group, yet they also showed discrepancies in scores on subtests of the Detroit Tests of Learning Aptitude (Baker & Leland, 1967). Participants with Prader-Willi syndrome had relatively low scores on tasks assessing auditory attention and recall for words and high scores on tasks measuring visual attention and recall for objects and letters. Gabel et al. (1986) concluded that youngsters with Prader-Willi syndrome may have strengths in visual processing relative to auditory processing.

Further work details certain aspects of the apparent visual-processing strength. Administering the K-ABC to 21 participants, Dykens et al. (1992a) found that simultaneous processing was better developed than was sequential processing. High scores were noted in tasks assessing perceptual closure (e.g., inferring a picture from a few parts), long-term memory, spatial organization, attention to visual detail, and visual-motor inclusion. Among the sequential processing tasks, which rely on short-term memory, participants showed particular difficulties with visual-motor and auditory-visual short-term memory. A profile is thus suggested for some individuals with Prader-Willi syndrome of relative strengths in perceptual organization and difficulties in visual and other short-term memory tasks.

Consistent with these strengths, many people with Prader-Willi syndrome show an unusual facility with jigsaw puzzles. This skill is so striking that it is noted as a supportive finding in the consensus diagnostic criteria for Prader-Willi syndrome (see Table 6.1). Clinically, we observe that many adolescents and young adults also have a strong propensity for "word search" puzzles; we have even seen them carrying their word-find books to school or work. Although preliminary, we found that participant performance on a visual memory task was correlated with parental reports of partic-

Additional studies are needed to better relate facility with puzzles to cognitive profiles and to determine exactly how widespread jigsaw puzzle skills are in the Prader-Willi population.

ipant interest and facility with jigsaw and word search puzzles. Additional studies are needed to better relate facility with puzzles to cognitive profiles and to determine exactly how widespread jigsaw puzzle skills are in the Prader-Willi population.

Table 6.2. Summary of cognitive processing studies in people with Prader-Willi syndrome

Study	Tests	Number and age of participants (in years)	Salient findings
Curfs et al., 1991	Wechsler Intelligence Scale for Children–Revised (WISC–R)	26, 7–15	Performance IQ greater than Verbal IQ in 10 individuals; Verbal IQ greater than Performance IQ in 3 individuals. Block Design high in 9 individuals.
Dykens et al., 1992a	Kaufman Assessment Battery for Children (K–ABC) WISC–R or Stanford-Binet	21, 13–26 31, 5–30	Simultaneous > Sequential Processing. Strengths: visual-perceptual; weaknesses: visual, motor short-term memory. Stable IQ in childhood and adulthood.
Gabel et al., 1986	Battery, including Detroit Tests of Learning Aptitude	15, Mean age = 12 15 typical controls	Controls > Prader-Willi syndrome on all measures. For PWS on Detroit, visual recall of objects, letters > auditory recall of words.
Taylor, 1988	WISC–R	Unspecified PWS, Obese, retarded controls	PWS > controls on Block Design only.

From Dykens, E.M. (1999). Prader-Willi syndrome. In H. Trager-Flusberg (Ed.), *Neurodevelopmental disorders: Contributions to a framework from the cognitive sciences* (p. 140). Cambridge: MIT Press; reprinted by permission.

Cognitive Trajectories

Work has begun to describe how IQ relates to the child's increasing chronological age. A study conducted in the late 1960s of eight children with Prader-Willi syndrome reported that IQ declines in early childhood (Dunn, 1968). It was unclear, however, if these declines were assessed by formal IQ tests or by participants' not reaching certain developmental milestones. Using standardized IQ scores, Dykens et al. (1992a) conducted both cross-sectional and longitudinal analyses of IQ change in children and adults. IQ scores were cross-sectionally examined in 21 adolescents and adults, and longitudinal analyses included 31 participants ages 5–30 years who had been given the same IQ test twice. IQ scores showed nonsignificant fluctuations in both cross-sectional and longitudinal analyses, with no evidence of IQ declines in childhood or early adulthood. Although longitudinal studies in very young children or older adults have not yet been done, overall IQ scores appear relatively stable in school-age children and young adults. Further longitudinal work needs to clarify this stable trajectory, as it differs from the trajectories of intelligence seen in some other genetic syndromes, such as Down syndrome (Hodapp & Zigler, 1990) or fragile X syndrome (Dykens, Hodapp, & Leckman, 1994).

Correlates of Cognition

In addition to strengths and weaknesses and trajectories of intelligence, several other factors have been correlated with levels of intellectual functioning in people with Prader-Willi syndrome. We briefly describe three of the most important of these hypothesized correlates.

Weight Early work in Prader-Willi syndrome suggested a significant, inverse correlation among IQ and weight (Crnic, Sulzbacher, Snow, & Holm, 1980), with lower IQ scores associated with increased weight. But common lore within the Prader-Willi syndrome community suggests the opposite relation—that brighter individuals may be more clever or ingenious about obtaining food and are thus at increased risk of obesity. However, other data do not support either hypothesis. Dykens et al. (1992a) found no significant relationships among IQ and body mass indices (a measure of obesity). People with relatively high versus low IQ scores thus seem similarly vulnerable to the syndrome's problems with obesity and weight control.

Behavioral Problems The central issue here is whether high IQ scores might serve as a protective factor against some of the syndrome's more troublesome maladaptive behaviors. Comparing 43 participants with relatively high IQ scores (i.e., mean IQ of 79) with 43 participants with lower IQ scores (i.e. mean IQ of 59), Dykens and Cassidy (1995) found no significant differences in either the type or severity of maladaptive behavior across groups. These data, which are consistent with clinical observations, have important service delivery implications. In particular, state or other agencies that use low IQ scores (usually below 70) as a service-eligibility requirement may exclude higher functioning people who have similar treatment needs as lower functioning people. In Prader-Willi syndrome, then, IQ may be a less meaningful entry point into state or other systems of care than are the behavioral and dietary concerns of the person being served.

Genetic Status　A final issue concerns whether people with the two most common genetic causes of Prader-Willi syndrome—paternal deletion and maternal UPD—differ in their intellectual abilities. Although this question remains unresolved, it does appear that people with UPD may display slightly higher cognitive skills than those with the more common paternal deletions. Comparing 23 people with deletions to 23 age and gender-matched individuals with disomy, Dykens, Cassidy, and King (1999) found that the UPD group had average IQ scores of 71, whereas those with deletions averaged 63. Similarly, Thompson et al. (1999) found lower Verbal (but not Performance) IQ scores in participants with paternal deletions. More work is needed to delineate the exact areas in which the two groups differ; however, these studies indicate that people with the paternal deletion may, on average, show slightly lower cognitive functioning. Although such observations facilitate genotype-phenotype research, these data probably have less of an impact on the overall quality of life of people with the syndrome and their families.

Linguistic Functioning

Although language is a relatively unexplored area, the syndrome's few language studies find no distinctive linguistic profile in Prader-Willi syndrome. Branson (1981) found no common features in the language profiles of 21 children with Prader-Willi syndrome. Similarly, Kleppe, Katayama, Shipley, and Foushee (1990) found a variety of linguistic profiles in 18 children. Differences were seen across participants' severity of speech and language problems, and in the range of their intelligibility, fluency, and voice problems. Kleppe et al. (1990) did, however, find some common speech-language characteristics, primarily hypernasality, errors with certain speech sounds and complex syntax, and reduced vocabulary skills relative to age expectations. More recent work clarifies these early observations, underscoring the high-pitched, nasal speech qualities of many with the syndrome, as well as no striking strengths or weaknesses in grammar, vocabulary, or language comprehension (Akefeldt, Akefeldt, & Gillberg, 1997). Speech and articulation difficulties are likely associated with hypotonia, and perhaps thick, viscous saliva (Kleppe et al., 1990). Speech problems, primarily with articulation and intelligibility, were also noted by 33 of 43 parents of children with Prader-Willi syndrome ages 4–19 years (Dykens & Kasari, 1997). In addition, parents reported that individuals with Prader-Willi syndrome often talk too much and verbally perseverate on a narrow range of topics (Dykens, Leckman, & Cassidy, 1996). It remains unknown, however, how perseveration relates to linguistic features such as pragmatics, discourse, and the social uses of language.

ADAPTIVE FUNCTIONING AND PERSONALITY

Despite its prominence in definitions of mental retardation (see Hodapp & Dykens, 1996), little is known about the adaptive strengths and weaknesses of people with specific syndromes, including those with Prader-Willi syndrome (Dykens, 1995c). In one study of adolescents and adults with Prader-Willi syndrome, relative strengths were found on the daily living skills domain of the Vineland Adaptive Behavior Scales (VABS; Sparrow, Balla, & Cicchetti, 1984), especially in domestic skills such as cooking and cleaning (Dykens et al., 1992a). These same participants showed significant relative weaknesses in socialization skills, notably in their abilities to cope with the frustrations and demands of everyday living.

Although distinctive, these profiles are not unique to Prader-Willi syndrome. Males with fragile X syndrome, for example, show relative strengths in daily living skills (Dykens, 1995a; Dykens, Ort, et al., 1996), and females with fragile X syndrome have relative weaknesses in socialization (Freund, Reiss, & Abrams, 1993). But the reasons for these similar profiles likely differ across syndromes. In Prader-Willi syndrome, individuals' strengths in cooking or cleaning seem consistent with their interests in food, whereas these same skills exhibited by males with fragile X may be related to the repetitive, rote nature of these daily living tasks (Dykens, 1995a). Weaknesses in socialization and coping skills in people with Prader-Willi syndrome are likely associated with the syndrome's characteristic impulsivity, temper tantrums, and compulsivity (Dykens & Cassidy, 1995). Among females with fragile X syndrome, however, problems with socialization are seen primarily in the interpersonal domain and are likely related to that syndrome's proneness to shyness, gaze aversion, and social anxiety (Freund et al., 1993). VABS profiles may thus be similar across these or other syndromes, but factors associated with these profiles may differ.

Although adaptive behavior scores and IQ are often correlated in people with Prader-Willi syndrome, this relation is far from absolute, and the adaptive performances of many individuals fall well below their measured IQ. Even people with relatively high IQ scores in borderline to low average ranges struggle to meet the social and practical demands of everyday living. Although hyperphagia is partly to blame, so too are a distinctive personality, a host of maladaptive behaviors, and specific psychiatric vulnerabilities often experienced by those who have Prader-Willi syndrome.

Personality

Are there "characteristic" personality traits in people with Prader-Willi syndrome? As in other chapters, we again acknowledge the many difficulties posed in the study of personality. Such as most physical or behavioral characteristics, not every person will have any syndrome's "characteristic" behaviors (Dykens, 1995c). Equally important, a clear, accepted definition of "personality" remains somewhat elusive.

This difficulty in pinpointing a characteristic Prader-Willi personality is seen in several different studies. For example, several studies have examined personality in children with Prader-Willi syndrome using Costa and McRae's (1998) "Big Five" personality characteristics. These include the level of one's 1) extroversion, 2) openness to experience, 3) neuroticism, 4) agreeableness, and 5) conscientiousness. Across many studies of children and adults from a variety of cultures, Costa and McRae (1998) have validated these five characteristics as encompassing distinct, stable personality traits.

Some researchers have found Big Five personality differences in children with Prader-Willi syndrome relative to typical children without mental retardation. Comparing 22 children with Prader-Willi syndrome with 28 chronologically matched typically developing children, Curfs, Hoondert, van Lieshout, and Fryns (1995) found that children with Prader-Willi syndrome scored lower on Big Five domains of agreeableness, conscientiousness, and openness to experience. Children with Prader-Willi syndrome also scored lower on scales of motor activity and higher on measures of irritability and dependency. In a second study using the same measures, van Lieshout, de Meyer, Curfs, and Fryns (1998) found similar profiles of personality among children with Prader-Willi syndrome and age-matched controls. Children with Prader-Willi syndrome in this study also showed more irritability than children with either fragile X syndrome or Williams syndrome.

Another line of personality work has used Reiss and Havercamp's (1998) Reiss Profiles. This personality measure has a 15-factor structure based on the participant's motivational strengths and styles. Comparing 35 people apiece with Prader-Willi syndrome, Williams syndrome, and nonspecific mental retardation, Dykens and Rosner (1999b) found differences on several factors. Compared with the nonspecific group (Williams syndrome findings are presented in Chapter 4), adolescents and adults with Prader-Willi syndrome showed higher scores on five domains: Food, Order, Help Others, Rejection, and Frustration; they scored lower in Social Contact, Sex (i.e., sex drive), and Physical Activity. More informative, however, were specific items that differentiated the groups. Individuals with Prader-Willi syndrome were more motivated, for example, by jigsaw puzzles, concerns for order, and a strong maternal/paternal streak. Table 6.3 summarizes mean scores on representative items from each domain, and we discuss many of these in the next section of this chapter.

Table 6.3. Personality characteristics in individuals with Prader-Willi syndrome versus those with nonspecific mental retardation

Domain and highly discrepant items	Prader-Willi	Nonspecific
Domains in which Prader-Willi syndrome > nonspecific groups		
Food	27.17 (mean)	18.65 (mean)
Enjoys eating more than most	4.77	3.20
Always thinking about food	4.40	2.42
Very hearty appetite	4.57	3.34
Order	20.82	17.22
Upset with changes in routine	3.71	2.80
Does things in precise manner	3.63	2.95
Strong need to put things in order	3.09	2.05
Help Others	26.77	23.60
Strong maternal/paternal instincts	3.51	2.74
Rejection	26.40	22.77
Low tolerance for teasing	4.28	2.71
Frustration	24.63	19.71
Low frustration tolerance	3.88	3.02
Impatient with delays	3.77	2.60
Domains in which Prader-Willi syndrome < nonspecific groups		
Social Contact	24.11	27.63
Has many friends	2.57	3.68
Sex	7.65	10.46
Strong sex drive	1.60	2.37
Above average interest in sex	1.71	2.68
Physical Activity	14.08	18.31
Very energetic	1.96	3.25
Likes sports/athletics	2.31	3.26

Adapted from Dykens & Rosner, 1999.

Range and Severity of Maladaptive Behavior

Behavior problems in Prader-Willi syndrome are so salient that they have earned a place as minor diagnostic criteria in the consensus clinical criteria for this disorder (Holm et al., 1993). Indeed, as summarized in Table 6.4, people with Prader-Willi syndrome struggle with both externalizing and internalizing problems. Table 6.4 depicts salient problems in 100 people with Prader-Willi syndrome ages 4–46 years, as assessed by the Child Behavior Checklist (CBC; Achenbach, 1991). In addition to food-related difficulties, we found high rates of tantrums, impulsivity, stubbornness, arguing with others, disobedience, stealing food or money to buy food, lability, skin picking, compulsions, withdrawal, worry, and anxiety. Findings are remarkably consistent with our earlier studies and samples, including one study examining 43 children and adolescents ages 4–19 years (Dykens & Kasari, 1997), and another based on 61 adolescents and adults ages 13–49 years (Dykens

Table 6.4. Percentage of 100 individuals with Prader-Willi syndrome ages 4–46 years showing maladaptive behaviors on the Child Behavior Checklist

Maladaptive behavior	Percentage
Overeats	98
Skin picks	97
Stubborn	95
Obsessions	94
Tantrums	88
Disobedient	78
Impulsive	76
Labile	76
Excessive sleep	75
Talks too much	74
Compulsions	71
Anxious, worried	70
Prefers being alone	67
Gets teased a lot	65
Peers don't like	60
Hoards	55
Steals (food, money for food)	54
Withdrawn	53
Unhappy, sad	51

& Cassidy, 1995). Other groups of researchers also find a similar range and frequency of problem behaviors in their samples (e.g., Clarke, Boer, Chung, Sturmey, & Webb, 1996).

In addition to their wide scope, these maladaptive behaviors often reach clinically significant levels. Among the 43 children and adolescents that we examined, the vast majority (72%) had CBC *T*-scores consistent with Achenbach's (1991) clinically referred sample (Dykens & Kasari, 1997). Among the 61 adolescents and adults, 85% had one or more clinically elevated subtest scores on the Reiss Screen for Maladaptive Behavior (Reiss, 1988), with most (72%) showing two or more clinical elevations (Dykens & Cassidy, 1995). Maladaptive behaviors thus often reach a point in which further clinical evaluation and interventions are necessary (Dykens & Hodapp, 1997).

Specific Maladaptive and Psychiatric Features

Although each of the maladaptive features noted in Table 6.4 deserves further study, research to date clusters into three different problem areas or categories, including 1) overeating and food issues; 2) obsessions and compulsions; and 3) other maladaptive and psychiatric vulnerabilities, such as impulse control and affective disorders, and psychosis. We take up each category in turn.

Overeating and Food Issues As previously suggested, hyperphagia in Prader-Willi syndrome is likely related to a hypothalamic dysfunction that may involve a specific set of oxytocin-secreting neurons in the paraventricular nucleus of the hypothalamus; presumably these neurons are related to satiety (Swaab, Purba, & Hofman, 1995). Contrary to popular belief, then, overeating in Prader-Willi syndrome is not a result of a lack of willpower or self-control but instead stems from an impaired satiety response, or an abnormality of the brain in sending out signals of being full. On closer look, it appears that people with Prader-Willi syndrome show significant delays in their satiety responses. Holland, Treasure, Coskeran, and Dallow (1995) found that, when given free access to food, most of their 13 participants with Prader-Willi syndrome eventually indicated that they were full, but at a much

> *Contrary to popular belief, then, overeating in Prader-Willi syndrome is not a result of a lack of willpower or self-control, but instead stems from an impaired satiety response, or an abnormality of the brain in sending out signals of being full.*

later time than controls, and only after eating a large amount of food. Furthermore, these adults with Prader-Willi syndrome stated that they were hungry again much sooner than typical control participants.

Such observations have led to questions of whether people with Prader-Willi syndrome are so hungry that they eat indiscriminately. Such as anyone else, however, people with Prader-Willi syndrome have distinct food preferences. Early researchers found that adults with Prader-Willi syndrome showed a preference for sweet foods relative to salty, plain, or sour foods (Caldwell & Taylor, 1983; Taylor & Caldwell, 1985). More recent investigators found that people with Prader-Willi syndrome prefer high carbohydrate foods, and that this preference is distinct from individuals with either typical weight or who are obese (Fieldstone, Zipf, Schwartz, & Berntson, 1997).

Furthermore, although some individuals with the syndrome "just eat," others have certain rituals or rules that govern their eating (Dykens, Leckman, & Cassidy, 1996). Although findings are preliminary, examples of rituals include eating all of one food type before moving onto the next, based on

- Color (e.g., all green food first, then brown)
- Texture (e.g., hardest to softest)
- Caloric content (e.g., highest to lowest)
- Type (e.g., meat, then vegetables)
- Desirability (most to least preferred)

Some individuals need to have their food cut or served in particular ways, or their utensils arranged in "just the right spot" before eating. As discussed below, these food rituals are just one part of a larger picture of compulsivity in Prader-Willi syndrome.

Food preferences or rituals do not necessarily prevent many with the syndrome from making poor food choices, such as eating food from the floor or garbage can, or eating unusual or unpalatable items, such as frozen meat or pet food. Dykens (in press) recently administered visually based food choice tasks to 50 adults with Prader-Willi syndrome as well as to individuals with and without mental retardation. Most adults with Prader-Willi syndrome had similar understanding as typically developing individuals about the fate and purpose of food. Despite these well-developed perceptions, participants with Prader-Willi syndrome were much more likely than either comparison group to endorse eating contaminated food (e.g., cake with a bug on it) and unusual food combinations (e.g., hot dog with whipped cream, pizza with chocolate sauce). Table 6.5 summarizes percentages in each group

Table 6.5. Percentages of participants by group who endorsed eating various food combinations

Food	Prader-Willi syndrome	Mental retardation	Typically developing individuals
Hot dog and whipped cream	60	24	12
Steak and ice cream	54	16	12
Cheerios and ketchup	25	07	0
Cake with grass	36	02	04
Cheese with bugs	28	0	02
Three slices pizza with chocolate sauce versus a regular slice	35	05	02
Three scoops of ice-cream with mustard versus one regular scoop	26	07	0

Adapted from Dykens (in press).

For all examples, individuals with Prader-Willi syndrome had significantly higher frequency scores than remaining groups, all χ^2 values $p < .001$.

that endorsed eating various food combinations. As suggested by Table 6.5, some individuals with Prader-Willi syndrome endorsed eating inedible substances such as bugs or grass, when these were presented in combination with food. All participants, however, rejected eating these and other nonfood substances when these were presented alone. Pica (or eating nonfood substances) may thus be dependent on certain contextual cues in those with this syndrome. Findings suggest novel adjuncts to traditional dietary approaches, including teaching people with Prader-Willi syndrome about contamination and germs, and helping to instill in them a sense of disgust.

Obsessions and Compulsions   A second clustering of studies has identified increased risks of obsessions and compulsions in people with Prader-Willi syndrome. Most with the syndrome are "obsessed" about food to varying degrees. Yet these studies actually point to a host of compulsive behaviors outside of the food arena. Examining 91 children and adults, Dykens, Leckman, and Cassidy (1996) found high rates of specific symptoms on the Yale-Brown Obsessive Compulsive Scale (Y-BOCS; Goodman et al., 1989). These included hoarding (e.g., toiletries, paper, pens); ordering and arranging items by color, shape, or size, or until they were "just right"; needing to tell or say things (e.g., repeated questioning); being concerned with symmetry or exactness; and redoing things (e.g., tying and untying shoes, rewriting homework, recutting coupons until the lines were perfect). For 45%–80% of the sample, these symptoms were time consuming, distressful, or caused adaptive impairment, suggesting high probable rates of full-blown obsessive-compulsive disorder (OCD). Although the exact prevalence of OCD in the Prader-Willi population is unknown, rates are likely to be many times higher than the 1%–3% of people with heterogeneous mental retardation and comorbid OCD (e.g., Meyers, 1987; Vitiello, Spreat, & Behar, 1989).

Ties among Prader-Willi syndrome and OCD were seen as well in a follow-up study comparing 43 adults with Prader-Willi syndrome to 43 individuals without mental retardation but with OCD (Dykens, Leckman, et al., 1996). The two groups showed the same number and severity of compulsive symptoms on the Y-BOCS; as shown in Table 6.6, each group showed about four different nonfood compulsions. Table 6.6 also shows both similarities and differences in types of symptoms across groups, with the Prader-Willi group more likely to hoard and need to tell or say things and the group with OCD more likely to have checking compulsions.

Interestingly, these compulsive behaviors are even found in toddlers with Prader-Willi syndrome. Dimitropoulos, Feurer, Thompson, and Butler (1999) examined compulsive symptoms in eighty-nine 2- to 6-year-old children with Prader-Willi syndrome, 77 typically developing children, and 55 children with Down syndrome. Although both comparison groups showed age-related declines in compulsive behaviors (see also Evans et al., 1997), children with Prader-Willi syndrome did not do so. Skin picking in particular stood out among these young

Table 6.6. Yale-Brown Obsessive-Compulsive Scale (Y-BOCS) symptoms in 43 adults with Prader-Willi syndrome (PWS) versus individuals with obsessive-compulsive disorder (OCD)

Symptom	PWS	OCD
Mean number of compulsions	3.74	4.02
Mean severity of compulsions	10.77	9.09
Types of compulsions (percentage)		
Cleaning	33%	37%
Checking	16%	55%
Repeating rituals	40%	54%
Counting	19%	28%
Ordering/arranging	29%	28%
Hoarding	79%	7%
Need to tell, ask	51%	23%

Adapted from Dykens, Leckman, et al., 1996.

Table 6.7.   Compulsive symptoms in individuals with Prader-Willi syndrome and various comparison groups

Symptom	PWS	DS	NS	WS	PWS-like
Obsessions	1.61	.61	.61	1.31	1.27
Compulsions	1.29	.39	.51	.50	.44
Hoarding	.96	.21	.28	.47	.25
Skin picking	1.79	.26	.21	.71	.67

Note: PWS = Prader-Willi syndrome (N = 43); DS = Down syndrome (N = 43); NS = nonspecific mental retardation (N = 43); WS = Williams syndrome (N = 61); PWS-like = Prader-Willi syndrome-like patients (N = 8).

children; indeed, this behavior seems to persist over time, well into adulthood (Dykens et al., 1992a). Furthermore, skin picking can be severe, and detailed analyses of 61 participants find that the front of the head and legs are the most common targets for skin picking (Symons, Butler, Sanders, Feurer, & Thompson, 1999). Collectively, then, the skin picking and other obsessive-compulsive symptoms noted in Tables 6.5 and 6.6 are robust predictors of Prader-Willi syndrome in both childhood and the adult years.

Such compulsive features in Prader-Willi syndrome are elevated relative to others with mental retardation. Compared with those with Down syndrome, Smith-Magenis syndrome, Williams syndrome, and nonspecific mental retardation, individuals with Prader-Willi syndrome show higher rates of compulsive symptoms such as hoarding, repetitive rituals, talking too much, and skin picking (e.g., Dykens & Kasari, 1997; Dykens & Smith, 1998). Table 6.7 summarizes differences in obsessive-compulsive features across some of these groups, as measured by the CBC.

Compulsivity is even elevated in Prader-Willi syndrome relative to a particularly powerful contrast group of "Prader-Willi–like patients" (State, Dykens, Rosner, Martin, & King, 1999). These individuals had clinical diagnoses of Prader-Willi syndrome and consulted specialists at the Prader-Willi Syndrome Clinic at University of California at Los Angeles for care in the first months of the operation of the clinic. They had mental retardation, obesity, food preoccupations, and salient behavior problems, yet upon genetic testing, were methylation negative, and thus failed to show the Prader-Willi genotype. Comparing the eight Prader-Willi syndrome-like individuals with age- and gender-matched individuals with Prader-Willi syndrome due to paternal deletion, the two groups had similar IQ scores, degrees of obesity, and maladaptive behavior scores. Yet, although participants with Prader-Willi syndrome had an average of 6.25 symptoms on the Y-BOCS, the

Prader-Willi syndrome-like cases had a mean of just 1.37 symptoms. Similar patterns of findings were seen in Y-BOCS symptom severity scores. Obsessive-compulsive symptoms, then, can not be explained by mental retardation, obesity, or behavioral disturbance, and instead appear intrinsic to factors within the Prader-Willi genotype.

The pathogenesis of Prader-Willi syndrome thus appears to predispose many individuals to compulsivity, if not full-blown OCD. It may even be that the Prader-Willi critical region on chromosome 15 is associated with some forms of OCD in the general population, especially those cases characterized by hoarding and concerns with symmetry or exactness. Findings also bring advances in understanding and treating OCD to Prader-Willi syndrome. Individuals with non–tic-related OCD, for example, show elevated levels of cerebrospinal fluid oxytocin relative to typical controls (Leckman et al., 1994). Oxytocin is a neuropeptide implicated in a host of normative behaviors, such as grooming, aggression, appetite regulation, attachment, and reproduction (Leckman et al., 1994). As previously noted, decreased oxytocin-secreting neurons have been identified in the hypothalamic paraventricular nucleus of individuals with Prader-Willi syndrome (Swaab et al., 1995). In contrast, relative to typical individuals, high levels of cerebrospinal fluid oxytocin were recently found in five individuals with Prader-Willi syndrome (Martin, State, North, Hanchette & Leckman, 1998). Although the mechanisms are unclear, aberrant levels of oxytocin were seen in both studies. These anomalies may possibly mediate some of the compulsive features in Prader-Willi syndrome and perhaps other behaviors such as increased maternal/paternal instincts, and aggressive tendencies.

Other Maladaptive and Psychiatric Vulnerabilities   A third set of findings touch on other psychiatric conditions. In addition to OCD, impulse control and psychotic and affective disorders may also occur with increased frequency in people with Prader-Willi syndrome. Although impulsivity, temper tantrums, aggression, and stubbornness have long been considered hallmark features of the syndrome, they seem to vary widely in their severity. Although we found temper tantrums in 88% of 100 individuals with Prader-Willi syndrome (see Table 6.4), 42% engaged in property destruction and 34% physically attacked others. Stein, Keating, Zar, and Hollander (1994) found that 49% of 347 parents of offspring with Prader-Willi syndrome rated their children's temper tantrums as moderate or severe, although 41% indicated that tantrums were slight or mild. Some parents thus report mild tantrums and a "stubborn streak," although others report extreme rage reactions and property destruction. Although these more extreme symptoms may decline with age, temper tantrums and stubbornness do not (Dykens et al., 1992a). Further research needs to examine the extent to which the onset of symptoms are associated with the beginning of hyperphagia in childhood, as well as the possible genetic, biological, and psychosocial reasons for such wide variability in impulsive-aggressive symptoms.

Aggressive and compulsive symptoms seem more common than psychosis or affective disorders in people with Prader-Willi syndrome; yet a flurry of reports suggest a stronger than expected association among Prader-Willi syndrome and atypical psychosis. Several researchers have published a series of case studies of young adults with Prader-Willi syndrome with acute psychotic episodes (Beardsmore, Dorman, Cooper, & Webb, 1998, Clarke, 1993; Clarke et al., 1998; Clarke, Webb, & Bachmann-Clarke, 1995; Verhoeven, Curfs, & Tuinier, 1998). Many of these episodes were of sudden onset, and were characterized more by depression than by schizophrenia. Though many individuals responded well to pharmacotherapy and hospitalization, several showed vulnerabilities for disorganized thinking or behavior that persisted over the years.

Multiple reporting of single cases may be misleading in that they convey an impression of a stronger association than may actually be observed (Rutter, Bailey, Bolton, & Le Couteur, 1994). Moving away from case reports, however, Clarke (1998) administered a standardized checklist to parents of 95 adults with Prader-Willi syndrome and found that 6.3% showed psychotic symptoms in the previous month. Again based on parental reports, Stein et al. (1994) found visual or auditory hallucinations in 12.1% of 347 people with Prader-Willi syndrome. These rates are high even relative to rates in other people with mental retardation, and underscore the need for future research on possible associations between Prader-Willi syndrome and psychosis, especially among young adults. The extent to which people show distorted thinking independent of regressed behavior, or a bizarre or agitated presentation, also needs to be assessed.

These rates are high even relative to other people with mental retardation, and underscore the need for future research on possible associations between Prader-Willi syndrome and psychosis, especially among young adults.

In addition, depressive features, such as sadness and low self-esteem, as well as anxiety and worries, have been noted in various studies on maladaptive behavior associated with Prader-Willi syndrome (e.g., Dykens & Cassidy, 1995; Dykens et al., 1992b; Stein, et al., 1994; Whitman & Accardo, 1987). Table 6.4, for example, illustrates that of 100 participants examined, 51%–53% were unhappy, sad, or withdrawn, and 67% preferred being alone. Dykens and Cassidy (1995) found that advancing age in children with Prader-Willi syndrome ages 4–12 years was correlated with heightened internal distress and features of depression, including withdrawal, isolation, negative self-image, and pessimism. Among adults with Prader-Willi syndrome, Beardsmore et al. (1998) found that 17.4% of 25 young adults residing in the same county in the United Kingdom showed affective disorders, all with psychotic components. Still, symptoms of sadness and withdrawal seem more prevalent than full-blown affective disorder, and future work is needed to identify those factors that predispose some individuals to develop affective disorder.

In contrast to increased risks of OCD, impulse control, and perhaps psychotic and affective disorders as well, certain psychiatric disorders seem infrequent in those with Prader-Willi syndrome. Many people with Prader-Willi syndrome steal food and are impulsive and distractible, yet rates seem low for full-blown conduct disorder or attention-deficit/ hyperactivity disorder (ADHD). In contrast to those with Williams syndrome, fears or phobic disorders are infrequent in Prader-Willi syndrome (Beardsmore et al., 1998). And researchers have yet to observe people with Prader-Willi syndrome with co-morbid tic disorders or dementia.

Furthermore, unlike fragile X syndrome, Prader-Willi syndrome does not appear to include a heightened risk of autism spectrum disorder, beyond the risk due to mental retardation. As reflected in Table 6.4, many people struggle with peer and social relationships, and may be withdrawn or isolated at times. Many with the syndrome are accused of being self-centered, which may reflect an inward, obsessive style; rigidity related to compulsions; or difficulties taking the perspectives of others. Although these features, coupled with concerns for order and sameness, hint at autism, very few individuals show profound social indifference or are formally diagnosed with this disorder. Of the handful of people whom we have seen with both disorders (Dykens & Cassidy, 1999), all had maternal disomy of chromosome 15. Further work needs to carefully test these clinical observations, especially in light of newly identified associations among autism and chromosome 15 duplications involving the Prader-Willi/Angelman syndrome region (Battaglia et al., 1997; Cook et al., 1998).

Other Correlates of Maladaptive Behavior

Weight   Early work suggested that heavier adults with Prader-Willi syndrome were more slow-moving and antisocial than their thinner counterparts (Greenswag, 1987). Although some maladaptive behaviors may be related to weight, the general finding has been opposite to what one might expect. Dykens and Cassidy (1995) found that thinner adults (i.e., with lower body mass indices) had significantly higher maladaptive behavior scores than did heavier people (i.e., with higher body mass indices). Specifically, thinner participants showed more distressful affect and confused and distorted thinking, anxiety, sadness, fearfulness, and crying. Whitman and Accardo (1987) also found a nonsignificant trend of more psychiatric concerns among adults with good weight control. Longitudinal studies are needed, especially work that assesses if findings are related to the stress of losing weight, as well as to changes in brain chemistry and levels of physical activity.

Genetic Status Although preliminary, it seems that individuals with Prader-Willi syndrome due to maternal UPD versus paternal deletion may be susceptible to different levels of maladaptive behaviors. In the first such study, Dykens, Cassidy et al. (1999) compared 23 individuals with deletion with 23 individuals with disomy on the CBC and Y-BOCS. Compared with people with UPD, the group with deletions showed more symptom-related distress on the Y-BOCS and higher average scores on CBC Internalizing, Externalizing, and Total domains. The biggest differences occurred in the CBC narrow-band domains of Withdrawn and Other; the Aggressive domain approached significance. As shown in Table 6.8, as compared with the disomy group many more

Table 6.8. Differences in maladaptive behavior across 46 individuals with Prader-Willi syndrome due to paternal deletion or maternal uniparental disomy (UPD)

	Paternal deletion	Maternal UPD
Behavior		
Picks skin	100%	69%
Overeats	96%	65%
Hoards	65%	35%
Bites nails	61%	22%
Withdrawn	52%	17%
Symptom Severity		
Clinically elevated	83%	57%
Borderline clinical	17%	17%
Normal	0	26%
Intelligence		
K-BIT IQ score	63	71

Adapted from Dykens, Cassidy, & King (1999).

Note: Percentages based on the Child Behavior Checklist (Achenbach, 1991). All behaviors were significantly different across groups.

Key: K-BIT = Kaufman Brief Intelligence Test (Kaufman & Kaufman, 1990).

individuals from the deletion group were noted to be withdrawn and to overeat, hoard, bite their nails, sulk, and skin pick. Symons et al. (1999) also noted that skin picking is more frequent among those with deletions as opposed to UPD. Finally, as shown in Table 6.8, participants with deletions were more apt to have clinically elevated levels of maladaptive behavior on the Child Behavior Checklist.

The genetic mechanisms for such differences are currently under discussion. It may be that more genes are deleted than imprinted, or that imprinting is an imperfect, "leaky" process that allows for a low level of expression from both chromosome 15s (Dykens, Cassidy, et al., 1999). As with the IQ difference across the two genetic subtypes, it is unclear to what extent subtle differences in maladaptive behavior will affect the day-to-day living or quality of life for people with the syndrome and their families.

FAMILY ISSUES

Although families often have difficult times raising their children with Prader-Willi syndrome, only a few studies have specifically examined family issues. These studies, although different in many ways, nevertheless demonstrate that many of these families experience high levels of stress. They further show that certain characteristics of individual with Prader-Willi syndrome are associated with increased parental and family difficulties.

In the first study, Hodapp, Dykens, and Masino (1997) examined 42 families of 3- to 18-year-old children. Parents answered questionnaires about their child's maladaptive behavior, about themselves and their family, as well as about family stress and support. Families reported fairly high levels of social support, but also very high levels of parent and family problems and pessimism (two domains of family stress). Stress in Prader-Willi families was higher compared with other reports of stress in families of children with mental retardation due to mixed etiologies (see also Sarimski, 1997). The main correlate of parental stress was not the child's age, gender, weight, or even level of cognitive delay, but instead the child's degree of maladaptive behaviors.

Though different in its focus, design, and measures, van Lieshout, et al. (1998) reported similar results. These authors examined children's personalities, parent behaviors (control and anger), and family contexts (family stress, marital conflict, and parental consistency) in three groups of children and their families: those with Prader-Willi syndrome, fragile X syndrome, and Williams syndrome. Parents of children with Prader-Willi syndrome showed more (parent-reported) anger toward their children than did the parents of children with either fragile X syndrome or Williams syndrome. In addition, the main correlates of parental anger were aspects of the child's personality. Thus, more parental anger occurred when the child with Prader-Willi syndrome was less agreeable, less conscientious, less open, and more irritable. In these studies it is not clear which comes first—parental anger or children's maladaptive behavior. Although van Lieshout et al. (1998) considered the direction of effects to run from parent behavior to child personality, one could argue that this study actually demonstrates parental responses to the child's behavioral problems. Though the direction is uncertain, strong connections exist among the child's maladaptive behavioral and parental affect, and the parents of children with Prader-Willi syndrome do seem to experience high levels of stress.

INTERVENTION IMPLICATIONS

Prader-Willi syndrome is a "multisystem" disorder in which affected people have a wide variety of problems. Medically, these individuals can suffer from extreme, even life-threatening obesity. As has been discussed in this chapter, behaviorally, individuals often have difficulty controlling their hyperphagic and obsessive-compulsive behaviors, and impulsive, aggressive and other disruptive behaviors are also common. Families experience high levels of stress, and such stress seems related to the offspring's levels of behavioral problems.

It is often helpful for a health or mental health professional to follow the individual with Prader-Willi syndrome on a long-term basis to help maintain continuity of care and to coordinate services.

Given such a state of affairs, management becomes a critical issue in this syndrome. Coordinated care is typically needed from a wide variety of professionals. It is common for people with Prader-Willi syndrome to receive input from geneticists, primary care physicians, endocrinologists, nutritionists, psychologists, psychiatrists, special educators, speech-language therapists, occupational and physical therapists, families, group home staff, and other care providers. It is often helpful for a health or mental health professional to follow the individual with Prader-Willi syndrome on a long-term basis to help maintain continuity of care and to coordinate services. More detailed information on the management of Prader-Willi syndrome may be found in an edited volume written for care providers of all types (Greenswag & Alexander, 1995), as well as from the National Prader-Willi Syndrome Association (see Resources).

Medical Guidance

Obesity With good reason, weight and dietary management have long been the focus of intervention in Prader-Willi syndrome. Indeed, it is not uncommon for individuals to reach weights of 300 or even 400 pounds, even with heights at 5 feet or below. But experience shows that obesity can be prevented or already acquired weight can be reduced. Although many of these practices may seem obvious, long-term workers in the syndrome recommend the following for weight control in Prader-Willi syndrome:

- A well-balanced, low-calorie diet of about 1,000–1,200 calories/day (ensuring adequate calcium intake)
- Periodic weigh-ins (e.g., once per week)
- Regular exercise to increase muscle mass and thus efficiently burn calories (30 minutes per day is an appropriate goal)
- Environmental modification as needed, such as locking kitchen cabinets and the refrigerator
- Close supervision to prevent access to food; supervision of spending money; and supervision of meals in the school cafeteria, on the job, or in the community

Interventions should be continued even when people lose weight, have relatively high IQ scores, or show needs for less supervision in the nonfood parts of their lives

Although considered state of the art in treating hyperphagia in Prader-Willi syndrome, these techniques such as locking the cabinets and refrigerators or supervising spending money are often viewed as too restrictive by advocates in the developmental disabilities field. Many advocates feel that such practices limit the personal rights and choices of adults with Prader-Willi syndrome. Clinicians thus need to be aware of possible tensions among individuals' health concerns and personal rights (see Dykens, Goff, et al., 1997, for a discussion).

Clinicians thus need to be aware of possible tensions among individuals' health concerns and personal rights.

Despite widespread interest within the Prader-Willi syndrome community, no medication has yet shown long-term effectiveness in controlling appetites or in shifting the satiety responses of people with Prader-Willi syndrome. Thus, the most beneficial interventions continue to be a reduced-calorie diet and increased activity or exercise. Further, behavioral approaches are also effective in helping parents and other care providers set limits regarding food, and supporting individuals with Prader-Willi syndrome in the lifelong effort to prevent the health consequences of obesity (Dykens & Cassidy, 1996).

Other Medical Concerns The management of other of the syndrome's physical challenges is largely problem oriented. The use of growth hormone in Prader-Willi syndrome is still somewhat controversial, yet a series of recently published studies suggest cautious optimism in treating the short stature that is characteristic of Prader-Willi syndrome (Carrel, Myers, Whitman, & Allen, 1999; Hauffa, 1997; Lindgren et al., 1997). In addition to gains in height, growth hormone therapy appears to reduce the percentage of body fat and to increase muscle mass; children may also become more physically strong and agile.

Sex hormone replacement improves secondary sex characteristics and theoretically may improve symptoms of osteoporosis, but testosterone treatment is sometimes associated with an increase in aggressive behavior. No controlled trials of sex hormone replacement in people with Prader-Willi syndrome have yet been published.

Products to increase saliva production have proved of benefit in treating the dry mouth that is associated with Prader-Willi syndrome, and also likely improve dental hygiene and perhaps articulation as well. Speech-language therapy can be beneficial to people with Prader-Willi syndrome of all ages to address speech production abnormalities, and physical and occupational therapies have also proven helpful in treating hypotonia and poor coordination.

Educational Guidance

Most children with Prader-Willi syndrome need special education services to address their unique cognitive and behavioral concerns (Levine & Wharton, 1993). Although individualized education programs (IEPs) should be based on a careful assessment of each student's cognitive strengths and weaknesses, most IEPs include speech-language and physical therapies; supervision around food; and extra physical education classes or other ways of increasing physical activity during the school day (e.g., walking, taking stretch breaks, assisting teachers with "errands" that require walking).

It may also be possible for IEPs to capitalize on the specific cognitive profiles seen in many children with Prader-Willi syndrome. Instead of emphasizing short-term memory tasks for students with Prader-Willi syndrome, for example, teachers might rely on visual-perceptual cues or tasks, including pictures or models. Because many children with Prader-Willi syndrome are interested in jigsaw or word-search puzzles, these activities might themselves be used to teach words or concepts. Furthermore, Kaufman, Kaufman, and Goldsmith (1984) presented a variety of different intervention approaches to employ when one teaches a simultaneous learner as opposed to a sequential learner. By placing learning in an inclusive, visual context, educators can maximize the simultaneous processing strengths in children with Prader-Willi syndrome and avoid frustration with tasks that involve high levels of sequential processing and short-term memory (see Hodapp & Fidler, 1999, for further discussions).

In addition to considering how educational services are provided, one must also be concerned with the setting of such services. Currently, students with Prader-Willi syndrome are placed in a combination of inclusive and specialized or segregated educational settings. Given their behavior problems, many of these children are educated in more restrictive settings than suggested by their IQ scores alone. In one study, for example, almost two thirds of adults with Prader-Willi syndrome had attended special schools, even though their IQ levels were often at or above 70 (Waters, Clarke, & Corbett, 1990). Although educational practices have changed since this study was conducted, the bottom-line message remains the same: Because of their dietary and behavioral concerns, children with Prader-Willi syndrome more often require extra help and supervision across a variety of educational settings.

Another, less-often considered perspective comes from parents of children with Prader-Willi syndrome. In one study comparing parents of children with Prader-Willi syndrome with those with Down syndrome, the former group more often chose less-inclusive settings as their "ideal educational placement" (Hodapp, Freeman, & Kasari, 1998). Parents of children with Down syndrome often requested services that were more generic ("better trained teachers") or that were more community-based ("I want him in our community/placed in our neighborhood school"). In contrast, no parents of children with Prader-Willi syndrome showed these particular concerns. Instead, the parents of children with Prader-Willi syndrome requested specific educational aids for their child—greater amounts of occupational therapy, physical therapy, adapted physical education, reading, math, writing, and science. Also in contrast to parents of children with Down syndrome, parents of children with Prader-Willi asked that teachers be provided more knowledge about this particular syndrome; as one mother noted, "Professionals just are not educated about Prader-Willi syndrome."

Residential/Vocational Guidance

Just as children with Prader-Willi syndrome require more—and more specialized—educational services to help them succeed, so too do adults with Prader-Willi syndrome require help in coping with residential and vocational issues. Residentially, such help has come about in the form of "dedicated" Prader-Willi group homes that exist in many American communities. These are neighborhood group homes in which all residents have Prader-Willi syndrome; they are specifically designed to serve this population. Often featuring stricter controls on food and active exercise programs (in both the home and the community), such Prader-Willi group homes appear effective in reducing and maintaining individuals' weight over time, as well as in managing behavioral difficulties (Cassidy et al., 1994; Greenswag, 1987).

Similarly, when considering employment, people with Prader-Willi syndrome require more active intervention efforts. In a study comparing young adults with Prader-Willi syndrome with those with Down syndrome, Seguin and Hodapp (1999) found that individuals with Prader-Willi syndrome faced numerous difficulties in keeping their jobs. Compared with parents of young adults with Down syndrome, parents of young adults with Prader-Willi syndrome even reported more difficulties in qualifying for and receiving the transition services that might ease their child's shift from school to work. These parents also reported less satisfaction with their offspring's current vocational placement, and they held lower expectations for their children's future vocational achievements. Similar to parents of younger children, many parents of adults also felt that adult-service professionals need to be much better educated about Prader-Willi syndrome. Parents also struggled to convey to service providers that despite their offspring's relatively high IQ, they still needed fairly intensive supervision and supports (Seguin & Hodapp, 1998). Adults with Prader-Willi syndrome thus need careful vocational planning, as well as job coaches and extra supports to address food-seeking and other behavioral difficulties on the job.

> *Adults with Prader-Willi syndrome thus need careful vocational planning, as well as job coaches and extra supports to address food-seeking and other behavioral difficulties on the job.*

Behavioral/Psychiatric Guidance

Although food is a significant issue in Prader-Willi syndrome, maladaptive and psychiatric difficulties are likely to be the major reasons why many families seek professional help. Even as compared with food issues, obesity, age, or IQ level, the best predictors of family stress are maladaptive behaviors such as temper tantrums, compulsivity, and concerns for sameness in routine (Dykens, Leckman, et al., 1996; Hodapp, Dykens, et al., 1997). Improved behavior both at home and at school is often the result of strict reinforcement of behavioral limits, clear delineation of behavioral expectations, and establishment of regular routines. Establishing clear limits regarding food

Improved behavior both at home and at school is often the result of strict reinforcement of behavioral limits, clear delineation of behavioral expectations, and establishment of regular routines.

and behavior are especially important with the emergence of hyperphagia in the toddler or preschool years. Clinically, we find that setting behavioral limits when children are young paves the way for more successful responses to limit setting over the developmental and adolescent years.

But over the long-term, families often have difficulty constantly adhering to and enforcing behavioral and food limits. Some families benefit from respite care, from behavioral, family, and other therapists, as well as from the support of other families with a member who has Prader-Willi syndrome. Ongoing parent support groups are now offered through the state chapters of the Prader-Willi Syndrome Association, as well as through state and national meetings, and the Internet. These formal and informal parent-to-parent support mechanisms are often of enormous help to families.

Maladaptive behaviors may wax and wane over the course of development, and the causes of these shifts are not always readily apparent. In some cases, a clear environmental precipitant is the culprit; young adults may, for example, experience increased behavioral difficulties when they leave home and move into a group home setting, or when they make a transition from one job to another. Although planning for transitions is helpful, some families find that planning too early for events leads to increased perseveration, anxiety, and constant questioning about the issue. If so, containment tactics often work best (i.e., providing a brief reassuring response, ensuring that the child has understood the answer, and then moving onto another topic).

In addition, many people with Prader-Willi syndrome need extra help getting "unstuck" from their obsessions and compulsions. Indeed, tantrums and stubbornness in people with Prader-Willi syndrome often seem related to their being "stuck" and not being able to move from one activity or thought to the next. Consistent limit setting across home and school settings often help reduce tantrums, as do predictable daily routines. Other tantrums may be circumvented by distraction, and by giving individuals ample warning about transitions, including special auditory or visual transitional cues. If tantrums are inevitable, it is typically helpful for parents or teachers to avoid talking about the issue until well after the individual has settled down.

Instead of aiming to eliminate certain compulsive behaviors, it may be more helpful for teachers or parents to try to limit them to a certain part of the day, or to use them as a reward for on-task behavior (e.g., rewriting in a notebook after completing a lesson). Furthermore, some obsessive-compulsive features may have an adaptive component that can be reframed and perhaps put to constructive use. One individual, for example, has capitalized on his good visual-spatial skills and his need to order his collections by working in a library reshelving books. A young woman has made the most of her obsessions with food coupons by earning money from cutting coupons for her neighbors. Another man with Prader-Willi syndrome makes very creative use of his eye for detail and his love of animals in his artwork. A sample of his work is depicted in Figure 6.2. Featured in galleries throughout New England, this successful artist has an obsessive style that was characterized by a Boston Globe art critic as "a complex layering and overlapping of images . . . an almost cubist arrangement of planes in some of the works . . . the edges of the pictures can barely contain all of the activity compacted within them" (Kelley, 1991). Although this artist is unique in his talent, he is nonetheless a model for putting an "obsessive" style to creative and productive use.

In addition to environmental interventions, obsessive-compulsive and depressive features often respond well to pharmacotherapies. Medications may also help reduce the frequency or severity of aggressive outbursts. Several case studies reported that specific serotonin reuptake inhibitors (SSRIs) have helped some individuals gain better control of tantrums and compulsive symptoms such as skin picking (Benjamin & Buot-Smith, 1993; Dech & Budow, 1991; Hellings & Warnock, 1994; Warnock & Kestenbaum, 1992). Others, however, have found that medications do not generally help with skin picking over the long-term (Hanchett, 1998). Although SSRIs are currently quite popular for use with the Prader-Willi syndrome community, controlled studies have yet to be published.

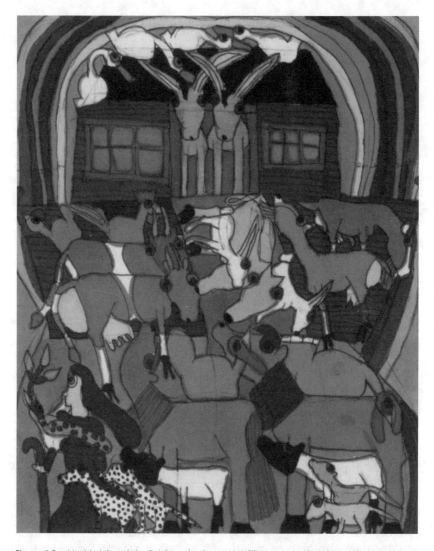

Figure 6.2.   Noah's Ark and the Rainbow, by Stuart H. Williams, Artist, Peterborough, New Hampshire. Stuart writes narratives for all his pieces, and for this one he notes, "Here are the animals that stay with Noah: Two goats, two ducks, two pigs, two cows, two chickens, two donkeys, two geese, two turkeys, two sheep, two horses, two dogs, two cats. The rainbow is coming down over the ark. Noah's ark is resting on the mountain Ararat. Noah has a dove in the palm of his hand and the dove is holding an olive leaf in her beak. The rainbow was the sign from God that the flood was over and his covenant that such a flood would never happen again."

Finally, many people benefit from school, clinic, or recreational programs that target improved self-esteem, social skills, and peer relations (Dykens & Cassidy, 1995; Levine & Wharton, 1993). As they develop, children with Prader-Willi syndrome may be particularly vulnerable to increased negative self-evaluation and isolation (Dykens & Cassidy, 1995) Also, in another study peer teasing and rejection were experienced by 60%–65% of 100 individuals with Prader-Willi syndrome (see Table 6.4, "Peers don't like."). In addition to formal social skills-training curricula, enrollment in recreational programs such as Special Olympics may also facilitate peer relations and bolster esteem. Special Olympics also has the extra benefit of increasing individuals' physical activity and possibly reducing their weight (Dykens, 1995b).

NEXT STEPS

Despite decades of progress in Prader-Willi syndrome, behavioral and developmental understandings in the following areas still lag considerably behind dramatic genetic advances:

- Variability in behavior and development across people with paternal deletions versus maternal UPD
- Familial, genetic, and psychosocial reasons for within-syndrome variability in hyperphagia and other behaviors
- Brain correlates of hyperphagia, and behavioral and cognitive dysfunction, with special reference to the hypothalamus
- Cognitive and adaptive strengths, including jigsaw puzzle skills
- The impact of hyperphagia on young children's cognitive and behavioral schema
- The efficacy of various psychotropic medications and of growth hormone treatment over the long-term

To help close these gaps, future studies are greatly needed on these and other topics.

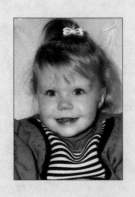

7

Five Other Intriguing Syndromes

*One aim of this chap-
ter is to spark more
research excitement
for some of these less-
understood or de-
scribed disorders.*

What do we know about behavior and development in the hundreds of other genetic syndromes that are associated with mental retardation? As detailed in this book's introductory chapter, precious few studies exist on the behavior of individuals with lesser-known genetic causes of mental retardation. One aim of this chapter is to spark more research excitement for some of these less-understood or described disorders.

With more than 750 known genetic syndromes associated with mental retardation, how did we select only five to include in this chapter? Our first rule was to only review those syndromes associated with mental retardation, as opposed to learning disabilities or adjustment difficulties. For example, although females with Turner syndrome (who are missing an X chromosome) show salient weaknesses in visual-spatial functioning, they do not have mental retardation. We thus elected not to review Turner syndrome, despite intriguing genetic advances showing an imprinting effect in this disorder (involving lower verbal IQ and social cognition scores in females with maternally derived X chromosomes; see Skuse et al., 1997).

Second, we have selected syndromes for review that either have behavioral research momentum or preliminary work hinting at specific behavioral or psychiatric outcomes. Thus, a flurry of work is now emerging on specific psychiatric vulnerabilities in people with velocardiofacial syndrome, and preliminary data in Rubinstein-Taybi syndrome also suggest ties to certain psychiatric disorders. Furthermore, recent studies on Smith-Magenis syndrome describe an unusual set of maladaptive behaviors, as well as salient sleep anomalies. Finally, we elected to review Angelman and 5p- syndromes, as more refined data are now emerging on genotype–phenotype relationships in both of these disorders. Both Angelman and 5p- syndrome feature new data that call into question previous assumptions about the prognosis of individuals who have these syndromes. Also, our list of five syndromes is a by-product of our own individual interests and clinical experiences.

This chapter, then, discusses salient features—physical, medical, genetic, cognitive, behavioral, and adaptive—in children and adults with

1. Velocardiofacial syndrome
2. Rubinstein-Taybi syndrome
3. Smith-Magenis syndrome
4. Angelman syndrome
5. 5p- (cri du chat) syndrome

As is apparent in this chapter, data are uneven across these five syndromes. Some syndromes feature a cluster of work on maladaptive behavior and no research on cognition or language; others show an opposite pattern. Although findings are sketchy, we adopt the same general structure as in previous chapters, first discussing what is known about physical and medical issues, then cognition and language (levels, profiles, and trajectories), followed by personality and/or adaptive behavior and maladaptive behavior or psychopathology. Next steps for research are offered throughout, and, when information is available we also discuss treatment implications.

VELOCARDIOFACIAL SYNDROME

Velocardiofacial syndrome (sometimes known as *Shprintzen syndrome*) affects approximately 1 in 4,000 people, making it the most common known microdeletion disorder (Papolos et al., 1996).

Physical, Genetic, and Medical Issues

The velocardiofacial phenotype is complex and variable, with four central features: 1) a cleft palate or *velopharyngeal incompetence;* 2) cardiac anomalies; 3) mental retardation or learning difficulties; and 4) characteristic facial features (e.g., Motzkin, Marion, Goldberg, Shpritzen, & Saenger, 1993). As depicted in Figure 7.1, these facial features include a long face with a "flat" expression; long, featureless philtrum; thin upper lip; small mouth; prominent nasal root; large nose with large tip; narrow, "squinting" eyes; and small ears with thick, overfolded helixes. Although these four central features are often considered key symptoms of velocardiofacial syndrome, the phenotype actually varies considerably and includes at least 40 other clinical symptoms that vary in both severity and prevalence. Table 7.1 summarizes some of these features, as well as their estimated prevalence rates.

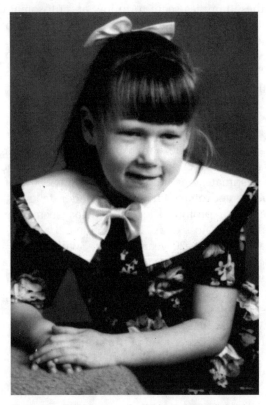

Figure 7.1. Facial features of a child with velocardiofacial syndrome.

Table 7.1. Medical features associated with velocardiofacial syndrome

Feature	%
Immunodeficiencies	77
Palate anomalies	69
Cardiac anomalies	74
Hearing loss/otitis media	39
Renal abnormalities	37
Feeding difficulties	30
Hypocalcemia	20

From McDonald-McGinn et al., 1999.

Velocardiofacial syndrome is caused by a microdeletion on the long arm of chromosome 22 (22q11.2), and most cases are now identified through flourescent *in situ* hybridization (FISH) analyses (see Chapter 2). Most cases are sporadic, or *de novo*, yet about 12% are familial, and these families seem to follow an autosomal dominant inheritance pattern (Driscoll et al., 1993). Though the size of the deletion may vary, the vast majority of cases have the same large deleted region encompassing two to three megabases and at least 20–30 genes (Lindsay et al., 1995). With one exception described in the next section, the function of these genes is unknown.

Cognitive Levels and Profiles

Overall IQ scores in people with velocardiofacial syndrome run the gamut from average functioning to moderate levels of mental retardation. Though estimates vary, approximately 40%–50% of people with velocardiofacial syndrome show mild to moderate levels of mental retardation; severe or profound levels of delay seem rare (McDonald-McGinn et al., 1999; Moss et al., 1999; Swillen et al., 1997). Examining 37 individuals as old as 20 years of age, Swillen et al. (1997) found higher IQ scores among *de novo* cases as opposed to familial cases; mean IQ scores were 80 versus 63, respectively.

Overall IQ scores, however, mask an intriguing cognitive profile highly suggestive of a nonverbal learning disability. In particular, many individuals with velocardiofacial syndrome show a significant IQ "split," with verbal IQ scores higher than performance IQs. Using the Wechsler Intelligence Scales for Children–Third Edition, (Wechsler, 1991), for example, Swillen et al. (1997) reported a mean verbal IQ of 78 and performance IQ of 70 in 20 children with velocardiofacial syndrome.

Problems with nonverbal reasoning are seen as well in the Wechsler-based factor scores of verbal comprehension versus perceptual organization factor scores. Moss et al. (1999) tested 26 children ages 6–17 years old with the WISC–III (Wechsler, 1991), and found a significant difference among participants' mean verbal comprehension score of 79 and perceptual organization score of 68. Children's scores were lower in subtests tapping their perceptual planning, visual-spatial problem-solving, and nonverbal reasoning. Conversely, they performed better in tasks assessing processing speed and acquired information. On achievement testing, these same children scored higher in reading comprehension and decoding relative to arithmetic skills; this profile is another hallmark feature of a nonverbal learning disability.

Further work is needed to specify exactly which aspects of arithmetic and visual-spatial functioning are most problematic for these individuals, and how these evolve over the course of development. In the meantime, many children with velocardiofacial syndrome may benefit from interventions commonly used with students with nonverbal learning disabilities (Rourke, 1995). Working intensively with six students with velocardiofacial syndrome, Kok and Solman (1995) found interactive computer instruction to be particularly effective in promoting reading, spelling, and math skills, as well as in bolstering self-confidence and self-esteem.

Language and Speech

Although language development has yet to be systematically examined, children with velocardiofacial syndrome appear to show delays in expressive language (Golding-Kushner, Weller, & Shprintzen, 1985; Pike & Super, 1997). Performance on language tasks requiring abstract reasoning may be dampened in children with this disorder, and children may also show reduced length of utterances, poor responsiveness to questions, and a reliance on nonverbal communication. Among older children, immature syntax and grammar have also been noted (Golding-Kushner et al., 1985). Administering the Clinical Evaluation of Language Fundamentals–Revised (CELF–R; Wiig, Secord, & Semel, 1992) to 20 children with velocardiofacial syndrome, Moss et al. (1999) found that both receptive and expressive language scores (70.6 and 66.4, respectively) fell significantly below participants' mean verbal IQ score of 78. Specific language impairments were reported in 50% of their sample. The frequency and nature of these language impairments need further study, especially in light of the apparent strengths in reading shown by many children with this disorder.

Both children and adults with velocardiofacial syndrome invariably have hypernasal speech associated with their cleft palate or other anomalies. In addition to a hypernasal quality, articulation and clarity of speech may be compromised. Typical speech may be attained by children who receive a pharyngoplasty, or pharyngeal flap surgery, followed by speech-language therapy. These interventions may be particularly effective in the preschool years (Lipson et al., 1991). It is unclear how many children with velocardiofacial syndrome receive this corrective surgery and to what extent changes in speech affect their expressive language, social interactions, and self-esteem.

Personality, Maladaptive Behavior, and Psychopathology

Though formal studies of personality or maladaptive behavior in velocardiofacial syndrome are sparse, children with this syndrome have been described in seemingly contradictory ways. On one hand, they have been depicted as impulsive, easily aroused, and inattentive (Golding-Kushner et al., 1985). Examining 25 children, adolescents, and young adults with velocardiofacial syndrome, Papolos et al. (1996) found that 24% ($n = 9$) met the *Diagnostic and Statistical Manual of Mental Disorders, Fourth Edition* (DSM-IV: 1994), American Psychiatric Association criteria for attention-deficit/hyperactivity disorder (ADHD) or attention-deficit disorder without hyperactivity. On the other hand, these children are also depicted as shy and withdrawn, and most children with this syndrome also show blunted or inappropriate affect (Golding-Kushner et al., 1985).

Some of these early impressions were confirmed by Swillen et al. (1997), who administered the Dutch version of the Child Behavior Checklist (CBC) (Achenbach, 1991) to 17 children with velocardiofacial syndrome. This group found elevated scores on the social and attention problems scales of the CBC. Inattention and impulsivity were present even in younger children, and older children were more apt to show social withdrawal and anxiety/depression. Yet even the six toddlers in this study exhibited social withdrawal and shyness, as well as problems with eating and constipation. This childhood presentation of blunted affect, and of being simultaneously withdrawn and impulsive, needs further study, especially as it relates to adjustment later in life.

Several studies and case reports point to specific maladaptive and psychiatric difficulties, primarily psychosis in older adolescents and adults (see Table 7.2). Examining 14 adolescents and adults with velocardiofacial syndrome, Pulver et al. (1994) found that 29% ($n = 4$) met clinical criteria for schizophrenia or schizoaffective disorder. Psychosis was also found in the distant relatives of these four cases. These four

Table 7.2. Personality and psychiatric features
found in people with velocardiofacial syndrome

Withdrawal, shyness

Impulsivity, inattention

Bland affect

Monotone speech

Flat affect

Psychosis/schizophrenia

Bipolar disorders

Attention-deficit/hyperactivity disorder (ADHD)

Social phobia

Personality disorders

individuals with velocardiofacial syndrome showed thought disorder, auditory hallucinations, and delusions, and all had received previous psychiatric treatment. Classic symptoms of schizophrenia were seen as well in two individuals with velocardiofacial syndrome reported by Chow, Bassett, and Weksberg (1994) and in 10 individuals described by Bassett et al. (1998). These 10 people, ascertained through a psychiatric facility, were also apt to have temper tantrums and aggressive outbursts and were less likely to show the salient cardiac or palatal anomalies characteristic of velocardiofacial syndrome.

The association among velocardiofacial syndrome and schizophrenia has generated considerable excitement among researchers, as a gene involved in the susceptibility to schizophrenia has been found on chromosome 22q in some families (Pulver et al., 1994). Further, relative to controls, individuals with schizophrenia are more likely to show minor physical anomalies, including a high palate and malformed ears (O'Callaghan, Larkin, Kinsella, & Waddington, 1991). Studies linking the 22q11 region to psychiatric illness are currently underway, yet in the meantime findings have immediate applications for screening purposes.

To this aim, Murphy, Jones, Griffiths, Thompson, and Owen (1998) screened 265 people with mental retardation living in two facilities who showed any of the following:

- Psychosis
- Family history of psychosis
- Facial dysmorphism

- Cleft palate
- Congenital heart disease
- History of hypocalcemia

Among the 75 adults who showed one or more of these symptoms, and subsequently underwent FISH analyses, 2 manifested deletions at 22q11. As both people had mild levels of mental retardation and psychosis, Murphy et al. (1998) suggested that velocardiofacial syndrome may be undetected in some portion of people with mild mental retardation and psychosis.

Papolos et al. (1998), however, called into question findings linking velocardiofacial syndrome to psychosis or schizophrenia. These researchers administered standard psychiatric interviews to 25 individuals with velocardiofacial syndrome ages 5–34 years old who were primarily identified as a result of their craniofacial anomalies or hypernasal speech. None met criteria for schizophrenia. Yet a full 64% (n = 16) met DSM-IV criteria for bipolar spectrum disorders, a rate considerably higher than the 1%–2% found in the general population. Furthermore, compared with mean age of onset of bipolar disorder in the general population (24 years), the individuals with velocardiofacial syndrome exhibited symptoms much younger, at a mean age of 12 years. As some young adults also had psychotic symptoms, Papolos et al. (1998) attributed diagnostic discrepancies across studies to confusion in differentiating schizophrenia from psychotic forms of mood disorders. Such diagnostic issues are further complicated by certain characteristics of the velocardiofacial phenotype, primarily concrete thinking, expressionless speech, and flat or blunted affect and facial expression.

Considerable work thus remains in sorting out the nature of psychiatric vulnerabilities in children and adults with velocardiofacial syndrome. If future research confirms associations between velocardiofacial syndrome and bipolar spectrum disorders or schizophrenia, such findings help narrow the search for genes involved in these complex psychiatric disorders among people in the general population.

Studies are also needed within the velocardiofacial population that identify which people with this syndrome are at greatest risk for developing severe psychiatric illness. Also, further research needs to be conducted on the relationship between velocardiofacial syndrome

Studies are also needed within the velocardiofacial population that identify which people with this syndrome are at greatest risk for developing severe psychiatric illness.

and neurotransmitters. Intriguingly, the deletion in velocardiofacial syndrome includes the gene for catechol-o-methyltransferase. Hemizygosity of this gene may reduce the metabolism of dopamine, noradrenaline, and adrenaline, and altered levels of these neurotransmitters are associated with a greater susceptibility to psychotic and other psychiatric disorders. Even so, not all people with velocardiofacial syndrome develop severe psychiatric illness, raising intriguing questions about how emotional and behavioral difficulties might relate to other deleted or modifying genes in the 22q11 region, as well as to psychosocial and developmental factors.

RUBINSTEIN-TAYBI SYNDROME

First recognized in 1963 by Rubinstein and Taybi, this syndrome is now thought to occur in approximately 1 in 125,000 live births (Hennekam, Boogaard, & Doorne, 1991).

Physical, Medical, and Genetic Issues

The salient features of Rubinstein-Taybi syndrome include mental retardation, short stature, microcephaly, and broad thumbs and first toes (thumbs may also be radially deviated). As shown in Figure 7.2, a characteristic facial appearance is also found, involving a downward slanting of palpebral fissures (i.e., openings of the eyes), a prominent and beaked nose, and a small mouth with a pouting lower lip (Rubinstein, 1990). Many of these physical features change with development. Newborns may have upslanting palpebral fissures, an abundance of scalp hair, and a puffy appearance, all which dissipate over time, and the syndrome's characteristic beaked nose does not generally appear until middle childhood (Allanson, 1990).

Many medical concerns have been routinely observed in people with Rubinstein-Taybi syndrome; rates of these problems in a cohort of 50 individuals are summarized in Table 7.3. These and other problems lead children with this disorder to have approximately 10 times the rate of hospitalizations and surgeries as do typically developing children; many surgeries correct undescended testes and thumb and toe anomalies (Stevens, Carey, & Blackburn, 1990). Infants who have Rubinstein-Taybi syndrome often show feeding difficulties, reflux, poor weight gain, and severe constipation. Constipation may persist into the adult years. Many adults are also prone to being overweight. Routine cardiac and opthalmology exams are recommended, as are orthopedic evaluations to assess radially deviated thumbs (Stevens et al., 1990).

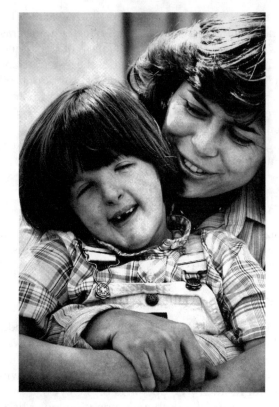

Figure 7.2.   Facial features of a child with Rubinstein-Taybi syndrome.

The genetic cause of some cases of Rubinstein-Taybi syndrome has now been linked to submicroscopic deletions on the short arm of chromosome 16, at 16p13.3 (Lacombe, Sabra, Taint & Batten, 1992). To date, one gene has been mapped to this region, CBP (a binding protein; Chen & Korenberg, 1995), and some individuals with Rubinstein-Taybi syndrome have point mutations in the CBP gene. Yet deletions on chromosome 16 account for just 12% of individuals with clinical diagnoses of Rubinstein-Taybi syndrome (Wallerstein et al., 1997), suggesting that other mechanisms are involved in the etiology of this syndrome. Cases with confirmed deletions at 16p13.3 do not appear to be clinically distinct from those without detectable deletions (Wallerstein et al., 1997).

Cognitive Levels and Profiles

Early reports suggested that most people with Rubinstein-Taybi syndrome were relatively low functioning, with average IQ scores in the

Table 7.3.   Salient medical features in individuals with Rubinstein-Taybi syndrome

Feature	%
Undescended testes	100
Broad thumbs and first toes	100
Palate abnormalities	92
Ocular problems	84
Dental problems	66
Frequent ear infections	52
Severe constipation	48
Overweight	47
Congenital heart defects	38
Urinary tract problems	28

Adapted from Stevens, Carey, & Blackburn, 1990.

30s and 40s (e.g., Padfield, Partington, & Simpson, 1968). Yet, these studies were conducted among people living in institutions, and more recent reports of individuals raised at home find they tend to have higher IQ scores. Reviewing IQ scores from 29 noninstitutionalized individuals, Stevens et al. (1990) reported IQ scores that ranged from 30 to 79, with a mean of 51. Hennekam et al. (1992) found a relatively low mean IQ score among 36 of 40 individuals with Rubinstein-Taybi syndrome, yet their sample consisted of 18 institutionalized and 22 home-reared participants. If these two groups are examined separately, an IQ disparity is evident; the mean IQ is 29.5 in the institutionalized group, and 45.5 in home-reared participants.

Although the performance IQ may exceed the verbal IQ score in some individuals with Rubinstein-Taybi syndrome (Hennekam et al., 1992), this finding is not consistent, and further studies are needed on specific areas of cognitive strength and weakness. Cross-sectional analyses suggest that IQ scores decline with advancing age, particularly in terms of verbal skills (Hennekam et al., 1992), yet longitudinal studies are needed to replicate these findings.

Language and Speech

Most people with Rubinstein-Taybi syndrome (up to 90%) show delays in speech acquisition, yet relatively few (10%) have severe articulation problems (Stevens et al., 1990). Assessing 40 individuals with this disorder, Hennekam et al. (1992) reported that although many participants had abnormal nasal air emission (a hypernasal quality), as well as palatal abnormalities, most showed relatively intact speech. Furthermore, articulation and intelligibility were described as good.

Language skills were also assessed in this same cohort of 40 participants with Rubinstein-Taybi syndrome (Hennekam et al., 1992). Receptive vocabulary was slightly better developed than expressive vocabulary, and most language indices were consistent with IQ expectations. Syntax was simple, with a mean length of utterance of 3.3, and concepts were generally concrete. Even so, these researchers found remarkably good levels of communication skills in their sample, with most people able to use their language to engage others, control actions, make comments, and get their needs met. These observations encourage further studies on the pragmatic skills of people with Rubinstein-Taybi syndrome, including to what extent their social uses of language may exceed mental age (MA) expectations.

Personality, Maladaptive Behavior, and Psychopathology

Although formal studies are sparse, the personality of people with Rubinstein-Taybi syndrome has been anecdotally described as loving, friendly, and happy, with many individuals also showing interest in music (e.g., Hennekam et al., 1992; Stevens et al., 1990). Consistent with this congenial style, most people do not seem to show clinically significant levels of maladaptive behavior. Stevens and colleagues (1990), for example, found that just 10% of 50 participants with Rubinstein-Taybi syndrome had serious problems with maladaptive behavior as assessed by the Inventory for Client and Agency Planning, a standardized survey (Bruininks, Hill, Weatherman, & Woodcock, 1986). Even so, 90% were described as having a short attention span and 65% as engaging in self-stimulatory behaviors such as body rocking or hand flapping. Sensitivities to sounds were reported in 46%, particularly loud sounds associated with crowds.

Although formal studies are sparse, the personality of people with Rubinstein-Taybi syndrome has been anecdotally described as loving, friendly, and happy, with many individuals also showing interest in music.

Similar concerns were observed by Hennekam et al. (1992), who administered the Dutch version of the CBC to parents of 37 people with Rubinstein-Taybi syndrome. As shown in Table 7.4, frequent problems were noted in concentration, attention-seeking, impulsivity, and social withdrawal. Across both studies, then, primary concerns in this population appear to be inattention, social withdrawal, attention-seeking, and stereotypies. Though temper tantrums were noted in up to 40% of

Table 7.4.   Salient behavioral features in individuals with
Rubinstein-Taybi syndrome

Feature	%
Short attention span	90
Inability to concentrate	76
Poorly coordinated, clumsy	73
Clings to adults	70
Likes to be alone	68
Speech problems	65
Self-stimulatory behaviors	65
Daydreams	62
Demands much attention	62
Nervous	57
Impulsive	54
Sound dislikes, sensitivities	46
Sudden changes in mood	46
Overweight	46

Adapted from Hennekam et al., 1992, and Stevens et al., 1990.

the Hennekam et al. (1992) sample, aggressive or acting-out behavior
has rarely been reported. It is unclear how any of these maladaptive
features relate to age, IQ, or 16p13.3 deletion status.

In contrast to these early studies of maladaptive behavior, Levitas
and Reid (1998) reported provocative findings on a possible association
among Rubinstein-Taybi syndrome and a specific clustering of psychiatric disorders. Examining 13 adults with
Rubinstein-Taybi syndrome who were
attending a psychiatric clinic, unusually
high rates were found of mood and
tic/obsessive-compulsive spectrum disorders. Given their method of ascertainment, the researchers expected to find
significant difficulties among these adults;
what was unexpected was the pattern of
these problems, with 61% manifesting
mood disorders, and 31% showing tic/

*Adults with Rubinstein-
Taybi syndrome may thus
be at heightened risk for
bipolar and tic/obsessive-
compulsive spectrum dis-
orders. . .*

obsessive-compulsive spectrum disorders. Of these, 46% had neu-
roleptic-induced movement disorders; given this high rate, Levitas and
Reid (1998) cautioned against use of neuroleptics in the Rubinstein-
Taybi population. Adults with Rubinstein-Taybi syndrome may thus be
at heightened risk for bipolar and tic/obsessive-compulsive spectrum

disorders, and future work is needed that compares a larger, more representative sample of people with Rubinstein-Taybi syndrome with others with delay. It is also unclear how these problems develop, and to what extent the social withdrawal, impulsivity, and lability in children serve as harbingers of difficulties later in life. If the bipolar and tic/obsessive-compulsive findings are replicated, this will encourage future research on the Rubinstein-Taybi locus and possible genes in this area that might regulate certain neurotransmitters (e.g., serotonin, dopamine) involved in these major psychiatric disorders.

SMITH-MAGENIS SYNDROME

Although Smith-Magenis syndrome was first identified in the early 1980s (Smith et al., 1986; Smith, McGavran, Waldstein, & Robinson, 1982), researchers have only recently appreciated that this disorder has a wide array of intriguing physical and behavior problems. At present, the syndrome may also be underdiagnosed, although this situation may be changing (Chen, Potocki, & Lupski, 1996).

Physical, Medical, and Genetic Issues

People with Smith-Magenis syndrome show a range of minor physical and facial anomalies. They are described as having a flat mid-face and a flat head shape. In addition, the face is often characterized by a broad nasal bridge and an upper lip shaped like a "cupid's bow" (Greenberg et al., 1991; see Figure 7.3). These individuals are also often short in stature, and have short, small hands; ear anomalies; and a deep, hoarse voice.

In addition to having such physical characteristics, many of these individuals exhibit a wide variety of medical issues. As summarized in Table 7.5, individuals with Smith-Magenis syndrome often experience visual problems, ranging from squints and near-sightedness (i.e., myopia) to detached retinas, which may be the result of the combination of myopia, overactivity, and self-injurious behaviors such as head banging (Finucane, Jaeger, Kurtz, Weinstein, & Scott, 1993). In addition, as many as 75% of people with this disorder have symptoms associated with peripheral neuropathy (Greenberg et al., 1996a). These symptoms include decreased sensitivity to pain or temperature, decreased deep tendon reflexes, scoliosis, and chest abnormalities (*pes cavus* or *pes planus*). Several of these physical-medical issues (most notably the decreased sensitivity to pain and temperature) may also relate to commonly observed maladaptive behaviors such as sticking foreign objects

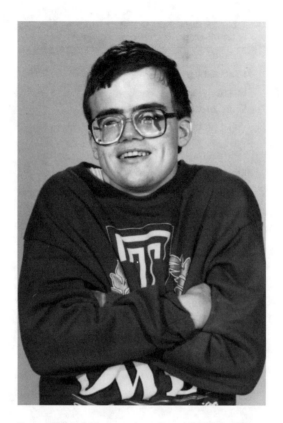

Figure 7.3.   Facial features of a young adult with Smith-Magenis syndrome.

into body orifices. Congenital heart defects, seizures, hearing impairments, and urinary tract anomalies are also seen in some people with Smith-Magenis syndrome (see Table 7.5).

Estimates of the prevalence of Smith-Magenis syndrome range from 1 per 50,000 (Colley, Leversha, Voullaire, & Rogers, 1990) to about 1 per 25,000 (Greenberg et al., 1991). Often considered a rarely occurring disorder, Smith-Magenis syndrome may actually be more prevalent than originally thought (Chen et al., 1996; Smith, Dykens, & Greenberg, 1998a). In addition to its recent discovery, missed or incorrect diagnoses may have resulted because this syndrome's physical characteristics are subtle. In addition, physical characteristics in some people partially overlap with other genetic mental retardation syndromes such as fragile X syndrome (Chen et al., 1996) or Prader-Willi syndrome (Greenberg et al., 1996b). As a result, many people with Smith-Magenis syndrome may remain either undiagnosed or misdiagnosed.

Table 7.5. Salient physical and medical features of Smith-Magenis syndrome

Feature	%
Midface hypoplasia	93
Brachycephaly	89
Short, broad hands	85
Visual problems	85
Myopia	42–80
Strabismus	32–100
Broad nasal bridge	84
Broad face	81
Middle ear/laryngeal anomalies	81
Hoarse voice	80
Peripheral neuropathy	75
Sleep abnormalities	75
Short stature	69
Hearing impairment	63–68
Scoliosis	42–65
Cardiovascular abnormalities	29–27
Renal abnormalities	28–35

Sources: Chen, Potocki, & Lupski, 1996; Finucane, Jaeger, Kurtz, Weinstein, & Scott, 1993; Greenberg et al., 1996a.

Another complication involves the nature of the syndrome's genetic etiology. It has long been known, for example, that Smith-Magenis syndrome is caused by a new (*de novo*) deletion on chromosome 17 derived from either the mother or the father. Although this deletion has been localized to a small (interstitial) region on the proximal short arm of chromosome 17 (at 17p11.2), the deletion is not always detectable cytogenetically. Until the more widespread use of FISH and other molecular genetic techniques, then, the small deletion causing the disorder often went undiagnosed.

Cognitive and Adaptive Functioning

Most people with Smith-Magenis syndrome function in the moderate to mild ranges of mental retardation, though a few individuals show more or less severe levels of delay (Greenberg et al., 1996a). In fact, Crumley (1998) reported a 12-year-old girl with Smith-Magenis syndrome who did not have mental retardation but showed the syndrome's characteristic behavior and sleep problems. Assessing 24 people ages 1–30 years old with a variety of tests, Greenberg et al. (1996a) found an average IQ score of 47.44, with no difference in verbal versus perform-ance IQ scores seen in the 18 participants receiving Wechsler-based tests (mean = 55.83 and 55.17, respectively).

Administering the Kaufman Assessment Battery for Children (K-ABC; Kaufman & Kaufman, 1984) to 10 people with Smith-Magenis syndrome, Dykens, Finucane, and Gayley (1997) found significant rel-ative weaknesses in sequential processing, and strengths in achievement. Participants did particularly well in tasks tapping long-term memory and acquired information, although they performed relatively poorly in subtests requiring auditory and visual short-term memory. All par-ticipants had Expressive One-Word Picture Vocabulary Test (EOWPVT; Gardner, 1991) age-equivalent scores that exceeded their K-ABC age scores by 1–5 years, with an average discrepancy of 2.29 years. Such findings speak to the relative strengths in acquired information shown by many with the syndrome.

Language and Speech

Although formal speech and language studies have yet to be reported, virtually all people with Smith-Magenis syndrome show delays in speech acquisition. Although 75% have a char-acteristic deep, hoarse voice, laryngeal anomalies do not appear to be widespread (Greenberg et al., 1991, 1996; Smith et al., 1998a). Speech-language therapy is re-commended, as is the use of sign lan-guage, as a means of building language skills and reducing frustration.

speech-language therapy is recommended, as is the use of sign language, as a means of building lan-guage skills and reducing frustration.

People with Smith-Magenis syn-drome appear to show adaptive skills that are commensurate with their levels of intellectual functioning. We found, for example, mean composite age-equivalent scores of 5.25 years on the Vineland Adaptive Behavior Scales (VABS; Sparrow, Balla, & Cicchetti, 1984) and 5.19 years on the K-ABC (Dykens, Finecone, et al., 1997). Similarly, Greenberg et al. (1996a) found an overall Vineland composite of 46.50 among 24 people with SMS, simi-lar to the average IQ of 47.44. No significant scatter among Vineland domains was found in either study, suggesting evenly developed com-munication, daily living, and social skills. It is unknown how cognitive and adaptive skills change over time, and to what extent the syndrome's salient maladaptive problems interfere with learning or optimal adaptive outcomes.

Maladaptive Behavior and Psychopathology

Many people with Smith-Magenis syndrome show a mixture of unusual maladaptive behaviors that pose a continual challenge for their families, teachers, and other caregivers (Smith et al., 1998a). These problems are often elevated even relative to others with genetic syndromes or mixed causes of delay (Clarke & Boer, 1998; Dykens & Smith, 1998). Many people with Smith-Magenis syndrome have problems with sleep, aggression, impulsivity, hyperactivity, and self-injurious behaviors (e.g., Colley, 1990; Greenberg et al., 1991; Stratton et al., 1986).

Examining these behaviors in more detail, Dykens and Smith (1998) administered the CBC to parents of 35 children and adolescents with Smith-Magenis syndrome, as well as to control participants with other causes for their delay. The children who have Smith-Magenis syndrome scored significantly higher than did their counterparts, with 89% having CBC scores in the clinically significant range, as opposed to 28% of those with mixed etiologies. As shown in Table 7.6, most children (75% –100%) showed hyperactivity, disobedience, temper tantrums, lability, poor concentration, stereotypies, self-injury, impulsivity, stubbornness, restlessness, property destruction, sleep problems, attention-seeking behaviors, and a tendency to cling to adults. Bed wetting and having bowel movements outside the toilet were seen in 50%–80% of children.

Stereotypies and Self-Injurious Behaviors Describing the nature of Smith-Magenis stereotypies and self-injurious behaviors in more detail, Dykens and Smith (1998) found that many stereotypies centered on the mouth (e.g., mouthing hands or objects). These behaviors may be related to the tendency for some with the syndrome to insert foreign objects into body openings, termed *polyembolokoilamania* by Greenberg et al. (1996a). Other unusual stereotypies include a characteristic "spasmodic upper body squeeze" or self-hug, seen especially when people are happy or excited (Finucane, Konar, Hass-Givler, Kurtz, & Scott, 1994). We also identified a highly persistent and unusual "lick-and-flip" repetitive behavior (i.e., inserting four fingers of hand into mouth and using the damp hand to flip the pages of a book), seen in 90% of our participants during their cognitive test sessions and in 51% of our larger sample (Dykens, Finucane et al., 1997; Dykens & Smith, 1998).

Although previous work suggested that many individuals with Smith-Magenis syndrome pull out their finger- or toenails (i.e., *onychotillomania;* Greenberg et al., 1996a), we found that just 25% of our sample

Table 7.6. Salient maladaptive behaviors
in Smith-Magenis syndrome

Behavior	%
Demands a lot of attention	100
Stereotypies	100
Mouthing	69
"Lick and flip"	51
Self-hug	46
Disobedient	97
Hyperactive	94
Sleeps less than others	94
Temper tantrums	94
Self-injury	92
Bites self	77
Hits self	71
Bangs head	68
Pulls out nails	30
Inserts objects	25
Labile	89
Can't concentrate	89
Destroys things	86
Impulsive	86
Wets bed	80
Argues a lot	80
Attacks people	57
Bowel movement outside toilet	50

Adapted from Dykens & Smith, 1998.

engaged in this form of self-injury (Dykens & Smith, 1998). As shown in Table 7.5, more commonly occurring self-injurious behaviors included self-biting and head-banging. All of these self-injurious behaviors are likely related to peripheral neuropathy, seen in as many as 75% of those with Smith-Magenis syndrome (Greenberg et al., 1996a).

Sleep Problems Sleep problems are salient in Smith-Magenis syndrome and include impairments in rapid eye movement sleep, difficulties falling asleep, shortened sleep cycles, frequent and prolonged nocturnal awakenings, snoring, and subsequent daytime sleepiness and napping (Smith, Dykens, & Greenberg, 1998b). These problems are among the most challenging to parents, who become exhausted because they are up most nights attending to their children; indeed sleep and other problem behaviors are strongly associated with heightened family stress (Hodapp, Fidler, & Smith, 1998). Sleep disturbance is a robust predictor of maladaptive behavior in children with Smith-Magenis syndrome, especially attentional, aggressive, and acting-out behaviors (Dykens & Smith, 1998). Conversely, improved sleep (and longer daytime naps) are associated with fewer acting out and other maladaptive behaviors (Dykens & Smith, 1998).

Sleep difficulties are so striking in this population that some have speculated that the Smith-Magenis syndrome critical region on chromosome 17 may contain a gene involved with REM sleep (Greenberg et al., 1996a). Others suggest that people with Smith-Magenis syndrome have aberrant levels of melatonin, leading them to have a disturbed biological clock and circadian rhythm (Smith et al., 1998b). Indeed, many parents report that over-the-counter melatonin helps improve sleep patterns (Smith et al., 1998b). Thus, studies assessing the efficacy of melatonin or other treatments are greatly needed in light of the negative impact that chronic sleep problems have on families.

ANGELMAN SYNDROME

Angelman syndrome was first identified in the mid-1960s by Harry Angelman (1965). The prevalence estimates for Angelman syndrome vary widely, from approximately 1 in 25,000 to 1 in 12,000 live births (Clayton-Smith & Pembrey, 1992; Kyllerman, 1995). Such variability may be associated with imprecise clinical diagnoses, which in past years have included an underdetection of the syndrome's occurrence in infants (due to their unremarkable facial features), as well as in older individuals residing in institutional settings (Buckley, Dinno, & Weber, 1998; Buntinx et al., 1995; Clayton-Smith & Pembrey, 1992; Jacobsen et al., 1998).

Physical, Medical, and Genetic Issues

Angelman syndrome is characterized by severe levels of developmental delay; absence of expressive speech; seizure disorders; bouts of spontaneous laughter; a happy demeanor; and an ataxic, jerky gait. Because of these last two qualities, this disorder was initially referred to as the "happy puppet" syndrome; because of its deprecatory overtones, this term is no longer used. As shown in Figure 7.4, people with Angelman syndrome tend to have long faces, prominent jaws, wide mouths and widely spaced teeth, protruding tongues, flat occiputs, deep-set eyes, and microcephaly.

Angelman syndrome has come under recent and intensive study from geneticists, in part because of its unique relationship with Prader-Willi syndrome. Prader-Willi syndrome is caused by paternally inherited anomalies of chromosome 15q11-q13; Angelman syndrome is associated with the opposite pattern, or maternally derived abnormalities in this same region of chromosome 15q. Most cases of Angelman syndrome, approximately 70%, are due to relatively large (four megabase), *de novo* maternal deletions of chromosome 15 (q11-q13). From 2%

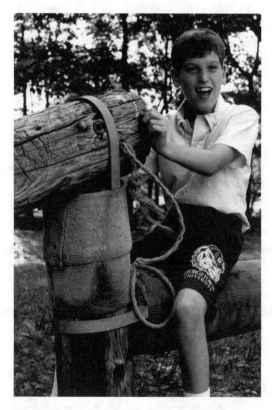

Figure 7.4.   Facial features of a child with Angelman syndrome.

to 5% of Angelman syndrome cases are attributed to paternal uni-parental disomy (UPD), which occurs when both copies of chromosome 15 are inherited from the father (Robinson et al., 1993). Either through maternal deletion or paternal UPD, then, imprinted information is missing from the mother in the Angelman syndrome critical region (the opposite is seen in Prader-Willi syndrome, in which 70% of cases are due to paternal deletion and 25% to maternal UPD).

Approximately 2%–3% of individuals with Angelman syndrome have imprinting defects, including deletions of the so-called "imprinting center" on chromosome 15 (Buiting et al., 1995; Saitoh et al., 1997). A handful of cases (1%) have other, unusual chromosomal re-arrangements involving chromosome 15 (Chan et al., 1993). The remaining 22%–25% of individuals with Angelman syndrome show none of these anomalies, and for a long time were an enigma to researchers. In recent breakthroughs, however, many of these cases were shown to have specific mutations in one of the genes in the Angelman/Prader-Willi critical region called UBE3A (Kishino, Lalande, & Wagstaff, 1997; Matsuura et al., 1997). UBE3A appears to be specifically expressed in the brain (Albrecht et al., 1997), yet it is unknown how the absence of UBE3A (which encodes for a protein ligase involved in intracellular protein processing) leads to the Angelman syndrome phenotype.

In addition to UBE3A, newly developed animal models point to other candidate genes that appear to play a role in the Angelman syndrome phenotype. The Angelman/Prader-Willi deletion region contains a gene called GABRA3, a subunit of $GABA_A$ receptors, which is implicated in epilepsy and is the target of certain anticonvulsive medications (Olsen & Avoli, 1997). DeLorey et al., (1998) found that disrupting the GABRA3 gene in mice caused electroencephalogram (EEG) abnormalities and seizures, as well as other key features of Angelman syndrome such as poor learning and motor coordination, hyperactivity, and disrupted rest—activity patterns. Disruptions of both the GABA3 and UBE3A genes are thus implicated in Angelman syndrome, although the relative contributions of each of these or other genes remain unknown.

Advances in classifying the various genetic subtypes of Angelman syndrome have critically important implications for genetic counseling, and for future phenotypic studies. In particular, the recurrence risk of Angelman syndrome is low in families with a child with a deletion or paternal disomy: less than 1% (Stalker & Williams, 1998). In contrast, as imprinting center mutations appear to be transmitted maternally, mothers who have these mutations have a 50% risk of having the syndrome recurr in future pregnancies. Finally, current estimates suggest that approximately half of cases with UBE3A defects are familial and half are *de novo,* leading to a probable recurrence risk of 50% for familial cases (Stalker & Williams, 1998). Given these complexities and the rapid advances in genetics, clinicians working with families with a member who has Angelman syndrome need to ensure that all family members have received up-to-date genetic counseling.

Furthermore, phenotypic differences appear to exist across these genetic sub-types, though to varying degrees. Those with the deletion show almost all of the "classic" features of Angelman syndrome. Examining 27 individuals with confirmed deletions, Smith et al., (1996) found that all had severe levels of mental retardation, ataxic movements, absent speech, abnormal EEG, a happy disposition, typical birth weight and head circumference at birth, and a large, wide mouth. These and other clinical features of people with paternal deletions are summarized in Table 7.7.

In contrast, a milder phenotypic picture is found among the relatively few individuals with Angelman syndrome due to paternal UPD (e.g., Bottani et al., 1994; Gillessen-Kaesbach, Albrecht, Passarge, & Horsthemke, 1995; Smith, Marks, Haan, Dixon, & Trent, 1997; Smith, Robson, & Buchholz, 1998). Relative to their counterparts with deletions, individuals with paternal UPD have better growth parameters;

Table 7.7. Salient clinical features of Angelman syndrome due to paternal deletions

Feature	%
Ataxic movements	100
Severe mental retardation	100
Absent language	100
Happy disposition	100
Normal birth weight	100
Normal head circumference at birth	100
Abnormal electroencephalogram (EEG)	100
Seizures	96
Large, wide mouth, large chin	92
Bouts of laughter	91
Sleeping problems	86
Protuding tongue	81
Feeding difficulties in infancy	77
Hypopigmentation	73
Hypotonia at birth	63
Microcephaly	53

Adapted from Smith et al., 1996.

and more subtle facial features; walk at earlier ages; and have less severe or frequent seizure disorders, less ataxia, and a greater facility with rudimentary communication such as signing or gesturing. Those with imprinting center mutations are less apt to show microcephaly or hypopigmentation, and they also appear to have less severe seizure disorders (Burger, Kunze, Sperling, & Reis, 1996; Minassian et al., 1998; Saitoh et al., 1997). Milder epilepsy is also noted among those with Angelman syndrome cases with UBE3A abnormalities (Minassian et al., 1998). Further studies are needed to assess a wider range of behavior across these genetic subtypes; a challenge given the rarity of some of these cases. Ultimately, data from different genetic subtypes have the potential to refine gene–behavior understandings as well as treatment and prognosis.

Cognition and Language

Although most researchers note that people with Angelman syndrome show severe levels of delay, studies have yet to document these delays using standardized testing. Indeed, many individuals are deemed "untestable," in part because of their inattention and lack of speech.

Yet many psychometrically sound measures now exist that assess nonverbal intelligence and prelinguistic communication. Recently, Penner, Johnston, Faircloth, Irish, and Williams (1993) administered some of these measures to seven institutionalized adults with Angelman syndrome. Using a series of Piagetian tasks, they found that 4 participants scored at sensory-motor Stage 2, two at Stage 3, and one between Stages 5 and 6. For all participants, their use of objects or means–ends were better developed than their vocal and gestural imitation skills. Indeed, none of the 7 engaged in imitative vocalizations or spontaneous speech-like babbling, as would be expected at this stage of development, and instead produced single-sound, open-mouth vowel-like sounds. As participants were also unable to imitate mouth motor acts, the researchers proposed that Angelman syndrome may involve an oral-motor or developmental verbal dyspraxia. Furthermore, 6 of 7 participants did not show joint attention, joint action on an object, or turn-taking; all are prerequiste skills for successful social interaction.

Additional developmental studies are imperative, especially with children who have received benefit of early intervention, which may have not been the case with Penner et al.'s (1993) older, institutionalized sample. Though many individuals with Angelman syndrome seem to show unfocused, non–goal-related actions and a lack of sustained attention to others, others show some babbling, use of gestures, turn-taking, and relatively well-developed receptive language skills (e.g., Williams et al., 1995). Clayton-Smith (1993), for example, found that 90% of 82 people with Angelman syndrome used some type of signing or gesturing, but only 20% could be taught standard (Makaton) sign language. Although 30% had no expressive vocabulary, most participants in this sample had from one to three words (especially "ma-ma," "hi-ya," "bath" and "'bye"). It is unknown how or if variations in developmental levels or skills are associated with age, early intervention, or genetic subtypes of this disorder.

Maladaptive Behavior and Neurological Findings

Beginning with Harry Angelman's (1965) first observations, data have been remarkably consistent in describing the behavior of people with Angelman syndrome. Speech delays are salient, as are inappropriate laughter or bouts of laughter unrelated to context, mouthing objects, problems falling or staying asleep, feeding problems during infancy, motoric hyperactivity and inattention, and stereotypies such as hand-flapping or twirling (e.g., Summers, Allison, Lynch, & Sandler, 1995; Summers & Feldman, 1999). Table 7.8 summarizes rates of these and other behaviors across various studies.

Though temper tantrums were noted in 45% of 11 children with Angelman syndrome (Summers et al., 1995), tantrums and irritability were significantly lower among 27 children with Angelman syndrome compared with age- and IQ-matched controls (Summers & Feldman, 1999). Children with Angelman syndrome in this study were also less likely

Table 7.8. Behavioral features of people with Angelman syndrome across studies

Behavior	%
Grabs people or things	100
Frequent smiling	96–100
Characteristic electroencephalogram (EEG)	92–100
Hand flapping	84
Inappropriate laughter	77–91
Excessive mouthing	75–100
Hyperactivity	64–100
Sleeping difficulty	57–100
Eating problem	45–64

Sources: Clayton-Smith, 1993; Laan, Boer, Hennekan, Reinera, & Brouwer, 1996; Summers, Allison, Lynch, & Feldman, 1995; Zori et al., 1992.

than age- and IQ-matched children with mental retardation to show social withdrawal; such findings are consistent with long-noted clinical observations of a happy disposition, marked by frequent smiling.

Although not formally studied, clinical observations suggest that
many people with Angelman syndrome love water (Clayton-Smith,
1993). Many children are drawn to water play, bathing, and swimming,
as well as to shiny objects such as mirrors or plastic. A fascination with
musical toys or objects that make loud sounds have also been anecdotally reported (Clayton-Smith, 1993). All of these interests are also seen
in others with mental retardation, including those with autism and 5p-
syndrome, and it is unknown if they are elevated in Angelman syndrome relative to other groups.

The seizure disorder associated with Angelman syndrome is fairly
well-understood. Many people with the disorder show a similar pattern of abnormal EEG findings involving
large amplitude slow-spike waves (Boyd,
Harden, & Patton, 1988). Seizures are not
typically seen before 1 year of age, with
most people showing an onset after 3
years of age (Zori et al., 1992). For many
children with Angelman syndrome, seizures are initially severe and hard to control, but they often become less severe
and more manageable over the course of
development (Zori et al., 1992). Diagnosis and treatment of seizures may be
complicated by the ataxic gait and trem-
ulous arm and leg movements shown by
most with the disorder. Williams et al.

> *Williams et al. (1995)
> warn that these features,
> as well as abnormal EEGs
> even when seizures are
> controlled, may lead some
> children to be overmed-
> icated.*

(1995) warned that these features, as well as abnormal EEGs even when
seizures are controlled, may lead some children to be overmedicated.
For most children with Angelman syndrome, they advocated only single use of the types of anticonvulsants used to treat minor as opposed
to major motor seizures (see also Laan, Boer, Hennekam, Reiner, &
Brouwer, 1996).

Some of the syndrome's characteristic behavioral and neurological
features may change over time. Hyperactivity may diminish with age,
and people may also calm down and show fewer sleep disturbances as
they get older (Buntinx et al., 1995; Clayton-Smith, 1993). Characteristics
such as unsteady gait, happy demeanor, bouts of laughter, and smiling
seem to persist; yet adults may have a less excitable overall presentation, including fewer bouts of laughter (e.g., Buckley, Dinno, & Weber,
1998; Laan et al., 1996).

Further, many individuals show improvement in their seizure disorders over time, with less frequent or severe involvement, and a subsiding of abnormal EEG patterns (Buntinx et al., 1995; Clayton-Smith, 1993). Laan et al. (1996), however, found that 82% of their sample of 28 adults with Angelman syndrome still manifested regular seizure activity. Others have identified individuals who have a more variable course, showing periods of inactivity or "silence," followed by a sudden re-emergence of hard-to-control seizures (Buckley et al., 1998; Buntinx et al., 1995).

Seizures aside, most adults enjoy good general physical health, suggesting the possibility of near-normal life expectancies (Buntinx et al., 1995). Relative to children, however, adults with Angelman syndrome may show increased risks of scoliosis, as well as decreased mobility leading to the need for wheelchair use (e.g., Buntinx et al., 1995; Laan et al., 1996). To avoid contractures and other problems, many recommend that adults with Angelman syndrome be keep active and mobile for as long as possible (Buckley et al., 1998; Buntinx et al., 1995; Clayton-Smith, 1993; Laan et al., 1996).

> *To avoid contractures and other problems, many recommend that adults with Angelman syndrome keep active and mobile for as long as possible.*

Although adaptive skills have yet to be assessed with standardized measures, several researchers find that many adults with Angelman syndrome perform basic dressing, toileting, and feeding tasks. As many as 85% of 28 institutionalized adults in Laan et al.'s (1996) study used a fork and spoon and made their wants and concerns known, 80% used gestures and followed simple commands, and 50%–60% undressed themselves and had achieved daytime continence. Rates of these skills may vary among younger or noninstitutionalized people; however, most people with the disorder require close, long-term supervision and care.

5p- (CRI-DU-CHAT) SYNDROME

Affecting about 1 in 50,000 births, this syndrome was initially named by a group of French physicians after one of its cardinal features—a high-pitched, infantile, cat-like cry (Lejune et al., 1963). Though still commonly referred to as cri-du-chat syndrome (translated from French as "cry of the cat"), many parents and researchers have opted to use the more neutral 5p- syndrome, which refers to the disorder's underlying genetic etiology.

Physical, Medical, and Genetic Issues

Medically, most all individuals with classic 5p- syndrome show early hypotonia, with about 50% showing hypertonia and also some limited range of motion in their later years (Carlin, 1990). Other common concerns include feeding problems, a poor suck, regurgitation, and frequent respiratory and ear infections. As summarized in Table 7.9, many people with 5p- syndrome also have severe constipation, especially with advancing age, as well as dental malocclusion and ocular problems (Carlin, 1990; Wilkins, Brown, Nance, & Wolf, 1983). Seizure disorders are relatively rare.

The exact cause of the high-pitched, cat-like cry in 5p- syndrome remains unknown; however, some hypotheses have focused on abnormalities of the larynx and others on a particular genetic makeup, as is discussed later. A small larynx or minor structural anomalies of the larynx have been found in some individuals, although others show a normal larynx (see Neibuhr, 1978, for a review). In light of this variability, some researchers speculate that the cat-cry is associated with central nervous system dysfunction. Regardless of the etiology, the cry seems to be both perceptually and acoustically similar to a kitten's meow (see Sohner & Mitchell, 1991).

The cat-cry is depicted in the literature as occurring predominantly in newborns and infants, and as dissipating over time (e.g., Breg et al., 1970). Others, however, suggest that even though the cry may change in form or be less frequent with advancing age, the quality of the cry remains abnormal (e.g., Neibuhr, 1978). A longitudinal study of one infant with 5p- syndrome appears to bear out this hypothesis

Table 7.9. Salient medical features of 5p-syndrome

Feature	%
Frequent infections	100
Early hypotonia	100
Voice hypernasality	100
Regurgitation	92
Dental malocclusion	53
Strabismus/myopia	44–47
Constipation	37
Hypertonia	35
Cardiac abnormalities	29–40

Sources: Carlin, 1990, and Wilkins, Brown, Nance, & Wolf, 1983.

(Sohner & Mitchell, 1991). Both the cry and noncry vocalizations of this child were similarly high-pitched, and remained so from ages 8 months through 26 months. Although large-scale studies are needed, the voices of many older children have been informally noted as being high-pitched in tone.

Although occasionally associated with parental translocations (see Chapter 2), most cases of 5p- syndrome are attributed to a deletion on the tip of the short arm of chromosome 5. Recent developments have localized the deletion to 5p15, but with some fascinating twists (Overhauser et al., 1994). People with deletions that encompass a portion of 5p15.2 typically show the syndrome's characteristic features of severe mental retardation and distinct round face with epicanthal folds, downslanting palpebral fissures, microcephaly, and low-set, malformed ears (see Figure 7.5) (e.g., Wilkins et al., 1983). Yet, in recent years a small group of individuals have been identified who have the syndrome's

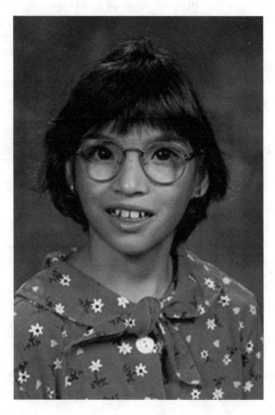

Figure 7.5.   Facial features of a child with 5p- syndrome.

characteristic high-pitched cry, but do not show the syndrome's typical facial features or mental retardation. These people have deletions at 5p15.3 (Church et al., 1995; Gersh et al., 1995, 1997).

A cat-like cry in a newborn may thus lead to two very different clinical outcomes, depending on which areas of the 5p15 region are deleted. Diagnostic tools have now been developed that allow clinicians to make distinctions among the classic cri-du-chat syndrome, which encompasses both critical regions (5p15.2, 5p15.3) versus those with just the cat-cry, which encompasses deletions only at 5p15.3 (Gersh et al., 1997).

Cognition and Language

Historically, virtually all people with 5p- syndrome were depicted as having severe to profound levels of mental retardation, and many families were told not to expect their children to walk or talk. Although many older people residing in long-term care facilities were indeed nonambulatory or nonverbal, more recent findings of noninstitutionalized people paint a more variable and optimistic picture.

On formal IQ testing, many children with 5p- syndrome show severe levels of mental retardation. Examining 26 children ages 6–15 years old with the WISC-III (Wechsler, 1991), Cornish, Bramble, Munir, and Pigram (1999) found that 21 of these children had Full-Scale IQ scores of 50 or less, with 5 participants showing moderate delay. The average IQ score for the 22 children who scored above the test floor (IQ 40) was 47.81. Similarly, as measured by the Battelle Developmental Inventory (BDI; Newborg, Stock, Wnek, Guidubaldi, & Svinicki, 1988), Dykens, Hodapp, Ly, & Rosner (2000) found severe levels of developmental delay in 20 individuals with 5p- syndrome ages 3–20 years old, with an overall MA of 17.26 months.

Yet some individuals score in the moderate and even mild ranges of mental retardation. Smith et al., (1990) reported two such cases: a 7-year-old girl with an IQ score of 66, and a 21-month-old girl with a developmental age of 19.6 months. An 11-year-old female with an IQ score of 72 was also reported (Cornish, 1996).

Genetic Implications Early reports suggested that the size of the 5p- deletion may be associated with some of the variability in cognitive level, such that higher-functioning people might have smaller deletions (Wilkins et al., 1983). But these three high-functioning people all had the large deletions typically seen in those with syndrome. Indeed, Marinescu, Johnson, Dykens, Hodapp, and Overhauser (1999) found no correlation among deletion size and developmental level in 50 participants with 5p- syndrome. Thus, other as-yet unidentified genetic factors likely mediate the expression of cognitive involvement in 5p-syndrome.

In this vein, people with 5p- syndrome due to unbalanced translocations are generally lower functioning than their counterparts with deletions—a likely consequence of two chromosomes (5p and one other) being disrupted in these cases. Relative to those with deletions, Wilkins et al. (1983) found that 15 participants with various types of translocations had lower IQs and more medical complications. Similarly, compared with age- and gender-matched participants with deletions, Dykens and Clarke (1997) found lower adaptive behavior scores among 13 participants with translocations. In striking contrast to the friendly and social orientation of those individuals with deletions, these 13 participants with translocations were more withdrawn, hard to reach, uncommunicative, and unresponsive. Although autism-like features were once thought to be characteristic of 5p- syndrome, these symptoms seem to only apply to those with translocations.

Cognitive/Linguistic Profiles At first glance, the cognitive profile in 5p- syndrome appears relatively flat. Cornish et al. (1999) found no significant scatter in WISC–III sub-test scores in their sample of 26 children with 5p- syndrome, and we also found no profile of salient strengths or weaknesses in Battelle domain scores in 20 children. Within the Battelle Communication domain, however, participants showed significantly better developed receptive than expressive language. Using measures of receptive and expressive language, children in the Cornish et al. (1999) sample showed mean receptive scores that were two years in advance of their expressive abilities. Finally, administering the VABS to parents of 100 individuals with 5p- syndrome ages 1–31 years (mean age = 9 years, 6 months), we found that approximately 30% routinely used 50 or more words, and that 21% used sentences of 4 or more words (See Table 7.8). In contrast, virtually all 100 participants demonstrated a receptive understanding of 10 or more words. Across various studies and measures, then, a consistent profile emerges of better developed receptive than expressive language abilities in people with 5p- syndrome.

What is less clear in these language assessments is how signing affects expressive language skills. Carlin (1990) found that although 50% of 80 people with 5p- syndrome had some expressive speech, 75% used some form of sign language, including their own idiosyncratic signs. Among 27 children, Cornish and Pigram (1996) found that 48% used a nonverbal method of some sort to communicate, with only 2 participants (7%) using a formal sign or symbol system. The efficacy of other techniques, such as the use of communication boards, has yet to be formally studied.

Adaptive Behavior

Relative to their communication, daily living, and motor skills, people with 5p- syndrome appear to have strengths in socialization skills. Using the VABS, we found an average standard score of 47 in the Socialization domain, as opposed to mean scores of 40, 33, and 36 in the domains of Communication, Daily Living, and Motor, respectively (Dykens et al., 1999). As summarized in Table 7.10, the vast majority of participants were aware of family members versus others, responsive to praise, and orientated to peers, and they imitated others. Such strengths debunk a persistent myth that people with 5p- syndrome are socially withdrawn, or even have autism.

Findings from other VABS domains also cast a more optimistic prognosis than early depictions of the syndrome. Approximately 70% of individuals in our study walked as their primary means of getting around; similarly, Cornish and Pigram (1996) found that 80% of 27 children were mobile. We found that 80% of our sample showed adequate pincer grasp, and from 40% to 70% actively participated in dressing and/or toileting activities (see Table 7.10).

Table 7.10.   Selected adaptive skills in 100 individuals with 5p- syndrome

Adaptive skill	%
Aware of family members versus others	97
Understands at least 10 words	95
Responsive to praise	95
Imitates actions of others	94
Interested in peers	82
Picks up objects with pincer grasp	80
Dresses self with help	70
Walks as main way to get around	68
Opens doors with knobs	68
Climbs on play equipment	54
Knows hot things are dangerous	45
Asks to use toilet	40
Puts things away when asked	40
States first and last name	37
Alternates feet on stairs	33
States 50 or more words	30

Source: Dykens, Hodapp, Ly, & Rosner, 1999.

On average, people showed slow but steady gains in their adaptive skills over time, with modest increases in VABS age-equivalent scores seen both cross-sectionally and longitudinally (Dykens et al., 2000). Correlating chronological age with VABS standard scores, however, strong negative correlations were found in all domains (from –.65 to –.75). Although further work is needed, these findings suggest some individuals who have 5p- syndrome show a slowing in their rate of adaptive skill acquisition over time. Most people continue to learn new adaptive skills but do so at a slower and slower rate relative to their advancing chronological age.

Although further work is needed, these findings suggest that some individuals who have 5p- syndrome show a slowing in their rate of adaptive skill acquisition over time.

Maladaptive Behavior and Psychopathology

Many of the maladaptive features observed in 5p- syndrome are also seen in people in general with severe levels of mental retardation. Carlin (1990) reported self-stimulatory behaviors in 96% of 62 people, and these repetitive behaviors were seen as well in most of the 80 participants in the Wilkins et al. (1983) sample. Cornish and Pigram (1996) found repetitive movements and self-injurious behavior in 70% of 27 children with 5p- syndrome. Examining 130 people with deletions, Dykens and Clarke (1997) found that increased stereotypies and self-injury were related to lower cognitive-adaptive levels. Though temper tantrums were noted in 67% of this large sample, these problems may not necessarily involve severe outbursts or aggression aimed at others.

High rates of hyperactivity and inattention are often noted clinically (Carlin, 1990; Wilkins et al., 1983), and ADHD symptoms are also found in formal studies using standardized instruments. Administering the Aberrant Behavior Checklist (ABC; Aman, Burrow, & Wolford, 1995) to parents or caregivers of 146 participants, Dykens and Clarke (1997) found that hyperactivity was significantly elevated relative to other problems. Furthermore, hyperactivity was the only scale on the ABC that was significantly elevated in 5p- participants relative to two other comparison groups of participants with mental retardation. Interestingly, a dopamine transporter gene, called *DAT1*, has been strongly implicated among children with ADHD in the general population, and is located on the tip of chromosome 5 (e.g., Gill, Daly, Heron, Hawi, & Fitzgerald, 1997). It is unclear how or if the DAT1 gene might play a role in the elevated levels of ADHD symptoms seen in

Table 7.11. Salient behavioral concerns in people with 5p- syndrome

Behavior	%
Easily distracted, can't concentrate	85–90
Can't sit still	75–59
Demands a lot of attention	73–90
Impulsive	68–71
Temper tantrums	67
Disobedient	64–68
Aggressive, destructive	63–70
Injures self	60
Stereotypies	52

Sources: Dykens & Clarke, 1997; Dykens, Hodapp, Ly, & Rosner, 2000.

people with 5p- syndrome. Specific rates of ADHD symptoms and other behavioral problems are summarized in Table 7.11.

Collectively, the behaviors noted in Table 7.11 are strong predictors of family stress. Examining 99 families of offspring with 5p- syndrome, Hodapp, Wijma, and Masino (1997) found that relative to the child's age or IQ, maladaptive behavior was the best predictor of family stress. Siblings in 44 of these families were also interviewed about their perceptions of family life. Siblings rarely reported feeling ignored by their parents or wishing that their parents would spend more time with them rather than their siblings with 5p- syndrome. Parents, however, rated these issues as significantly more troubling for their unaffected offspring than did the siblings themselves. Future work is needed to clarify if parents' perceptions of how their unaffected children are faring is another source of stress and concern to them.

Research also needs to examine the effect of the unusual cat-cry on parental responses. Frodi and Senchak (1990) found that high-pitched infantile cries were associated with less than optimal responses from adults, including ignoring the cry. These researchers compared adult responses to low-pitched cries (from a typically developing infant and an infant with Down syndrome) versus high-pitched cries (from an infant with 5p- syndrome or an infant with brain injury). Adults were more responsive to low-pitched cries, less apt to report hearing high-pitched cries, and more apt to interpret the cry of the 5p- infant as reflecting illness. It is unknown how the high-pitched cry in 5p- syndrome might affect parent–child interactions over the course of time.

III

NEW DIRECTIONS

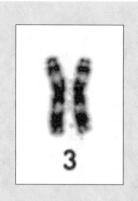

3

8

Next Steps for Research

We take stock of etiology-based research, and highlight certain methodological considerations for future work on behavioral phenotypes.

Etiology-based research is burgeoning in the field of mental retardation. Our sense—which writing this book has confirmed—is that many more etiology-based studies are appearing in a variety of journals, even since our "two cultures" article appeared in 1994 (Hodapp & Dykens, 1994). But it is not always clear how best to conduct etiology-based studies. As one of our final goals of this book, we take stock of etiology-based research, and highlight certain methodological considerations for future work on behavioral phenotypes.

HOW SHOULD ETIOLOGY-BASED RESEARCH BE PERFORMED?

As described in previous chapters, etiology-based studies vary in many ways. Topics range from cognition and language, to adaptive and maladaptive behavior, to parents' perceptions of their child's best educational or adult placements. Infants, children, adolescents, and adults have been examined, with some studies separating participants by age, and others combining two or more of these age groups. Different types of control or contrast groups—or no groups at all—have characterized this research.

To impose some order on what has become a dizzying array of research approaches, we identify in the next section six separate research questions centered on two different themes. One theme involves between-group studies that help characterize a syndromic group as a whole; between-group issues are taken up in Questions 1–3 that follow. The second theme touches on various within-group factors that help explain individual differences within a particular etiological group. Within-group issues are discussed in Questions 4–6.

1. Which group should be designated the control or contrast group(s)?

Ideally, researchers select a control or comparison group that best enables them to answer a question. Often, however, selecting one type of comparison group means answering one question at the expense of another, and researchers often struggle with the fact that no one control group is perfectly suited to answer all of their questions about a given syndrome. Thus, different contrast groups have strengths and weaknesses that need to be taken into account in planning a study. Using several syndromes as examples, in this section we describe the strengths and weaknesses of the most common approaches to control or contrast groups that we encountered in researching this book.

Often, however, selecting one type of comparison group means answering one question at the expense of another, and researchers often struggle with the fact that no one control group is perfectly suited to answer all of their questions about a given syndrome.

No Control Group The no-control-group strategy compares each person's scores on one domain of functioning with his or her own scores on other domains of the same measure. In this approach, which often uses repeated measures ANOVA's or *t*-tests, each person acts as his or her own "control," providing the baseline functioning to which that person's functioning in other areas can be compared.

Many examples exist of this self-as-control strategy. Our early studies examined individuals' domain scores on the Kaufman Assessment Battery for Children (an IQ test, K-ABC; Kaufman & Kaufman,

1983) within a sample of boys with fragile X syndrome (Dykens, Hodapp, & Leckman, 1987) and within children with Prader-Willi syndrome (Dykens, Hodapp, Walsh, & Nash, 1992a). In both cases, weaknesses were found in sequential processing versus simultaneous process and achievement. Another example is Miller's (1992) study showing that children with Down syndrome have better receptive than expressive language. Yet another is Mervis, Morris, Bertrand, and Robinson's (1999) use of the Differential Abilities Scale (DAS; Elliot, 1990) to delineate cognitive-linguistic strengths and weaknesses in children with Williams syndrome.

Many benefits can be derived from this self-as-control strategy. If used with a single, standardized instrument, the researcher can identify cognitive, linguistic, adaptive, or other strengths and weaknesses that characterize a particular group. In addition, new statistical techniques are now being developed that involve "profile analyses" for these single-group studies (Mervis & Robinson, 1999). These analyses go beyond the use of standard repeated-measures statistics; they simultaneously determine the group's degree of strength or weakness as well as the percentage of individuals within the group exhibiting the syndrome's profile. Until now, one could only perform the "group" and "individual" analyses separately.

Strictly speaking, however, the no-control-group approach can only be used when certain conditions are met. The scores of a group (and of the individuals within that group) can only be compared across domains or sub-domains of the same test, which has been normed on the same sample. More obviously, one can only perform this type of analysis on results from standardized, normed instruments, and these are more common in certain areas of psychology (e.g., cognition, language) than in others (e.g., interaction, emotion).

It is also important to acknowledge what the no control group strategy does not reveal. Because no control or contrast groups are used, one cannot be certain of the degree to which people with the disorder are similar to people with other genetic disorders or even to groups with mixed or heterogeneous causes for their mental retardation. The self-as-control strategy tells us only about strengths or weaknesses of a particular etiological group, not how unique or shared such strengths or weaknesses are when compared with other groups.

Control Group(s) of Typical Children The practice of using control groups of typical children is among the most widely used research designs in the disabilities field; however, various methods are used within this type of design, and each has its proponents. Researchers of different philosophical orientations have argued for years about the merits of comparing groups of individuals with mental retardation with individuals of the same chronological age (CA-matched design) versus of the same mental age (MA-matched design). For example, "defect theorists"—those who feel that all mental retardation arises from a single defect—have long argued for CA-matched designs. To these researchers, impaired functioning relative to CA-matched controls is evidence for a specific defect. Developmentalists counter that many areas of functioning are impaired in people with mental retardation; to quote Cicchetti and Pogge-Hesse, "We know that they are retarded; the important and challenging research questions concern the developmental process" (1982, p. 279).

Two recent complications make the use of control groups of typical children—matched either on CA or MA—even more interesting. The first involves "noncognitive" domains, or tasks that do not directly assess cognition per se. For these domains, one might predict that an individual's accumulated life experience—essentially contained within his or her CA—is more important than the person's overall level of intellectual functioning (MA). With advancing age, for example, a person might learn certain adaptive daily living or social skills based on practicing these skills every day over an extended period of time. To determine if people are performing at the level of their MA or CA (or somewhere in between), then, *two* groups of typically developing individuals are necessary, one of the same MA, the other of the same CA.

A second issue concerns the "intactness" question. In recent years, seemingly striking skills have been discovered in a few genetic etiologies. Children with Williams syndrome have been thought to have intact language skills and, possibly, musical abilities; some children with Prader-Willi are thought to have high-level jigsaw puzzle skills. Throughout these discussions, one must distinguish between a skill that is "relatively strong" and one that is "intact." A relative strength occurs in comparison to one's overall MA. If children with Prader-Willi syndrome show relative strengths in jigsaw puzzles, then, as a group, these children show puzzle abilities significantly above their overall mental ages. In contrast, if these children have skills in puzzles that are intact, or truly spared, then they perform at or very near their CA levels.

Throughout these discussions, one must distinguish between a skill that is "relatively strong" and one that is "intact."

For most groups, relative strengths—and not intact skills—are probably seen in most children. Thus, children with Williams syndrome show receptive vocabulary and grammatical skills that are better than expected for their overall MAs, but such skills are not at the same level as they are in others of the child's same CA. In Mervis et al.'s (1999) study, for example, children with Williams syndrome had standard scores averaging 66.50 in receptive vocabulary (Peabody Picture Vocabulary Test–Revised, or PPVT–III; Dunn & Dunn, 1981) and 73.12 in receptive grammar (Test for Reception of Grammar, or TROG; Bishop, D, 1983). Granted, a few individuals with Williams syndrome scored near or even above levels predicted by their CAs (i.e., standard scores around 100), but the group as a whole showed only relative strengths in these domains (see Bellugi, Mills, Jernigan, Hickok, & Galaburda, 1999, and Mervis et al., 1999, for discussions). Though less studied, jigsaw puzzle skills in individuals with Prader-Willi syndrome are in most cases probably relatively strong (versus overall MA) but also somewhat impaired (versus CA). All such debates, however, involve comparisons with both typical children of comparable MAs and of comparable CAs (or, as in the Mervis et al., 1999, study, to age-norms of various tests).

As in the no-control-group design, comparing with typical children cannot tell us the degree to which the behavior of a certain etiological group is found in other groups with mental retardation. Strengths or weaknesses in any one area may be unique to the etiological group under consideration, or shared by a few other etiological groups, or common to most people with mental retardation. Because the comparisons are to typically developing children, we cannot know for certain.

Control Group of People with Mixed, Heterogeneous or Nonspecific Mental Retardation   In contrast to the self-as-control and typically developing control cases, comparisons with groups with mixed etiologies directly test whether a behavioral feature is characteristic of people with mental retardation in general or instead to the specific etiological group under study. Examples include Meyers and Pueschel's (1991) comparison of maladaptive behavior in children and adults with Down syndrome or Dykens and Rosner's (1999) examination of personality characteristics in children with Williams syndrome and Prader-Willi syndrome. In both instances, researchers employed a group with mixed or heterogeneous mental retardation in order to show that etiology-related behaviors were not simply characteristic of mental retardation in general.

Although often considered the appropriate way to perform etiology-based research, using a mixed or heterogeneous control group also presents some vexing problems. The first is practical: How does one find a group of people with "mixed mental retardation"? Most researchers favor approaching different service systems, such as public or private schools or vocational or recreational programs (e.g., summer camp, supported employment) run by large-scale programs such The Arc (formerly The Association for Retarded Citizens), Easter Seals, or state departments of mental retardation. But it is impossible to know just how representative participants of any of these organizations are compared with the entire population of people with mental retardation.

A second issue concerns the changing nature of the mixed group itself. Generally, when studying Down syndrome, one compares the group with Down syndrome with a "mixed but not Down syndrome" group; when examining Prader-Willi syndrome, one compares to a "mixed but not Prader-Willi syndrome" group. The mixed group thus changes depending on the etiology being studied. Using a "literature control group" (published data from other researchers) somewhat avoids this problem, as in Dykens and Clarke's (1997) comparisons of Aberrant Behavior Checklist data from individuals with 5p- syndrome to the normative group used to develop this measure (Aman, Burrow, & Wolford, 1995). But issues then arise as to how similar the etiological and normative, mixed groups were in other ways, such as socioeconomic status (SES), living status (home, group home), or the method of administering the measure.

A third issue concerns the difference between a "mixed or heterogeneous" group and a "nonspecific" group. Although the terms are often used synonymously, in a mixed or heterogeneous group the individuals have many different causes for their mental retardation; in a nonspecific group individuals have no obvious cause for their delay. This last group is similar to the "familial" or "cultural-familial" group described by Zigler (1967, 1969). As such, the familial or cultural-familial group might be more likely to be of lower socioeconomic status and of minority status than the etiologies to which they are being compared (Hodapp, 1994).

Control Group of People with Down Syndrome In addition to research focused on people with Down syndrome themselves, this group has often served as the control or contrast group in studies of other conditions. Some studies have compared people with Down syndrome with those with other genetic etiologies, whereas others have compared them with children or adults with autism or even other psychiatric disorders.

Using a Down syndrome contrast group makes sense in some ways, but not in others. As the most common known chromosomal cause of mental retardation, Down syndrome is diagnosed at birth and has many active parent groups; people with this disorder are therefore relatively easy to recruit. Any possible effects for a genetic disorder would seem to be controlled for. And in contrast to diverse types of participants obtained through social services agencies, one has a fuller understanding of who comprises the control or contrast group.

As we are increasingly appreciating, however, researchers may know less than they think about their Down syndrome control groups. As we have detailed in Chapter 3, Down syndrome itself has a specific behavioral phenotype—ignoring this phenotype may invite over- or under-interpretations of one's findings. To take a recent controversy, the "intactness" of language in Williams syndrome may have been oversold partly because of the way in which most studies contrasted children with Williams syndrome to those with Down syndrome (see Mervis et al., 1999; Mervis & Robinson, 1999). Children with Down syndrome have relative weaknesses in grammar and in other areas of language. As such, language studies of people with Down syndrome versus with Williams syndrome compare one group with a relative weakness (Down syndrome) with another with a relative strength (Williams syndrome) in the domain of interest. Still, people with Down syndrome serve as the control or contrast group in much etiologically oriented research.

As we see it, the problem does not arise in the use of Down syndrome as a contrast group per se, but rather in how one understands one's study. Children with Down syndrome display their own behavioral strengths and weaknesses—the most important etiology-specific behaviors seem to involve heightened sociability, visual processing strengths, language problems, and a relative lack of maladaptive behavior—psychopathology (see Chapter 3). One can even compare children with some other syndrome to those with Down syndrome because of one or more of these characteristics. A possible study, then, might compare friendship qualities in people of similar overall MA levels in which language is a relative weakness (Down syndrome) versus a relative strength (Williams syndrome). Or, another study might compare the school placement of people with a syndrome featuring low levels of maladaptive behaviors (Down syndrome) versus one with high levels of maladaptive behavior (Prader-Willi syndrome). The important point to acknowledge is that individuals with Down syndrome differ from "most people with mental retardation" on certain aspects of behavior; one then needs a mixed or heterogeneous group to distinguish such behavior from people with mental retardation in general.

Control Group of Etiology that Is the "Same but Different" Another strategy that is currently underutilized is to compare two or more etiological groups on a domain in which the two groups are superficially similar. Historically, for example, geneticists often remarked on the "friendly and pleasant" demeanors of people with many different syndromes; formal studies have since confirmed some of these early observations in, for example, Williams syndrome and Down syndrome. Other syndromes feature preliminary behavioral studies, often based on a global rating scale, pointing to syndrome-specific problems with "anxiety," "aggression," or "inattention." Although often reasonably accurate, such general descriptors are also often similar across two or more syndromes, such as inattention in fragile X or 5p- syndromes.

This "similar but different" approach works best when the two or more etiologies are similar in terms of behavior, not genetics.

Given this state of affairs, researchers can more clearly delineate behavioral characteristics of one versus another genetic mental retardation etiology by comparing two or more groups that would seem, at first glance, to be identical. In one study, Dykens and Rosner (1999b) examined the ways in which adolescents and adults with Prader-Willi syndrome and those with Williams syndrome showed their anxiety. In both syndromes, previous work had noted increased levels of anxiety, relative to others with delay. In this case, however, children with Williams syndrome demonstrated increased levels of fears and phobias; those with Prader-Willi syndrome showed increased obsessions and compulsions. This type of study alone cannot determine the degree to which fears/phobias or obsessions/compulsions are characteristic of most people with mental retardation. But this approach can help researchers attain more fine-grained understandings of "similar but different" behaviors across two or more syndromes. This "similar but different" approach works best when the two or more etiologies are similar in terms of behavior, not genetics. In recent years, an occasional published paper compares two or more disorders that fall within the same genetic class. Thus, several studies have compared groups in which all people have different deletion syndromes. To us, this strategy makes little sense behaviorally. As shown by the syndromes examined in this book, few commonalities exist among the behaviors of different disorders, even those of the same genetic class. For example, Williams syndrome, 5p- syndrome, and (most cases of) Prader-Willi syndrome all involve deletions on various chromosomes; each also varies greatly in characteristic behaviors.

Specialized Control Group without Mental Retardation A final research strategy uses groups chosen because of their similarity in behavior to a group with a genetic etiology of mental retardation, but who themselves do not have retardation. As in the design comparing two or more "same but different" genetic etiologies, the goal is to better characterize etiology-specific behavior.

Although this approach has been used only rarely, Dykens, Leckman, and Cassidy (1996) presented one good example by comparing children and adults with Prader-Willi syndrome to people without mental retardation, but who do have obsessive-compulsive disorder (OCD). This study showed that the two groups were fairly similar in both the nature and severity of their obsessions and compulsions. It also revealed a few interesting differences. For example, the OCD group without mental retardation showed higher rates of religious obsessions and of checking compulsions; the Prader-Willi group showed higher rates of hoarding and needing to ask or tell. But overall, by comparing individuals with Prader-Willi syndrome with a group with OCD only, this study demonstrated that obsessions and compulsions may indeed reach clinically significant levels in many people with Prader-Willi syndrome.

Although rarely utilized by most researchers, other examples could also be considered. How, for example, do the fears and anxieties of children with Williams syndrome differ from the fears and anxieties of typically developing children with phobias, panic disorder, or other anxiety disorders? How does food ideation in Prader-Willi syndrome differ from the food ideation of people with eating disorders such as bulimia nervosa or anorexia nervosa? In what ways do children with fragile X syndrome or Prader-Willi syndrome differ from other "simultaneous learners" (Kaufman, Kaufman, & Goldsmith, 1984)? How are the hyperverbal behaviors of people with Williams syndrome the same or different from hyperverbal behaviors of children with spina bifida and hydrocephaly (c.f. Hodapp, 1998)? Using this type of control group gets us closer to understanding the exact manifestations of different strengths, weaknesses, or maladaptive behaviors.

Although intriguing, using a specialized control group of participants without mental retardation also presents some problems. Specifically, such studies generally involve "no difference" findings. By trying to show how a particular syndrome leads to a particular psychiatric condition or learning style, one designs a study in which the group with the syndrome is not predicted to differ from the specialized group of participants who do not have mental retardation. Although not fatal, this limitation should cause researchers to think closely about the goals of their studies.

How, then, should one perform etiology-based behavioral research? As the previous discussion shows, every approach has its strengths and weaknesses. Each also relates to what, exactly, the study is designed to determine. Table 8.1 summarizes the different strengths and weaknesses of each of these research approaches.

Table 8.1. Strengths and weaknesses of common etiology-based research approaches

Control group	Characteristics	Strengths	Weaknesses
None	Performance "against self"	Shows etiology strength	Unclear if profile is unique, partially shared on different domains of a test or weakness, or similar to all persons with MR
Typical	Equated on mental age (MA)	Shows relative strength	Unclear if strength (or intactness) is unique, partially shared, or similar to all persons with MR
	Equated on chronological age (CA)	Shows intact functioning	
Mixed mental retardation (MR)	Mixed causes of MR	Shows that etiological strength weakness is not due to MR	Participants hard to find; control group changes acrossstudies; mixed does not equal non-specific
Down syndrome (DS)	DS	Shows behavior not due to genetic MR; easy to find	DS has its own behavioral characteristics; may lead to inaccurate conclusions
Same but different MR	Etiology similar in behavior to group of interest	Highlights fine-grained differences in behavior to make contrast meaningful	Two or more etiologies must have similar behaviors
Special non-MR	Group w/ special behavioral characteristic(s)	Shows ways that etiology is same or different	A "no-difference" design, but useful in identifying behavioral similarities or differences from genetic to non-MR group

Adapted from Hodapp & Dykens, 2000.

2. What can examining behavior in different etiological groups tell us about typical development?

Throughout the 20th century, developmentally oriented researchers have realized that children with any disability can tell us much about typical development. Vygotsky (1927/1993), for example, considered deaf (nonsigning) children as a good way to understand the thought–language connection; Piaget and Inhelder (1947) showed that even children with mental retardation proceeded in order through Piagetian stages (albeit with more regressions and oscillations); and Werner and Strauss (1939) used findings from children with (mild) mental retardation to help formulate the distinction between performance and competence (see Hodapp, 1998, for reviews). Within the modern-day field of developmental psychopathology, it has become an article of faith that "We can learn more about the typical functioning of an organism by studying its pathology, more about its pathology by studying its normal condition" (Cicchetti, 1984, p. 1).

Until recent years, however, this interplay among typical and atypical development has remained more a mantra than a practical, day-to-day research strategy. Yet, this state of affairs may be changing. We detail in the next sections some issues about which recent etiology-based findings are shedding light on typical development.

Cross-Domain Relations As best shown in Chapter 4, Williams syndrome is at the heart of many discussions of the "modularity" of language. Briefly, the linguist Jerry Fodor (1983) proposed that language is a "modular" system, operating separately from other, nonlinguistic aspects of cognition. In contrast to Piaget (1954), then, who espoused a pattern of cognitive-linguistic development in which many separate areas were closely intertwined, Fodor considers language a separate system.

Since the studies of Bellugi and her colleagues in the late 1980s (e.g., Bellugi, Marks, Bihrle, & Sabo, 1988), Williams syndrome has appeared to be a good case of the separation among language and nonlinguistic cognitive skills. Indeed, Bellugi et al. have shown that some children display high levels of language relative to their overall mental ages. More recently, Mervis et al. (1999) have shown strong correlations among certain aspects of language—particularly grammatical abilities—and short-term memory skills.

Given the debates among these researchers, it remains an open question as to just how separable language and cognition are in Williams syndrome. These children do, however, provide several developmental lessons. First, children with Williams syndrome demonstrate relative strengths and weaknesses across various domains of cognition and language. Just as children with Down syndrome show visual strengths and those with fragile X syndrome and Prader-Willi syndrome show simultaneous strengths (and sequential weaknesses), cognition may not be as "all of a single piece" as originally thought by Piaget.

Data on Williams syndrome also illustrate what different etiological groups can tell us about typical development (Hodapp & Burack, 1990). These groups can tell us whether something can occur. Is it possible for one's levels of language to be 5 or 7 or more years ahead of one's levels of visual-spatial skills? An additional usage involves replication. Mervis et al. (1999) noted that the strong correlations among short-term memory and linguistic grammar are similar to connections found in both typical adults (Kemper, Kynette, Rash, & O'Brien, 1989) and in children with Down syndrome (Chapman, 1995; Rondal, 1995). Especially when shown in several different groups, such findings would seem to indicate the necessity of cross-domain connections in human development.

Critical Age Hypotheses   Across a variety of disability conditions and exceptional individuals, a "critical" or at least a "sensitive" period seems likely for certain aspects of language. Thus, Genie—a girl who was so severely neglected from birth through early puberty that her intelligence was virtually untestable—was never able to develop in grammar (Curtiss, 1977). Similarly, late learners of American Sign Language (ASL) rarely become as grammatically proficient as earlier learners (Newport, 1990). Although the "critical age" for language learning may not be as immutable as Lenneberg (1967) thought—and may relate more to grammar than to other aspects of language—some lessening in one's abilities to acquire high levels of grammar generally occurs in most groups after the pubertal years.

As noted previously, however, Chapman, Seung, Schwartz, & Kay-Raining Bird (1998) findings on adolescents and young adults with Down syndrome may be an exception to this general finding. From Chapman's cross-sectional studies, adolescents and young adults with Down syndrome do seem to continue developing in linguistic grammar. If this finding holds, one must ask why Down syndrome, a disorder noted for its relative weakness in linguistic grammar (Fowler, 1990), is somehow spared from the sensitive period.

Brain–Behavior Connections   In making "gene–brain–behavior" connections, one assumes that certain brain changes are associated with certain behavioral strengths, weaknesses, developments, or other characteristics. Although connections among brain changes and etiology-specific behaviors are just beginning to be discovered, this area promises to reveal interesting findings over the next few decades.

Part of the difficulty in these studies relates to the meaning of *brain changes*. Which aspects of the brain are most responsible for which behavior(s)? In each instance, should one be looking for changes in the brain's structure, its size, its connections from one part to another, its neurochemistry, or something else?

Even so, findings from different genetic etiologies are telling us much about which aspects of brain structure or function relate to which particular behaviors. In Williams syndrome, many individuals have difficulties with visual-motor action and construction—this particular skill seems associated with parietal lobe (i.e. dorsal stream) functioning. In Down syndrome, certain brain changes may relate to certain behavioral strengths and weaknesses. Witness the temporal lobe anomalies related to these children's difficulties in short-term memory (and grammar), and the coordination problems involved in expressive language and verbal fluency that may relate to the decreased width of certain parts of the corpus callosum (Wang, 1996). Although such findings are currently suggestive, future research will inevitably discover particular brain changes underlying most etiology-specific behaviors.

Compensation   Both physically and psychologically, human beings are dynamic and constantly changing. Although many such changes occur from birth through adolescence, the adult years involve changes related to aging. Throughout life, one can conceptualize change as occurring in response to any mismatch among the person and the demands placed on that person.

This mismatch among the person and environmental demands often brings forth compensatory mechanisms (Dixon & Baeckman, 1994). As adults age, for example, we get slower in our physical-motor reactions. Yet in studies of skilled typists, Salthouse (1984) found that older skilled typists were equally as proficient as younger typists. Even though they were slower in their physical keystrokes, these older typists had adopted a strategy of looking further ahead in the to-be-typed material, thereby preparing themselves earlier to type each letter. As a result, even though older typists became slower on the component motor behaviors used in typing, they effectively employed strategies that enabled them to maintain their earlier typing rates.

Similarly, people with specific syndromes might react to their own weaknesses by compensating for or accommodating them (although the technical meanings of the two terms differ slightly, here we use them interchangeably). In response to their difficulties in performing difficult tasks, for example, children with Down syndrome try to "charm their way" out of performing these tasks (Pitcairn & Wishart, 1994). As individuals who have Williams syndrome draw, they often engage in verbal me di ation, perhaps telling a story about the

Similarly, people with specific syndromes might react to their own weaknesses by compensating for or accommodating them.

drawing, or using verbal prompts that guide them through an otherwise arduous task. Although as yet unstudied, similar accommodations might be found in other syndromes as well.

Unlike aging typists, however, such accommodations may not always be totally successful for children with mental retardation. Children with Down syndrome, for example, demonstrate levels of early social skills that exceed those shown by MA-matched typically developing children. Compared with typical controls, these children show more frequent (but shorter) glances at others during interactions, as opposed to glances toward objects or to ongoing events (Kasari et al., 1990; 1995). But as preschoolers with the syndrome get older they perform increasingly below typical MA-matched children on social tasks such as labeling the emotions of others. Moreover, examined longitudinally, preschoolers with Down syndrome show little development in their ability to label emotions (Kasari, et al., 2000). Children with Down syndrome may thus try to use their social strengths to circumvent their cognitive-linguistic weaknesses, but such attempts may be less successful at later ages. As children age, it seems, even predominantly social tasks (e.g., understanding and labeling the emotions of others) increasingly involve skills in cognition and language.

3. What about indirect effects?

Given the preponderance of research on families, mother–child interactions and friends using mixed etiological groups, little work currently exists on the indirect effects of different genetic mental retardation disorders. With few exceptions, then, indirect effects constitute the unexamined part of the etiology story.

Even given such limitations, several important research issues have arisen. A first concerns the difference between CA- and MA-matching. As a general rule, most family studies compare families of children with one or another genetic mental retardation syndrome to typically developing CA-matched children, or to children with mixed or different etiologies who are both MA- and CA-matched. The family of a 10-year-old child with mental retardation (of whatever type) is considered most comparable to a family of a typically developing 10-year-old, not to a family of a child who is at the same MA (e.g., of a typically developing 5-year-old). In mother–child studies, however, the opposite seems the case. In this area, most studies compare behaviors of mothers of, for example, 4-year-old children with Down syndrome with mothers of 2-year-old (MA-matched) children without mental retardation.

As in the CA- versus MA-matching discussion above, the issue concerns which variables are most important. Is one's accumulated life experience most important, as in most family issues? If so, then CA-comparisons seem appropriate. Conversely, is the most important variable others' responses to the child's level of functioning? In this case, MA-matching seems appropriate. Yet, such easy distinctions may not always be foolproof. Examples of troublesome cases include "delayed launching" (Seltzer & Ryff, 1994), when the young adult with mental retardation does not leave home such as most typical young adults, or the effects of the child's slowing rates of development on mothers of older children with either Down syndrome or fragile X syndrome. In such cases, both CA and MA matches might be necessary.

A second troublesome issue concerns disentangling different genetic disorders' indirect versus "associated" effects. Simply stated, do others react differently to individuals of one versus another genetic syndrome because the people themselves differ, or are differential reactions instead due to circumstances merely associated with the syndrome? Consider Down syndrome. As noted in Chapter 3, parents, families, and siblings cope well—often better than parents, families, and siblings of children with different etiologies. We have assumed that such differences reflect others' reactions to behavioral characteristics of children with Down syndrome. At the same time, however, Down syndrome is widely known to the public at large; parents of these children are often older, of higher SES, and more experienced as parents, and the syndrome features several active parent groups that provide both information and support (Cahill & Glidden, 1996). Are, then, lower levels of parent and family stress due to the indirect effects of the child's behaviors, or to the associated effects of having a child with Down syndrome?

A third issue concerns direction of effects. The very term "indirect" or "child" effects assumes that children affect parents, in ways described by Bell (1968) and other interactional researchers (see Hodapp, 1999, for a review). But a connection among, for example, parental stress and child maladaptive behaviors is just that—a connection. It remains possible that parental stress in some sense "fosters" child maladaptive behaviors. Even more likely is a system in which a continuing cycle occurs. Child maladaptive behaviors might increase parental stress, which further elicits more child maladaptive behavior, that in turn leads to even greater levels of parental stress (as in conduct disorders; Lytton, 1990). Currently, sophisticated path analyses are typically lacking in studies of indirect effects of different genetic mental retardation syndromes.

A final issue involves the acknowledgment that, although rarely stated explicitly, the model for most indirect-effects research involves typical development. The best example here might be sibling reactions.

As described by Stoneman (1998), studies of typically developing siblings show that inter-sibling problems are most likely to arise when one sibling displays a difficult temperament, lower levels of competence, secondary disabilities, and chronic health problems (necessitating repeated hospitalizations). Because each characteristic is more often found in certain etiologies than others, one would expect sibling reactions to differ across etiologies. The typical developmental model—in this case, the usual reactions of one typically developing sibling to another—underlies much thinking about how indirect effects might operate.

4.   What about individual differences within a group?

Many researchers erroneously assume that people with a specific genetic syndrome are all alike. But, as noted in Chapter 1, behavioral phenotypes generally do not involve certainties that a specific behavioral characteristic will occur. Indeed, few (possibly no) syndromes show a particular behavior in every affected person, and the strength of a given behavior may also vary considerably. Weaknesses in linguistic grammar are found in most people with Down syndrome, for example, but an occasional person with trisomy 21 shows relatively intact language skills (e.g., Françoise, a 32-year-old woman with Down syndrome described by Rondal, 1995). Similarly, in most other genetic syndromes, an "etiology-specific" behavioral characteristic is usually—but not always—noted.

But why does a particular behavior or profile show itself in some individuals, but not in others? Although preliminary, studies are now addressing behavioral differences associated with genetic factors. Recent advances in fragile X syndrome, for example, show how certain aspects of the cognitive and behavioral phenotype are directly associated with the amount of fragile X protein produced (see Chapter 5). In other examples, people with Prader-Willi syndrome due to paternal deletion have slightly lower IQ scores (possibly only verbal IQ scores) than those with the maternal UPD; similarly, individuals with the deletion show higher levels of withdrawal, overeating, hoarding, sulking and skin-picking (see Chapter 6). Similarly, people with Angelman syndrome due to paternal UPD have better growth parameters, fewer seizure disorders, and better communication skills than their counterparts with maternal deletions (see Chapter 7). Gene–behavior relationships are also being actively studied in 5p- syndrome, Williams syndrome, and other mental retardation disorders.

In addition to genetic factors, within-group behavioral differences may also be associated with environmental and psychosocial variables. There may, for instance, be "treatment by person interactions," such that different people respond differently to different environments. In one study, Hauser-Cram et al. (1999) showed a strong predictive relation among several family characteristics and the social and intellectual development of young children with Down syndrome. Using growth-curve analyses, more cohesive families produced children who showed faster rates of development in social skills (23% of variance), communication (14.3%), and daily living skills (6.3%). As the authors note, cohesive families who better stimulate their children "have children who, over time, demonstrate significant benefits in communicating and socializing with others and in their ability to engage in independent self-care tasks" (p. 985).

But such treatment by people interactions might also occur in more specific skills. To what extent, for example, is a child with Prader-Willi syndrome's jigsaw puzzle skills related to that child's opportunity to do puzzles, or early (versus later) exposure to puzzles, or even to parental interest and encouragement in puzzles? To what extent are children with Down syndrome's reading skills related to whether, when, and how long they have been instructed in reading? In turn, to what extent do children with Down syndrome's abilities in reading relate to abilities in short- and long-term memory, vocabulary, and other abilities (Buckley, 1999; Laws, Buckley, Bird, MacDonald, & Broadley, 1995)? All are issues only beginning to be examined.

In a similar way, we are only beginning to examine the operations of within-group variance in studies of indirect effects. In one study, naïve observers overgeneralized immature personality traits and behaviors to more versus less "baby-faced" children even within the Down syndrome group (Fidler & Hodapp, 1999). So, too, might other child characteristics vary within any particular etiological group, thereby eliciting different amounts (or types) of reactions from others.

5. What about development?

Another "within-group" characteristic concerns development. Simply stated, behavioral phenotypes change over time. Indeed, it is probably the case that few behavioral phenotypes appear at birth. In this sense, the view that behavioral phenotypes are probabalistic, not determinative (Dykens, 1995c), is probably true of individuals as well. Thus, individuals are born with a propensity or predisposition to develop in a certain way, but the "full-blown" behavioral etiology will show itself more at certain ages than others.

Many examples exist of the developmental nature of behavioral phenotypes. In obvious examples, hyperphagia and food preoccupations in Prader-Willi syndrome generally appear after 2 years of age.

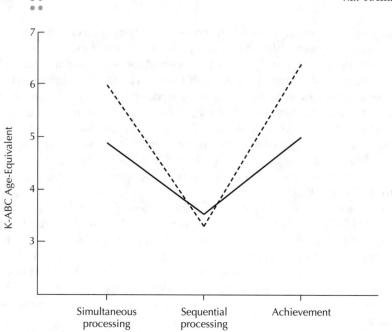

Figure 8.1. Average levels of simultaneous processing, sequential processing, and achievement for younger versus older males with fragile X syndrome. (Key: ——— < 11 years old, - - - - - > 11 years old.) (From Hodapp, Dykens, Ort, Zelinsky, & Leckman (1991). Changing patterns of intellectual strengths and weaknesses in males with fragile X syndrome. *Journal of Autism and Developmental Disorders, 21,* 508. New York: Kluwer Academic/Plenum Publishers; reprinted by permission.)

The linguistic weaknesses in Down syndrome and linguistic strengths in Williams syndrome only appear with the onset of language.

But in a more specific way, strengths and weaknesses also change in their salience as children get older. Boys with fragile X syndrome, for example, show relative weaknesses in sequential versus simultaneous processing and achievement. If one places these children's age-equivalent levels of sequential processing in the middle—among simultaneous processing and achievement—one gets a "V-like" line. But as these children get older, skills in both simultaneous processing and achievement show greater advances than do sequential processing skills. As a result, the original "V" becomes more "V-like" (Hodapp et al., 1991). As Figure 8.1 illustrates, the weakness in sequential processing is much more pronounced in males who are 11 years old or older; moreover, it appears that these sequential processing skills have not advanced from the pre-11-year to the post-11-year-period.

Such findings of slower developments in relatively weak domains have also recently been found in children with Williams syndrome. Bellugi et al. (1999) found that, cross-sectionally over the childhood years, receptive vocabulary skills (on the PPVT-R) and face-recognition skills show strong increases with advancing age. In contrast, these children's (nonfacial) spatial processing (the VMI) advanced only slightly across the childhood years. As in boys with fragile X syndrome, a weak area develops at a slower rate than originally stronger areas, producing greater and greater discrepancies from one domain to another. Many behavioral phenotypes, then, seem to evolve over time, with individuals growing into increasingly salient patterns of strength or weaknesses over the course of development.

6. What about intervention?

A final within-syndrome consideration relates to intervention research. Although such research is still in its infancy, a host of interesting questions are emerging.

What principles characterize etiology-based interventions? In evaluating whether etiology-based interventions "work," a description first seems necessary of some principles of such interventions. A preliminary, somewhat obvious, principle involves playing to the child's etiology-based strengths. This suggestion makes sense both intuitively and when examining the existing research. Intuitively, children who show relative strengths in a particular area should be able to utilize these skills to learn, to perform day-to-day behaviors, or to circumvent weaknesses (or to deal with maladaptive behaviors). Research, too, suggests that playing to strengths is important. If, for example, over time boys with fragile X syndrome develop quickly in their relatively strong area of simultaneous processing but slowly in their weak area of sequential processing, then it would seem beneficial to provide interventions aimed at helping them learn through the use of simultaneous skills. Similarly, if linguistic—but not visual–spatial—skills advance relatively quickly in Williams syndrome, then it would seemingly be beneficial to focus on linguistic skills.

Moreover, relative strengths might also be employed when intervening in otherwise weak areas. A recent example involves the use of visually based approaches to foster language development in Down syndrome. Although few good studies exist, it may be helpful to teach early language skills through sign language (or "total communication," the simultaneous use of both spoken and signed input; Freeman & Hodapp, 1999). Similarly, instruction in reading may be particularly helpful for children with Down syndrome (Buckley, 1999; Hodapp & Ly, in press). Moreover, Laws et al. (1995) even argue that the benefits of learning to read may spill over into other areas of language and cognition for these children. By intervening in a visual way, then, children with Down syndrome may become able to use one of their areas of strength to overcome other, relatively weak areas of behavior.

Other intervention principles also emerge from etiology-based behavioral research. For example, apropos of our discussion of "total versus partial specificity" in Chapter 1, two or more syndromes often show similar cognitive profiles or maladaptive behaviors. As a result, similar interventions would seem necessary. Thus, the hyperactivity often found in boys with fragile X syndrome and in children with 5p-syndrome might therefore both be treated with a combination of pharmocotherapy and behavioral interventions. Similarly, if two or more syndromes show a particular learning style—the "simultaneous learners" among children with Prader-Willi and fragile X syndromes—then both might receive similar educational interventions (Hodapp & Fidler, 1999).

How do etiology-based interventions change or influence phenotypes themselves? Assuming that etiology-based interventions are effective in helping individuals with different syndromes, how should one think about a phenotype? Here we differentiate symptoms (or profiles) from underlying predispositions. It is our intuitive sense that, for the most part, etiology-based interventions will most influence the manifestations of a person's behavior, not that behavior's underlying predisposition.

To take a few examples, it now seems likely that psychotropic medications may ultimately be used to target obsessive-compulsive symptoms in Prader-Willi syndrome, hyperactivity and inattention in fragile X syndrome, 5p- syndrome, and Williams syndrome, and salient sleep disturbance in Smith-Magenis syndrome. Similarly, in terms of educational approaches, promising interventions include phonetics in Williams syndrome (using these children's strengths in auditory short-term memory), or signing and reading in Down syndrome (using strengths in visual–motor short-term memory).

But have any of these interventions changed the underlying problems—or predispositions to such problems—in any of these groups? Our sense is no, that medications, therapies, or educational interventions generally address the symptoms, not the underlying causes, of etiology-based problems or learning styles. As a result, it may be necessary to adhere to such etiology-based interventions for long periods. Although symptoms or manifestations of etiology-based behavioral characteristics may be changed somewhat, underlying propensities are probably less easily affected.

How do interventions in people with mental retardation syndromes compare with interventions for people without mental retardation, but with similar problems?

Our sense is generally that similar problems require similar solutions. Thus, whether or not a person has Prader-Willi syndrome, symptoms of obsessive-compulsive disorder should be treated through similar drugs or therapies. Granted, people with mental retardation will not be as strong in cognitive or linguistic abilities as typically developing people, and interventions will need to be adapted as a result. In most other ways, however, one would hypothesize that identical interventions should help similar problems.

This principle should also work for different learning styles. Such as some typically developing children, children with fragile X syndrome or with Prader-Willi syndrome both show relative weaknesses in sequential processing and relative strengths in simultaneous processing. For both groups, then, appropriate educational strategies might be identical to those provided for "simultaneous learners" in general (Finucane, 1995, 1996; Hodapp & Fidler, 1999). Similar to recommendations for sequential or simultaneous learners without mental retardation (Kaufman et al., 1984), teachers could maximize the simultaneous processing strengths in children with Prader-Willi syndrome and fragile X syndrome by relying on visual-perceptual cues, including pictures or models. Reading might be taught by matching words to familiar objects in the child's surroundings (e.g., sight word reading such as pairing the word *stop* with the hexagonal stop sign) (Braden, 1989). By relying on their existing styles of learning, these children can presumably avoid being frustrated by tasks that involve high levels of sequential processing and short-term memory.

As the discerning reader has noted, virtually every discussion of etiology-based interventions has been stated tentatively. We simply do not know if the many etiology-based interventions described throughout this book are any more effective than more generic approaches. Although recommendations for intervention stem from well-established research findings, they have yet to be put to the test: Are particular drugs, therapies, educational strategies or even work or residential settings more suited to one versus another etiological group? Examining intervention outcomes with specific etiological groups is a field waiting to happen.

> *Our sense is generally that similar problems require similar solutions. Thus, whether or not a person has Prader-Willi syndrome, symptoms of obsessive-compulsive disorder should be treated through similar drugs or therapies.*

CONCLUSION

Reviewing the work discussed in this book, a mixed picture emerges on the state of the art in syndrome-specific behavioral studies. On one hand, etiology-based information has exploded in several different disorders. Although the amount of behavioral work in Down syndrome has probably increased somewhat in recent years, increases in other syndromes have been dramatic. From a handful of studies conducted during the 1980s, an impressive number of behavioral studies now exist in Williams syndrome, fragile X syndrome, and Prader-Willi syndrome. Growing numbers of behavioral studies are now occurring as well in several of those syndromes described in Chapter 7. Further, as described throughout the book, exciting advances are now being made in each of these and other syndromes that connect genes, brain, and behavior.

At the same time that these advances have occurred, we know little about many different genetic etiologies or about certain aspects of behavior. As Chapter 7 illustrates, less is known about these particular disorders, and even less about the remaining 750-plus syndromes associated with mental retardation. Indeed, it is probably the case that not one single behavioral article—or even, in most cases, an article with a substantial section on behavior—exists for most of these disorders. Similarly, the scope of our knowledge is also fairly narrow. For many disorders, behavioral information is limited to IQ scores and the researcher's informal, general impressions of personality or maladaptive behavior. For almost every disorder, we know little about families; peers; parent–child interactions; schools; work; early intervention; or the best therapeutic, educational, or other treatments.

On our journey to understand behavior in genetic disorders, then, we have a long way to go. One could almost argue that those examining various aspects of behavior are only now playing "catch up" compared with the quickly developing genetic and biomedical researchers. Our hope is that this book is seen as a foundation for the subsequent discoveries of other researchers in only a few years' time. If so, we will continue to learn a great deal about behavior in all genetic mental retardation syndromes, to the ongoing benefit of all.

References

Abbeduto, L., & Hagerman, R.J. (1997). Language and communication in fragile X syndrome. *Mental Retardation and Developmental Disabilities Research Reviews, 3,* 313–322.

Abrahamsen, A., Cavallo, M., & McCluer, J.A. (1985). Is the sign advantage a robust phenomenon?: From gesture to language in two modalities. *Merrill-Palmer Quarterly, 31,* 177–209.

Abrahamsen, A., Lamb, M., Brown-Williams, J., & McCarthy, S. (1991). Boundary conditions on language emergence: Contributions from atypical learners and input. In P. Siple & S.D. Fischer (Eds.), *Theoretical issues in sign language research* (Vol. 2, pp. 231–254). Chicago: University of Chicago Press.

Abrams, M.T., & Reiss, A.L. (1995). The neurobiology of fragile X syndrome. *Mental Retardation and Developmental Disability Research Reviews, 1,* 269–275.

Abrams, M.T., Reiss, A.L., Freund, L.S., Baumgardner, T.L., Chase, G.A., & Denckla, M.B. (1994). Molecular-neurobehavioral associations in females with the fragile X full mutation. *American Journal of Medical Genetics, 51,* 317–327.

Achenbach, T.M. (1991). *Manual for the Child Behavior Checklist/4-18 and 1991 profile.* Burlington: University of Vermont, Department of Psychiatry.

Akefeldt, A., Akefeldt, B., & Gillberg, C. (1997). Voice, speech and language characteristics of children with Prader-Willi syndrome. *Journal of Intellectual Disability Research, 41,* 302–311.

Albrecht, U., Sutcliffe, J.S., Cattanach, B.M., Beechey, C.V., Armstrong, D., Eichele, G., & Beaudet, A.L. (1997). Imprinted expression of the murine Angelman syndrome gene, ube3a, in hippocampal and Purkinje neurons. *Nature Genetics, 17,* 75–78.

Allanson, J.E. (1990). Rubinstein-Taybi syndrome: The changing face. *American Journal of Medical Genetics* (Suppl. 6), *6,* 38–41.

Allanson, J.E., O'Hara, P., Farkas, G., & Nair, R.C. (1993). Anthropometric craniofacial pattern profiles in Down syndrome. *American Journal of Medical Genetics, 47,* 748–52.

Aman, M.G., Burrow, W.H., & Wolford, P.L. (1995). The Aberrant Behavior Checklist-Community: Factor validity and effect of subject variables for adults in group homes. *American Journal on Mental Retardation, 100,* 283–292.

American Academy of Pediatrics (1994). Health supervision for children with Down syndrome. *Pediatrics, 93,* 855–859.

American Association on Mental Retardation (1992). *Mental retardation: Definition, classification, and systems of supports.* Washington, DC: Author.

American Psychiatric Association. (1994). *Diagnostic and statistical manual of mental disorders* (4th ed.). Washington, DC: Author.

American Society of Human Genetics/American College of Medical Genetics Report (1996). Diagnostic testing for Prader-Willi and Angelman syndromes: Report of the ASHG/ACMG Test and Technology Transfer committee. *American Journal of Human Genetics, 58,* 1085.

Angelman, H. (1965). "Puppet" children: A report of three cases. *Developmental Medicine and Child Neurology, 7,* 681–688.

Atkinson, J., King, J., Braddick, O., Nokes, L., Anker, S., & Braddick, F. (1997). A specific deficit of dorsal function in Williams syndrome. *Cognitive Neuroscience and Neuropsychology, 8,* 1919–1922.

Bailey, A., Bolton, P., Butler, L., Le Couteur, A., Murphy, M., Scott, S., Webb, T., & Rutter, M. (1993). Prevalence of the fragile X anomaly amongst autistic twins and singletons. *Journal of Child Psychology and Psychiatry and Allied Disciplines, 34,* 673–688.

Bailey, D.B., Hatton, D.D., & Skinner, M. (1998). Early developmental trajectories of males with fragile X syndrome. *American Journal on Mental Retardation, 103,* 29–39.

Bailey, D.B., Jr., Mesibov, G.B., Hatton, D.D., Clark, R.D., Roberts, J.E., & Mayhew, L. (1998). Autistic behavior in young boys with fragile X syndrome. *Journal of Autism and Developmental Disorders, 28,* 499–508.

Baird, P.A., & Sadovnick, A.D. (1987). Life expectancy in Down syndrome. *Journal of Pediatrics, 110,* 849–854.

Baker, H.J., & Leland, B. (1967). *Detroit Tests of Learning Aptitude.* Indianapolis, IN: Bobbs-Merrill.

Baron-Cohen, S. (1995). *Mindblindness: An essay on autism and theory of mind.* Cambridge: MIT Press.

Bassett, A.S., Hodgkinson, K., Chow, E.W., Correia, S., Scutt, L.E., & Weksberg, R. (1998). 22q11 deletion syndrome in adults with schizophrenia. *American Journal of Medical Genetics, 81,* 328–337.

Battaglia, A., Gurrieri, F., Bertine, E., Bellacosa, A., Pomponi, M.G., Paravatou-Petsotas, M., Mazza, S., & Neri, G. (1997). The inv dup(15) syndrome: A clinically recognizable syndrome with altered behavior, mental retardation, and epilepsy. *Neurology, 48,* 1081–1086.

Baumgardner, T.L., Reiss, A.L., Freund, L.S., & Abrams, M.T. (1995). Specification of the neurobehavioral phenotype in males with fragile X syndrome. *Pediatrics, 95,* 744–752.

Bawden, H.N., MacDonald, G.W., & Shea, S. (1997). Treatment of children with Williams syndrome with methylphenidate. *Journal of Child Neurology, 12,* 248–252.

Beardsmore, A., Dorman, T., Cooper, S.A., & Webb, T. (1998). Affective psychosis and Prader-Willi syndrome. *Journal of Intellectual Disability Research, 42,* 463–471.

Beery, K.E. (1989). *Developmental Test of Visual-Motor Integration* (3rd rev.). Cleveland, OH: Modern Curriculum Press.

Bell, R.Q. (1968). A reinterpretation of direction of effects in studies of socialization. *Psychological Review, 75,* 81–95.

Bell, R.Q. & Harper, L.V. (1977). *Child effects on adults.* Mahwah, NJ: Lawrence Erlbaum Associates.

Bellugi, U., Bihrle, A., Jernigan, T., Trauner, D., & Doherty, S. (1990). Neuropsychological, neurological, and neuroanatomical profile of Williams syndrome. *American Journal of Medical Genetics* (Suppl. 6), *6*, 115–125.

Bellugi, U., Lichtenberger, L., Mills, D., Galaburda, A., & Korenberg, J.R. (1999). Bridging cognition, the brain and molecular genetics: Evidence from Williams syndrome. *Trends in Neuroscience, 22,* 197–207.

Bellugi, U., Marks, S., Bihrle, A., & Sabo, H. (1988). Disassociation between language and cognitive functions in Williams syndrome. In D. Bishop & K. Mogford (Eds.), *Language development in exceptional circumstances* (pp. 177–189). Edinburgh U.K.: Churchill Livingston.

Bellugi, U., Mills, D., Jernigan, T., Hickok, G., & Galaburda, A. (1999). Linking cognition, brain structure, and brain function in Williams syndrome. In H. Tager-Flusberg (Ed.), *Neurodevelopmental disorders* (pp. 111–136). Cambridge: MIT Press.

Bellugi, U., Sabo, H., & Vaid, J. (1988). Spatial deficits in children with Williams syndrome. In J. Stiles-Davis, M. Kritchevesky, & U. Bellugi (Eds.), *Spatial cognition: Brain bases and development* (pp. 273–298). Mahwah, NJ: Lawrence Erlbaum Associates.

Bellugi, U., Wang, P., & Jernigan, T.L. (1994). Williams syndrome: An unusal neuropsychological profile. In S.H. Browman & J. Grafram (Eds.), *Atypical cognitive deficits in developmental disorders* (pp. 23–56). Mahwah, NJ: Lawrence Erlbaum Associates.

Benezech, M., & Noel, B. (1985). Fra(X) syndrome and autism. *Clinical Genetics, 28,* 93.

Benjamin, E., & Buot-Smith, T. (1993). Naltroxone and fluoxetine in Prader-Willi syndrome. *Journal of the American Academy of Child and Adolescent Psychiatry, 32,* 870–873.

Benton, A.L., Hamsher, K., Varney, N.R., & Spreen, O. (1983). *Test of Facial Recognition, Form SL.* New York: Oxford University Press.

Bernheimer, L.C., & Keogh, B. (1988). Stability of cognitive performance of children with developmental delays. *American Journal on Mental Retardation, 92,* 539–542.

Bernheimer, L.C., Keogh, B., & Guthrie, D. (1997). Stability and change over time in cognitive level of children with delays. *American Journal on Mental Retardation, 101,* 365–373.

Berry, P., Groeneweg, G., Gibson, D., & Brown, R.I. (1984). Mental development of adults with Down syndrome. *American Journal of Mental Deficiency, 89,* 252–256.

Bersu, E. (1981). Anatomical analysis of the developmental effects of aneuploidy in man: The Down syndrome. *American Journal of Medical Genetics, 5,* 399–420.

Bertelson, P. (1993). Reading acquisition and phemic awareness testing: How conclusive are data from Down's syndrome? (Remarks on Cossu, Rossini, & Marshall, 1993). *Cognition, 48,* 281–283.

Bertrand, J., & Mervis, C.B. (1996). Longitudinal analysis of drawings by children with Williams syndrome. *Visual Arts Research, 22,* 19–34.

Bertrand, J., Mervis, C.B., & Eisenberg, J.D. (1997). Drawing by children with Williams syndrome: A developmental perspective. *Developmental Neuropsychology, 13,* 41–67.

Beuren, A.J., Apitz, J., & Harmjanz, D. (1962). Supravalvular aortic stenosis in association with mental retardation and a certain facial appearance. *Circulation, 26,* 1235–1240.

Beuren, A.J., Schulze, C., Eberle, P., Harmjanz, D., & Apitz, J. (1964, April). The syndrome of supravalvular aortic stenosis, perihperal pulmonary stenosis, mental retardation, and similar facial appearance. *The American Journal of Cardiology*, 471–483.

Bishop, D. (1983). *Test for Reception of Grammar*. London: Medical Research Council.

Blackhurst, A.E., & Birdine, W.H. (1993). *An introduction to special education*. New York: HarperCollins.

Blomquist, H.K., Bohman, M., Edvinsson, S.O., Gillberg, C., Gustavson, K.H., Holgren, G., & Wahlstrom, J., (1985). Frequency of the fragile X syndrome in infantile autism: A Swedish multicenter study. *Clinical Genetics, 27*, 113–117.

Bockoven, J.R., Kaplan, P., Namey, T., & Gleasal, M. (1997). Williams syndrome: The first decade is crucial for cardiovascular monitoring. *Proceedings of the Greenwood Genetic Center, 16*, 134–135.

Bondy, C., Cohen, R., Eggert, D., & Luer, G. (1969). *Testbatterie fur Geistig Behinderte Kinder TBGB*. Weinheim: Beltz-Verlag.

Borghgraef, M., Fryns, J.P., Dielkins, A., Pych, K., & Van den Berghe, H. (1987). Fragile X syndrome: A study of the psychological profile in 23 prepubertal patients. *Clinical Genetics, 32*, 179–186.

Borghgraef, M., Fryns, J.P., & Van den Berghe. (1990). Psychological profile and behavioral characteristics in 12 patients with Prader–Willi syndrome. *Genetic Counseling, 38*, 141–150.

Bottani, A., Robinson, W.P., DeLozier-Blanchet, C.D., Engel, E., Morris, M.A., Schmitt, B., Thun-Hohenstein, L., & Schinzel, A. (1994). Angelman syndrome due to paternal uniparental disomy of chromosome 15: A milder phenotype? *American Journal of Medical Genetics, 51*, 35–40.

Boyd, S.G., Harden, A., & Patton, M.A. (1988). The EEG in early diagnosis of the Angelman (happy puppet) syndrome. *European Journal of Pediatrics, 147*, 508–513.

Braden, M.L. (1989). *Logo reading system*. (Available from the author, 219 E. Saint Vrain Street, Colorado Springs, CO 80903)

Braden, M. (1992). Educational interventions: new approaches. In Hagerman, R.J., & McKenzie, P. (Eds.), *1992 International Fragile X Conference Proceedings* (pp. 227–233). Dillon, CO: Spectra.

Branson, C. (1981). Speech and language characteristics of children with Prader-Willi syndrome. In V.A. Holm, S. Sulzbacher, & P. Pipes (Eds.), *The Prader-Willi syndrome* (pp. 179–183). Baltimore: University Park Press.

Breg, W.R., Steele, M.W., Miller, O.J., Warburton, D., DeCapoa, A., & Allderdice, P.W. (1970). The cri du chat syndrome in adolescents and adults: Clinical findings in 13 older patients with partial deletion of the short arm of chromosome No. 5(5p-). *The Journal of Pediatrics, 77*, 782–791.

Bregman, J.D., Leckman, J.F., & Ort, S.I. (1988). Fragile X syndrome: Genetic predisposition to psychopathology. *Journal of Autism and Developmental Disorders, 18*, 343–354.

Broder, K., Reinhardt, E., Ahern, J., Lifton, R., Tamborlane, W., & Pober, B. (1999). Elevated ambulatory blood pressure in 20 subjects with Williams syndrome. *American Journal of Medical Genetics, 834*, 356–360.

Broder, K., Reinhardt, E., Lifton, R., Timborlane, W., & Pober, B.R. (1995). Ambulatory blood pressure monitoring in Williams syndrome. *Genetic Counseling, 6*, 150–151.

Brown, R. (1973). *A first language*. Cambridge, MA: Harvard University Press.

Brown, F.R., Greer, M., Aylward, E., Fisch, G.S., Wolf-Schein, E.G., Gross, A., Waterhouse, L., Fein, D., Mason-Brothers, A., Ritvo, E., Ruttenberg, B.A., Bentley, W., & Castellas, S. (1986). Fragile X syndrome and autism: A multicenter study. *American Journal of Medical Genetics, 23,* 341–352.

Brown, F.R., Greer, M., Aylward, E., & Hunt, H. (1990). Intellectual and adaptive functioning in individuals with Down syndrome in relation to age and environmental placement. *Pediatrics, 85,* 450–452.

Brown, W.T., Jenkins, E.C., Friedman, E., Brooks, J., Wisniewski, K., Raguthu, S., & French, J. (1982). Autism is associated with the fragile X syndrome. *Journal of Autism and Developmental Disorders, 12,* 303–307.

Brugge, K.L., Nichols, S.L., Salmon, D.P., Hill, L.R., Delis, D.C., Aaron, L., & Trauner, D.A. (1994). Cognitive impairment in adults with Down's syndrome: Similarities to early cognitive changes in Alzheimer's disease. *Neurology, 44,* 232–238.

Bruininks, R.H., Hill, B.K., Weatherman, R.F., & Woodcock, R.W. (1986). *Inventory for Client and Agency Planning.* Itasca, IL: Riverside Publishing.

Brun, C., Obiols, J.E., Cheema, A., O'Connor, R., Riddle, J., DiMaria, M., Wright-Calamante, C., & Hagerman, R.J. (1995). Longitudinal IQ changes in fragile X females. *Developmental Brain Dysfunction, 8,* 230–241.

Buckley, S. (1995). Teaching children with Down syndrome to read and write. In L. Nadel & D. Rosenthal (Eds.), *Down syndrome: Living and learning in the community* (pp. 158–169). New York: Wiley-Liss.

Buckley, S. (1999). Promoting the cognitive development of children with Down syndrome: the practical implications of recent psychological research. In J.A. Rondal, J. Perera, & L. Nadel (Eds.), *Down's syndrome: A review of current knowledge* (pp. 99–110). London: Whurr Publishers.

Buckley, R.H., Dinno, N., & Weber, P. (1998). Angelman syndrome: Are the estimates too low? *American Journal of Medical Genetics, 80,* 385–390.

Buiting, K., Saitoh, S., Gross, S., Dittrich, B., Schwartz, S., Nicholas, R.D., & Horsthemke, B. (1995). Inherited microdeletions in the Angelman and Prader-Willi syndromes define an imprinting centre on human chromosome 15. *Nature Genetics, 9,* 395–400.

Buntinx, I.M., Hennekam, R.C.M., Brouwer, O.F., Stroink, H., Beuten, J., Mangelschots, K., & Fryns, J.P. (1995). Clinical profiles of Angelman syndrome at different ages. *American Journal of Medical Genetics, 56,* 176–183.

Burger, J., Kunze, J., Sperling, K., & Reis, A. (1996). Phenotypic differences in Angelman syndrome patients: Imprinting mutations show less frequently microcephaly and hypopigmentation than deletions. *American Journal of Medical Genetics, 66,* 221–226.

Butler, M.G. (1989). Hypopigmentation: A common feature of Prader-Willi syndrome. *American Journal of Human Genetics, 45,* 140–146.

Butler, M.G. (1990). Prader-Willi syndrome: Current understanding of cause and diagnosis. *American Journal of Medical Genetics, 35,* 319–332.

Byrne, A., Buckley, S., MacDonald, J. & Bird, G. (1995). Investigating the literacy, language and memory skills of children with Down's syndrome. *Down's Syndrome: Research and Practice, 3,* 53–58.

Byrne, B. (1993). Learning to read in the absence of phonemic awareness?: A comment on Cossue, Rossini, and Marshall (1993). *Cognition, 48,* 285–288.

Byrne, E.A., Cunningham, C., & Sloper, P. (1988). *Families and their children with Down's syndrome.* London: Routledge.

Cahill, B.M., & Glidden, L.M. (1996). Influence of child diagnosis on family and parent functioning: Down syndrome versus other disabilities. *American Journal on Mental Retardation, 101,* 149–160.

Caldwell, M.L., & Taylor, R.L. (1983). A clinical note on the food preference of individuals with Prader-Willi syndrome: The need for empirical research. *Journal of Mental Deficiency, 27,* 45–49.

Cantu, E.S., Stone, J.W., Wing, A.A., Langee, H.R., & Williams, C.A. (1990). Cytogenetic survey for autistic fragile X carriers in a mental retardation center. *American Journal on Mental Retardation, 94,* 442–447.

Capirci, O., Sabbadini, L., & Volterra, V. (1996). Language development in Williams syndrome: A case study. *Cognitive Neuropsychology, 13,* 1017–1039.

Carlin, M.E. (1990). The improved prognosis in cri du chat (5p-) syndrome. In W.I. Fraser (Ed.), *Proceedings of the 8th Congress of the International Association of the Scientific Study of Mental Deficiency* (pp. 64–73). Edinburgh, UK: Blackwell.

Carr, J. (1988). Six weeks to twenty-one years: A longitudinal study of children with Down's syndrome and their families. *Journal of Child Psychology and Psychiatry, 29,* 407–431.

Carr, J. (1994). Long-term outcome of people with Down's syndrome. *Journal of Child Psychology and Psychiatry, 35,* 425–439.

Carr, J. (1995). *Down's syndrome: Children growing up.* Cambridge: Cambridge University Press.

Carrel, A.L., Myers, S.E., Whitman, B.Y., & Allen, D.B. (1999). Growth hormone improves body composition, fat utilization, physical strength and agility, and growth in Prader-Willi syndrome: A controlled study. *Journal of Pediatrics, 134,* 215–221.

Cassidy, S.B. (1984). Prader-Willi syndrome. *Current Problems in Pediatrics, 14,* 1–55.

Cassidy, S.B., Devi, A., & Mukaida. C. (1994). Aging in Prader-Willi syndrome: 22 patients over age 30 years. *Proceedings of the Greenwood Genetics Center, 13,* 102–103.

Cassidy, S.B., Forsythe, M., Heeger, S., Nicholas, R.D., Schork, N., Benn, P., & Schwartz, S. (1997). Comparison of phenotype between patients with Prader-Willi syndrome due to deletion 15q and uniparental disomy 15. *American Journal of Medical Genetics, 68,* 433–440.

Chad, K., Jobling, A., & Frail, H. (1990). Metabolic rate: A factor in developing obesity in children with Down syndrome? *American Journal on Mental Retardation, 95,* 228–235.

Chan, C.T., Clayton-Smith, J., Cheng, X.J., Buxton, J., Webb, T., Pembrey, M.E., & Malcom, S. (1993). Molecular mechanisms in the Angelman syndrome: A survey of 93 patients. *Journal of Medical Genetics, 30,* 895–902.

Chapman, C.A., De Plessis, A., & Pober, B.R. (1996). Neurologic findings in children and adults with Williams syndrome. *Journal of Child Neurology, 11,* 63–65.

Chapman, R. (1995). Language development in children and adolescents with Down syndrome. In P. Fletcher & B. MacWhinney (Eds.), *The handbook of child language* (pp. 641–663). Oxford: Blackwell.

Chapman, R.S., Kay-Raining Bird, E., & Schwartz, S.E. (1990). Fast-mapping of words in event contexts by children with Down syndrome. *Journal of Speech and Hearing Disorders, 55,* 761–770.

Chapman, R.S., Seung, H.K., Schwartz, S.E., & Kay-Raining Bird, E. (1998). Language skills of children and adolescents with Down syndrome: II. Production deficits. *Journal of Speech, Language, and Hearing Research, 41,* 861–873.

Chen, K.S., Potocki, L., & Lupski, J.R. (1996). The Smith-Magenis syndrome [del(17)p11.2]: Clinical review and molecular advances. *Mental Retardation and Developmental Disabilities Research Reviews, 2,* 122–129.

Chen, X.N., & Korenberg, J.R. (1995). Localization of human CREBBP (CREB binding protein) to 16p13.3 by fluorescent *in situ* hybridization. *Cytogenetics and Cell Genetics, 71,* 56–57.

Chorney, M.J., Chorney, K., Seese, N., Owen, M.J., Daniels, J., McGuffin, P., Thompson, L.A., Detterman, D.K., Benbow, C., Lubinski, D., Eley, T., & Plomin, R. (1998). A quantitative trait locus associated with cognitive ability in children. *Psychological Science, 9,* 159–166.

Chow, E.W., Bassett, A.S., & Weksberg, R. (1994). Velo-cardio-facial syndrome and psychotic disorders: Implications for psychiatric genetics. *American Journal of Medical Genetics, 54,* 107–112.

Church, D.M., Bengtsson, U., Nielsen, K.V., Wasmuth, J.J., & Niebuhr, E. (1995). Molecular definition of deletions in different segments of distal 5p that result in distinct phenotypic features. *American Journal of Human Genetics, 56,* 1162–1172.

Cicchetti, D. (1984). The emergence of developmental psychopathology. *Child Development, 55,* 1–7.

Cicchetti, D., & Cohen, D.J. (Eds.). (1995). *Manual of developmental psychopathology* (Vols. 1–2). New York: John Wiley & Sons.

Cicchetti, D., & Ganiban, J. (1990). The organization and coherence of developmental processes in infants and children with Down syndrome. In R.M. Hodapp, J.A. Burack, & E. Zigler (Eds.), *Issues in the developmental approach to mental retardation* (pp. 169–225). New York: Cambridge University Press.

Cicchetti, D., & Pogge-Hesse, P. (1982). Possible contributions of the study of organically retarded persons to developmental theory. In E. Zigler & D. Balla (Eds.), *Mental retardation: The developmental-difference controversy* (pp. 277–318). Mahwah, NJ: Lawrence Erlbaum Associates.

Cicchetti, D., & Sroufe, L.A. (1976). The relationship between affective and cognitive development in Down syndrome infants. *Child Development, 47,* 920–929.

Clahsen, H., & Almazan, M. (1998). Syntax and morphology in Williams syndrome. *Cognition, 68,* 167–198.

Clarke, D.J. (1993). Prader-Willi syndrome and psychoses. *British Journal of Psychiatry, 163,* 680–684.

Clarke, D.J. (1998). Prader-Willi sysndrome and psychotic symptoms 2. A preliminary study of prevalence using the Psychopathology Assessment Schedule for Adults with Developmental Disability Checklist. *Journal of Intellectual Disability Research, 42,* 451–454.

Clarke, D.J., & Boer, H. (1998). Problem behaviors associated with deletion Prader-Willi, Smith-Magenis, and Cri du Chat syndromes. *American Journal on Mental Retardation, 103,* 264–271.

Clarke, D.J., Boer, H. & Webb, T. (1995). Genetic and behavioural aspects of Prader-Willi syndrome: A review with a translation of the original paper. *Mental Handicap Research, 8,* 38–53.

Clarke, D.J., Boer, H., Webb, T., Scott, P., Frazer, S., Vogels, A., Borghgraef, M., & Curfs, L.M.G. (1998). Prader-Willi syndrome and psychotic symptoms: 1. Case descriptions and genetic studies. *Journal of Intellectual Disability Research, 42,* 440–450.

Clarke, D.J., Boer, H., Chung, M.C., Sturmey, P., & Webb, T. (1996). Maladaptive behaviour in Prader-Willi syndrome in adult life. *Journal of Intellectual Disability Research, 40,* 159–165.

Clarke, D.J., Webb, T., & Bachmann-Clarke, J.P. (1995). Prader-Willi syndrome and psychotic symptoms: Report of a further case. *Irish Journal of Psychological Medicine, 12,* 27–29.

Clayton-Smith, J. (1993). Clinical research in Angelman syndrome in the United Kingdom: Observations on 82 affected individuals. *American Journal of Medical Genetics, 46,* 12–15.

Clayton-Smith, J., & Pembrey, M.E. (1992). Angelman syndrome. *Journal of Medical Genetics, 29,* 412–415.

Cohen, I.L. (1995a). Behavioral profiles of autistic and nonautistic fragile X males. *Developmental Brain Dysfunction, 8,* 252–269.

Cohen, I.L. (1995b). A theoretical analysis of the role of hyperarousal in the learning and behavior of fragile X males. *Mental Retardation and Developmental Disability Research Reviews, 1,* 286–297.

Cohen, I.L., Nolin, S.L., Sudhalter, V., Ding, X.H., Dobkin, C.S., & Brown, W.T. (1996). Mosaicism for the FMR1 gene influences adaptive skills development in fragile X-affected males. *American Journal of Medical Genetics, 64,* 365–369.

Cohen, I.L., Fisch, G.S., Sudhalter, V., Wolf-Schein, E.G., Hanson, D., Hagerman, R., Jenkins, E.C., & Brown, W.T. (1988). Social gaze, social avoidance, and repetitive behavior in fragile X males: a controlled study. *American Journal on Mental Retardation, 92,* 436–446.

Cohen, I.L., Vietze, P.M., Sudhalter, V., Jenkins, E.C., & Brown, W.T. (1991). Effects of age and communication level on eye contact in fragile X males and non-fragile X autistic males. *American Journal of Medical Genetics, 38,* 498–502.

Coleman, K. (1998). Music therapy and adapted music lessons. *Heart to Heart: Publication of the National Williams Syndrome Association, 15,* 10.

Collacott, R.A. (1992). The effect of age and residential placement on adaptive behavior of adults with Down's Syndrome. *British Journal of Psychiatry, 161,* 675–679.

Collacott, R.A., Cooper, S.A., & McGrother, C. (1992). Differential rates of psychiatric disorders in adults with Down's syndrome compared with other mentally handicapped adults. *British Journal of Psychiatry, 161,* 671–674.

Colley, A.F., Leversha, M.A., Voullaire, L.E., & Rogers, J.G. (1990). Five cases demonstrating the distinctive behavioral features of chromosome deletion 17(p11.2p11.2) (Smith-Magenis syndrome). *Journal of Paediatrics and Child Health, 26,* 17–21.

Comings, D.E. (1980). Presidential Address to the American Society of Human Genetics 31st Annual Meeting, New York.

Connolly, J.A. (1978). Intelligence levels on Down's sydrome children. *American Journal of Mental Deficiency, 83,* 193–196.

Cook, A.H., Courchesne, R.Y., Cox, N.J., Lord, C., Gonen, D., Guter, S.J., Lincoln, A., Nix, K., Haas, R., Leventhal, B.L., & Courchesne, E. (1998). Linkage-disequilibrium mapping of autistic disorder with 15q11–13 markers. *American Journal of Human Genetics, 62,* 1077–1083.

Cooley, W.C., & Graham, J.M. (1991). Down syndrome: An update and review for the primary pediatrician. *Clinical Pediatrics, 30,* 233–253.

Cooper, S.A. (1997). Epidemiology of psychiatric disorders in elderly compared with younger adults with learning disabilities. *British Journal of Psychiatry, 170,* 375–380.

Cooper, S.A., & Prasher, V.P. (1998). Maladaptive behaviours and symptoms of dementia in adults with Down's syndrome compared with adults with intellectual disability of other aetiologies. *Journal of Intellectual Disability Research, 42,* 293–300.

Cornish, K.M. (1996). The neuropsychological profile of cri du chat syndrome without significant learning disability. *Developmental Medicine and Child Neurology, 38,* 941–944.

Cornish, K.M., Bramble, D., Munir, F., & Pigram, J. (1999). Cognitive functioning in children with typical cri du chat (5p0) syndrome. *Developmental Medicine and Child Neurology, 41,* 263–266.

Cornish, K.M., & Pigram, J. (1996). Developmental and behavioural characteristics of cri du chat syndrome. *Archives of Diseases in Childhood, 75,* 448–450.

Cornwell, A., & Birch, H. (1969). Psychological and social development of home-reared children with Down's Syndrome (mongolism). *American Journal of Mental Deficiency, 74,* 341–350.

Cossu, G., Rossini, R., & Marshall, J.C. (1993a). Reading is reading is reading. *Cognition, 48,* 297–303.

Cossu, G., Rossini, R., & Marshall, J.C. (1993b). When reading is acquired but phonemic awareness is not: A study of literacy in Down's syndrome. *Cognition, 46,* 129–138.

Costa, P.T., & McRae, R.R. (1998). Trait theories of personality. In D.F. Barone, M. Hersen, & V.B. Van Hasselt (Eds.), *Advanced personality* (pp. 103–121). New York: Plenum.

Craddock, N., & Owen, M. (1994). Is there an inverse relationship between Down's syndrome and bipolar affective disorder? Literature review and genetic implications. *Journal of Intellectual Disability Research, 38,* 613–620.

Crisco, J.J. (1990). Rate of cognitive development in young children with Williams syndrome. *Clinical Research, 38,* 356A.

Crisco, J.J., Dobbs, J.M., & Mulhern, R.K. (1988). Cognitive processing of children with Williams syndrome. *Developmental Medicine and Child Neurology, 30,* 650–656.

Crnic, K.A., Sulzbacher, S., Snow, J., & Holm, V.A. (1980). Preventing mental retardation associated with gross obesity in the Prader-Willi syndrome. *Pediatrics, 66,* 787–789.

Crowe, S., & Hay, D. (1990). Neuropsychological dimensions of the fragile X syndrome: Support for a non-dominant hemisphere dysfunction hypotheses. *Neuropsychologia, 28,* 9–16.

Crumley, F.E. (1998). Smith-Magenis syndrome [Letter to the editor]. *Journal of the American Academy of Child and Adolescent Psychiatry, 37,* 1131–1132.

Cunningham, C.C. (1987). Early intervention in Down's syndrome. In G. Hoskins & G. Murphy (Eds.), *Prevention of mental handicap: A world view* (pp. 169–182). London: Royal Society of Medicine Services.

Curfs, L.M.G. (1992). Psychological profile and behavioral characteristics in Prader-Willi syndrome. In S.B. Cassidy (Ed.), *Prader-Willi syndrome and other 15q deletion disorders* (pp. 211–222). Berlin: Springer-Verlag.

Curfs, L.M.G., Hoondert, V., van Lieshout, C.F.M., & Fryns, J.P. (1995). Personality profiles of youngsters with Prader-Willi syndrome and youngsters attending regular school. *Journal of Intellectual Disability Research, 39,* 241–248.

Curfs, L.G., Wiegers, A.M., Sommers, J.R., Borghgraef, M., & Fryns, J.P. (1991). Strengths and weaknesses in the cognitive profile of youngsters with Prader-Willi syndrome. *Clinical Genetics, 40,* 430–434.

Curtiss, S. (1977). *Genie: A psycholinguistic study of a modern-day "wild child."* New York: Academic Press.

Dalton, A.J., & Crapper-McLachlan, D.R. (1984). Incidence of memory deterioration in aging persons with Down syndrome. In J.M. Berg (Ed.), *Perspectives and progress in mental retardation* (Vol. 2, pp. 55–62). Baltimore: University Park Press.

Davies, M., Howlin, P., & Udwin, O. (1997). Independence and adaptive behavior in adults with Williams syndrome. *American Journal of Medical Genetics, 70,*188–195.

Davies, M., Udwin, O., & Howlin, P. (1998). Adults with Williams syndrome. *British Journal of Psychiatry, 172,* 273–276.

de Vries, B.B., Wiegers, A.M., Smits, A.P., Mohkamsing, S., Duivenvoorden, H.J., Fryns, J.P., Curfs, L.M., Halley, D.J., Oostra, B.A., van den Ouweland, A.M., & Niermeijer, M.F. (1996). Mental status of females with an FMR1 gene full mutation. *American Journal of Human Genetics, 58,* 1025–1032.

Dech, D., & Budow, L. (1991). The use of fluoxetine in an adolescent with Prader-Willi syndrome. *Journal of the American Academy of Child and Adolescent Psychiatry, 30,* 298–302.

DeLorey, T.M., Handforth, A., Anagnostaras, S,G., Homanics, G.E., Minassian, B.A., Asatourian, A., Fanselow, M.S., Delgado-Escueta, A., Ellison, G.D., & Olsen, R.W. (1998). Mice lacking the B_3 subunit of the $GABA_A$ receptor have the epilepsy phenotype and many of the behavioral characteristics of Angelman syndrome. *The Journal of Neuroscience, 18,* 8505–8514.

Dereymaeker, A.M., Fryns, J.P., Haegeman, J., Deroover, J. & Van den Berghe, H. (1988). A genetic-diagnostic survey in an institutionalized population of 158 patients. The Viaene experience. *Clinical Genetics, 34,* 126–134.

Devenny, D.A., Silverman, W.P., Hills, A.L., Jenkins, E., Sersen, E.A., & Wisniewski, K.E. (1996). Normal ageing in adults with Down's syndrome: A longitudinal study. *Journal of Intellectual Disability Research, 40,* 208–221.

Dietz, H.C., Cutting, G.R., Pyeritz, R.E., Maslen, C.L., Sakai, L.Y., Corson, G.M., Puffenberger, E.G., Hamosh, A., Nanthakumar, E.J., Currisitn, S.M., Stetten, G., Meyers, D.A., & Frandomano, C.A. (1991). Marfan syndrome caused by a recurrent de novo missense mutation in the fibrillin gene. *Nature, 352,* 337–339.

Dilts, C.V., Morris, C.A., & Leonard, C.O. (1990). Hypothesis for development of a behavioral phenotype in Williams syndrome. *American Journal of Medical Genetics,* (Suppl. 6), *6,* 126–131.

Dimitropoulos, A., Feurer, I., Thompson, T., & Butler, M. (1999, July). *Compulsive behavior and tantrums in children with Prader-Willi syndrome, Down syndrome, and typical development.* Presentation to the 14th Annual Prader-Willi Syndrome Scientific Conference, San Diego.

Dixon, R.A., & Baeckman, L. (1994). Compensatory mechanisms. In R. Sternberg (Ed.), *Encyclopedia of human intelligence* (pp. 279–283). New York: Macmillan.

Doll, E.A. (1953). *Measurement of social competence: A manual for the Vineland Social Maturity Scale.* Circle Pines, MN: American Guidance Service.

Down, H.L. (1866). Observations on an ethnic classification of idiots. *London Hospital Clinical Lecture and Report, 3,* 259–262.

Drash, P.W. (1992). The failure of prevention or our failure to implement prevention knowledge. *Mental Retardation, 38,* 93–96.

Driscoll, D.A., Salvin, J., Sellinger, B., Budarf, M.L., McDonald-McGinn, D.M., Zackai, E.H., & Emanuel, B.S. (1993). Prevalence of 22q11 microdeletions in DiGeorge and velocardiofacial syndromes: Implications for genetic counseling and prenatal diagnosis. *Journal of Medical Genetics, 30,* 813–187.

Dunn, H.G. (1968). The Prader-Labhart-Willi syndrome: Review of the literature and report of nine cases. *Acta Paediatrica Scandanavica, 186,* 1–38.

Dunn, L., & Dunn, L. (1981). *Peabody Picture Vocabulary Test–Revised.* Circle Pines, MN: American Guidance Service.

Dunn, P.M. (1991). Dr. Langdon Down (1828–1896) and "mongolism." *Archives of Disease in Childhood, 66,* 827–828.

Dunst, C.J. (1988). Stage transitioning in the sensorimotor development of Down's syndrome infants. *Journal of Mental Deficiency Research, 32,* 405–410.

Dunst, C.J. (1990). Sensorimotor development of infants with Down syndrome. In D. Cicchetti & M. Beeghly (Eds.), *Children with Down syndrome: A developmental perspective* (pp. 180–230). New York: Cambridge University Press.

Dykens, E.M. (1995a). Adaptive behavior in males with Fragile X syndrome. *Mental Retardation and Developmental Disabilities Research Reviews, 1,* 281–285.

Dykens, E.M. (1995b). Benefits of Special Olympics for persons with Prader-Willi syndrome. *Prader-Willi Perspectives, 3,* 19–20.

Dykens, E.M. (1995c). Measuring behavioral phenotypes: Provocations from the "new genetics." *American Journal on Mental Retardation, 99,* 522–532.

Dykens, E.M. (1996a). DNA meets DSM: The growing importance of genetic syndromes in dual diagnosis. *Mental Retardation, 34,* 125–127.

Dykens, E.M. (1996b). The Draw-a-Person task in persons with mental retardation: What does it measure? *Research in Developmental Disabilities, 17,* 1–13.

Dykens, E.M. (1999). Direct effects of genetic mental retardation syndromes: Maladaptive behavior and psychopathology. *International Review of Research in Mental Retardation, 22,* 1–26.

Dykens, E.M. (1999). Prader-Willi syndrome. In H. Tager-Flusberg (Ed.)., *Neurodevelopmental disorders* (p. 137–154). Cambridge, MA: MIT Press.

Dykens, E.M. (2000). *Anxiety, fears, and phobias in Williams syndrome.* Manuscript submitted for publication.

Dykens, E.M. (in press). Contaminated and unusual food combinations: What do people with Prader-Willi syndrome choose? *Mental Retardation.*

Dykens, E.M. (Ed.). (in press). Special Issue: Behavioral phenotypes of genetic syndromes. *American Journal on Mental Retardation.*

Dykens, E.M., & Cassidy, S.B. (1995). Correlates of maladaptive behavior in children and adults with Prader-Willi syndrome. *American Journal of Medical Genetics, 60,* 546–549.

Dykens, E.M., & Cassidy, S.B. (1996). Prader-Willi syndrome: Genetic, behavioral, and treatment issues. *Child and Adolescent Psychiatric Clinics of North America, 5,* 913–927.

Dykens, E.M., & Cassidy, S.B. (1999). Prader-Willi syndrome. In S. Goldstein & C.R. Reynolds (Eds.), *Handbook of neurodevelopmental and genetic disorders in children* (pp. 525–554). New York: Guilford Press.

Dykens, E.M., & Cassidy, S.B., & King, B.H. (1999). Maladaptive behavior differences in Prader-Willi syndrome due to paternal deletion versus maternal uniparental disomy. *American Journal on Mental Retardation, 104,* 67–77.

Dykens, E.M., & Clarke, D.J. (1997). Correlates of maladaptive behavior in individuals with 5p- (cri du chat) syndrome. *Developmental Medicine and Child Neurology, 39,* 752–756.

Dykens, E.M., & Cohen, D.J. (1996). Effects of Special Olympics International on social competence in persons with mental retardation. *Journal of the American Academy of Child and Adolescent Psychiatry, 35,* 223–229.

Dykens, E.M., Finucane, B.M., & Gayley, C. (1997). Brief report: Cognitive and behavioral profiles in persons with Smith-Magenis syndrome. *Journal of Autism and Developmental Disorders, 27,* 203–211.

Dykens, E.M., Goff, B.J., Hodapp, R.M., Davis, L., Devanzo, P., Moss, F., Halliday, R.N., Shah, B., State, M., & King, B. (1997). Eating themselves to death: Have "personal rights" gone too far in Prader-Willi syndrome? *Mental Retardation, 35,* 312–314.

Dykens, E.M., & Hodapp, R.M. (1997). Treatment issues in genetic mental retardation syndromes. *Professional Psychology: Research and Practice, 28,* 263–270.

Dykens, E.M., Hodapp, R.M., & Evans, D.W. (1994). Profiles and development of adaptive behavior in children with Down syndrome. *American Journal on Mental Retardation, 98,* 580–587.

Dykens, E.M., Hodapp, R.M., Finucane, B.M., Shapiro, L., Ort, S.I., & Leckman, J.F. (1989). The trajectory of cognitive development in males with fragile X syndrome. *Journal of the American Academy of Child and Adolescent Psychiatry, 28,* 422–426.

Dykens, E.M., Hodapp, R.M., & Leckman, J.F. (1987). Strengths and weaknesses in intellectual functioning of males with fragile X syndrome. *American Journal of Mental Deficiency, 92,* 234–236.

Dykens, E.M., Hodapp, R.M., & Leckman, J.F. (1994). *Behavior and development in fragile X syndrome.* Newbury Park, CA: Sage Publications.

Dykens, E.M., Hodapp, R.M., Ly, T., & Rosner, B.A. (2000). *Profiles and trajectories of cognitive and adaptive behavior in persons with 5p- syndrome.* Manuscript in preparation.

Dykens, E.M., Hodapp, R.M., Ort, S.I., & Leckman, J.F. (1993). Trajectory of adaptive behavior in males with fragile X syndrome. *Journal of Autism and Developmental Disorders, 23,* 135–145.

Dykens, E.M., Hodapp, R.M., Walsh, K. & Nash, L.J. (1992a). Adaptive and maladaptive behavior in Prader-Willi syndrome. *Journal of the American Academy of Child and Adolescent Psychiatry, 31,* 1131–1136.

Dykens, E.M., Hodapp, R.M., Walsh, K.K., & Nash, L. (1992b). Profiles, correlates, and trajectories of intelligence in Prader-Willi syndrome. *Journal of the Academy of Child and Adolescent Psychiatry, 31,* 1125–1130.

Dykens, E.M., & Kasari, C. (1997). Maladaptive behavior in children with Prader-Willi syndrome, Down syndrome, and non-specific mental retardation. *American Journal on Mental Retardation, 102,* 228–237.

Dykens, E.M., & Leckman, J.F. (1990). Developmental issues in fragile X syndrome. In R.M. Hodapp, J. Burak, & E. Zigler (Eds.), *Issues in the developmental approach to mental retardation* (pp. 226–245). New York: Cambridge University Press.

Dykens, E.M., Leckman, J.F., & Cassidy, S.B. (1996). Obsessions and compulsions in Prader-Willi syndrome. *Journal of Child Psychology and Psychiatry and Allied Disciplines, 37,* 995–1002.

Dykens, E.M., Leckman, J.F., Paul, R., & Watson, M. (1988). Cognitive, behavioral, and adaptive functioning of fragile X and non-fragile X retarded men. *Journal of Autism and Developmental Disorders, 18,* 41–52.

Dykens, E., Ort, S., Cohen, I., Finucane, B., Spiridigliozzi, G., Lachiewicz, A., Reiss, A., Freund, L., Hagerman, R., & O'Connor, R. (1996). Trajectories and profiles of adaptive behavior in males with fragile X syndrome: multicenter studies. *Journal of Autism and Developmental Disorders, 26,* 287–301.

Dykens, E.M., & Rosner, B.A. (1999a). *Adaptive and maladaptive behavior in children and adults with Williams syndrome.* Manuscript in preparation.

Dykens, E.M., & Rosner, B.A. (1999b). Refining behavioral phenotypes: Personality-motivation in Williams and Prader-Willi syndromes. *American Journal on Mental Retardation, 104,* 158–169.

Dykens, E.M., Rosner, B.A., & Ly, T. (2000). *Drawings by individuals with Williams syndrome: Are people different from shapes?.* Manuscript submitted for publication.

Dykens, E.M., Shah, B., King, B.H., & Rosner, B.A. (1999). *Psychopathology and maladaptive behavior in Down syndrome: Clinic versus non-referred samples.* Manuscript in preparation.

Dykens, E.M., & Smith, A.C.M. (1998). Distinctiveness and correlates of maladaptive behavior in children and adolescents with Smith-Magenis syndrome. *Journal of Intellectul Disability Research, 42,* 481–489.

Dykens, E.M., & Volkmar, F.R. (1997). Medical conditions associated with autism. In D.J. Cohen & F.R. Volkmar (Eds.), *Handbook of autism and pervasive developmental disorders—2nd ed.,* (pp. 388–407). New York: John Wiley & Sons.

Einfeld, S.L., Molony, H., & Hall, W. (1989). Autism is not associated with the fragile X syndrome. *American Journal of Medical Genetics, 19,* 187–193.

Einfeld, S. L., Tonge, B. J., & Florio, T. (1994). Behavioral and emotional disturbance in fragile X syndrome. *American Journal of Medical Genetics, 51,* 386–391.

Einfeld, S.L., Tonge, B.J., & Florio, T. (1997). Behavioral and emotional disturbance in individuals with Williams syndrome. *American Journal on Mental Retardation, 102,* 45–53.

Elliott, C.D. (1990). *Differential Ability Scales.* San Antonio, TX: The Psychological Corporation.

Ellis, N.R. (1969). A behavioral research strategy in mental retardation: Defense and critique. *American Journal of Mental Deficiency, 73,* 557–566.

Erikson, M., & Upshure, C. (1989). Caretaking burden and social support: Comparison of mothers of infants with and without disabilities. *American Journal on Mental Retardation, 94,* 250–258.

Evans, D.W., Leckman, J.F., Carter, A., Reznick, S., Henshaw, D., King, R.A., & Pauls, D. (1997). Ritual, habit, and perfectionism: The prevalence and development of compulsive-like behavior in normal young children. *Child Development, 68,* 58–68.

Ewart, A.K., Morris, C.A., Atkinson, D., Jin, W., Sternes, K., Spallone, P., Stock, A.D., Leppert, M., & Keating, M.T. (1993). Hemizygosity at the elastin locus in a developmental disorder, Williams syndrome. *Nature Genetics, 5,* 11–16.

Farag, T.I., Al-Awadi, S.A., El-Badramary, M.H., Aref, M.A., Kasrawi, B., Krishna Murthy, S., El-Khalifa, M.Y., Yadav, G., Marafie, M.J., Bastaki, I., Wahba, R.A., Mohammed, F.M., Abul Hasan, S., Redha, A.A., Redha, M.A., Al-aboud, H., Al-Hijji, S., Al-Dighashem, D. Al-Hashash, N., Al-Jeeryan, L., Al-Khorafi, H., Qurban, E.A., & Al-Sulaiman, I. (1993). Disease profile of 400 institutionalized mentally retarded patients in Kuwait. *Clinical Genetics 44,* 329–334.

Ferrier, L.J., Bashir, A.S., Meryash, D.L., Johnston, J., & Wolff, P. (1991). Conversational skills of individuals with fragile X syndrome: A comparison of autism and Down syndrome. *Developmental Medicine and Child Neurology, 33,* 766–788.

Fidler, D.J., & Hodapp, R.M. (1998). Importance of typologies for science and service in mental retardation. *Mental Retardation, 36,* 489–495.

Fidler, D.J., & Hodapp, R.M. (1999). Craniofacial maturity and perceived personality in children with Down syndrome. *American Journal on Mental Retardation, 104,* 410–421.

Fidler, D.J., Most, D.E., Hodapp, R.M., & Dykens, E.M. (2000). *Stress in families of children with Williams syndrome: Child personality risk and protective factors.* Manuscript submitted for publication.

Fieldstone, A., Zipf, W.B., Schwartz, H.C., & Berntson, G.G. (1997). Food preferences in Prader-Willi syndrome, normal weight, and obese controls. *International Journal of Obesity and Related Metabolic Disorders, 21,* 1–7.

Finucane, B.M. (Ed.). (1995). Bridging the gap between genetic diagnosis and special education, *Genetwork, 1(1),* 1–12.

Finucane, B.M. (1996a). Should all pregnant women be offered carrier testing for fragile X syndrome? *Clinical Obstetrics and Gynecology, 39,* 772–782.

Finucane, B.M. (1996b). *What's so special about genetics? A guide for special educators.* Elwyn, PA: Elwyn.

Finucane, B.M., Jaeger, E.R., Kurtz, M.B., Weinstein, M., & Scott, C.I. (1993). Eye abnormalities in the Smith-Magenis continuous gene deletion syndrome. *American Journal of Medical Genetics, 45,* 443–446.

Finucane, B.M., Konar, D., Haas-Givler, B., Kurtz, M.D., & Scott, L.I. (1994). The spasmodic upper-body squeeze: A characteristic behavior in Smith-Magenis syndrome. *Developmental Medicine and Child Neurology, 36,* 78–83.

Fisch, G.S. (1992). Is autism associated with the fragile X syndrome? *American Journal of Medical Genetics, 43,* 47–55.

Fisch, G.S., Ariname, T., Froster-Iskenius, U., Fryns, J.P., Curfs, L.M., Borghgraef, M., Howard-Peebles, P.N., Schwartz, C.E., Simensen, R.G., & Shapiro, L.R. (1991). Relationship between age and IQ among fragile X males: A multicenter study. *American Journal of Medical Genetics, 38,* 481–487.

Fisch, G.S., Cohen, I.L., Wolf, E.G., Brown, W.T., Jenkins, E.C., & Gross, A. (1986). Autism and the fragile X syndrome. *American Journal of Psychiatry, 143,* 71–73.

Fisch, G.S., Simensen, R., Arinami, T., Borgfgraef, M., & Fryns, J. P. (1994). Longitudinal changes in IQ among fragile X females: A preliminary multicenter analysis. *American Journal of Medical Genetics, 51,* 353–357.

Fisch, G.S., Simensen, R., Tarleton, J., Chalifoux, M., Holden, J.J.A., Carpenter, N., Howard-Peebles, P.N., & Maddalena, A. (1996). Longitudinal study of cognitive abilities and adaptive behavior levels in fragile X males: A prospective multicenter analysis. *American Journal of Medical Genetics, 64,* 356–361.

Fisher, M.A., & Zeaman, D. (1970). Growth and decline of retardate intelligence. *International Review of Research in Mental Retardation, 4,* 151–191.

Fishler, K., Koch, R., & Donnell, G.N. (1976). Comparison of mental development in individuals with mosaic and trisomy 21 Down's syndrome. *Pediatrics, 58,* 744–74.

Flynt, J., & Yule, W. (1994). Behavioural phenotypes. In M. Rutter, E. Taylor, & L. Hersov (Eds.), *Child and adolescent psychiatry: Modern approaches* (3rd ed., pp. 666–687). London: Blackwell Scientific.

Fodor, J. (1983). *Modularity of mind: An essay on faculty psychology.* Cambridge: MIT Press.

Fowler, A. (1990). Language abilities in children with Down syndrome: Evidence for a specific syntactic delay. In D. Cicchetti & M. Beeghly (Eds.), *Children with Down syndrome: A developmental perspective* (pp. 302–328). New York: Cambridge University Press.

Fowler, A.E., Doherty, B.J., & Boynton, L. (1995). The basis of reading skill in young adults with Down syndrome. In L. Nadel & D. Rosenthal (Eds.), *Down syndrome: Living and learning in the community* (pp. 182–196). New York: Wiley-Liss.

Fowler, A., Gelman, R., & Gleitman, L.R. (1994). The course of language learning in children with Down syndrome. In H. Tager-Flusberg (Ed.), *Constraints on language acquisition: Studies of atypical children* (pp. 91–140). Mahwah, NJ: Lawrence Erlbaum Associates.

Frangiskakis, J.M., Ewart, A.K., Morris, C.A., Mervis, C.B., Bertrand, J., Robinson, B.F., Klein, B.P., Ensing, G.J., Everett, L.A., Green, E.D., Proschel, C., Gutowski, N.J., Noble, M., Atkinson, D.L., Odelberg, S.J., & Keating, M.T. (1996). LIM-kinase 1 hemizygosity implicated in impaired visuospatial constructive cognition. *Cell, 86,* 59–69.

Franke, P., Maier, W., Hautzinger, M., Weiffenbach, O., Gansicke, M., Iwers, B., Poustka, F., Schwab, S.G., & Froster, U. (1996). Fragile X females: evidence for a distinct psychopathological phenotype? *American Journal of Medical Genetics, 64,* 334–339.

Freeman, S.F.N., & Hodapp, R.M. (1999). Educating children with Down syndrome: Service needs and new educational strategies. *Down Syndrome Quarterly.*

Freeman, S.F.N., & Kasari, C. (2000). *Friendships of school-aged children with Down syndrome manuscript.* Submitted for publication.

Freeman, S.F.N., Kasari, C., & Alkin, M. (1999). Satisfaction and desire for change in educational placement for children with Down syndrome. *Remedial and Special Education, 20,* 143–151.

Freund, L.S., Peebles, C.D., Aylward, E., & Reiss, A.L. (1995). Preliminary report on cognitive and adaptive behaviors of preschool-aged males with fragile X. *Developmental Brain Dysfunction, 8,* 242–251.

Freund, L.S., & Reiss, A.L. (1991). Cognitive profiles associated with the fragile X syndrome in males and females. *American Journal of Medical Genetics, 38,* 542–547.

Freund, L.S., Reiss, A.L., & Abrams, M. (1993). Psychiatric disorders associated with fragile X in the young female. *Pediatrics, 91,* 321–329.5,

Freund, L.S., Reiss, A.L., Hagerman, R., & Vinogradov, S. (1992). Chromosome fragility and psychopathology in obligate female carriers of the fragile X chromosome. *Archives of General Psychiatry, 49,* 54–60.

Frith, U. (1985). Beneath the surface of developmental dyslexia. In K.E. Patterson, J.C. Marshall, & M. Coltheart (Eds.), *Surface dyslexia* (pp. 301–330). Mahwah, NJ: Lawrence Erlbaum Associates.

Frodi, A., & Senchak, M. (1990). Verbal and behavioral responsiveness to the cries of atypical infants. *Child Development, 61,* 76–84.

Fryns, J.P., Jacobs, J., Klecklowska, A., & Van den Berghe, H. (1984). The psychological profile of the fragile X syndrome. *Clinical Genetics, 25,* 131–134.

Fryns, J.P., & Van den Berghe, H. (1983). X-linked mental retardation and fragile Xq27 site. *Clinical Genetics, 23,* 203–206.

Gabel, S., Tarter, R.E., Gavaler, J., Golden, W., Hegedus, A.M., & Mair, B. (1986). Neuropsychological capacity of Prader-Willi children: General and specific aspects of impairment. *Applied Research in Mental Retardation, 7,* 459–466.

Galaburda, A.M., Wang, P.P., Bellugi, U., & Rossen, M. (1994). Cytoarchitectonic anomalies in a genetically based disorder: Williams syndrome. *Cognitive Neuroscience and Neuropsychology,* Neuroreport 5, 753–757.

Gardner, M.F. (1991). *Expressive One-Word Picture Vocabulary Test*. Novato, CA: Academic Therapy Publications.

Gath, A., & Gumley, D. (1986). Behaviour problems in retarded children with special reference to Down's syndrome. *British Journal of Psychiatry, 149*, 156–161.

Gersh, M., Goodart, S.A., Pasztor, L.M., Harris, D.J., Weiss, L., & Overhauser, J. (1995). Evidence for a distinct region causing a cat-like cry in patients with 5p deletions. *American Journal of Human Genetics, 56*, 1404–1410.

Gersh, M., Grady, D., Rojas, K., Lovett, M., Moyzis, R., & Overhauser, J. (1997). Development of diagnostic tools for the analysis of 5p deletions using interphase FISH. *Cytogenetics and Cell Genetics, 77*, 246–251.

Gibson, D. (1966). Early developmental staging as a prophesy index in Down's syndrome. *American Journal of Mental Deficiency, 70*, 825–828.

Gibson, D. (1978). *Down's syndrome: The psychology of mongolism*. Cambridge: Cambridge University Press.

Gill, M., Daly, G., Heron, S., Hawi, A., & Fitzgerald, M. (1997). Confirmation of association between attention deficit hyperactivity disorder and a dopamine transporter polymorphism. *Molecular Psychiatry, 2*, 311–313.

Gillberg, C., Persson, E., & Whalstrom, J. (1986). The autistic fragile X syndrome: A population-based study of 10 boys. *Journal of Mental Deficiency Research, 310*, 27–39.

Gillberg, C., & Rasmussen, P. (1994). Brief report: Four case histories and a literature of Williams syndrome and autistic behavior. *Journal of Autism and Developmental Disorders, 24*, 381–393.

Gillessen-Kaesbach, G., Albrecht, B., Passarge, E., & Horsthemke, B. (1995). Further patient with Angelman syndrome due to paternal disomy of chromosome 15 and a milder phenotype [Letter to the editor]. *American Journal of medical Genetics, 56*, 328–329.

Gillessen-Kaesbach, G., Robinson, W., Lohmann, D., Kaya-Westerloh, S., Passarge, E., & Horsthemke, B. (1995). Genotype-phenotype correlation in a series of 167 deletion and non-deletion patients with Prader-Willi syndrome. *Human Genetics, 96*, 638–643.

Glass, I.A. (1991). X-linked mental retardation. *Journal of Medical Genetics, 28*, 61–371.

Golden, J.A., & Hyman, B.T. (1994). Development of the superior temporal neocortex is anomalous in trisomy 21. *Journal of Neuropathology and Experimental Neurology, 53*, 513–520.

Goldfine, P.E., McPherson, P.M., Heath, G.A., Hardesty, V.A., Beauregard, L.J., & Gordon, B. (1985). Association of the fragile X syndrome with autism. *American Journal of Psychiatry, 142*, 108–110.

Golding-Kushner, K.J., Weller, G., & Shprintzen, R.J. (1985). Velo-cardio-facial syndrome: Language and psychological profiles. *Journal of Craniofacial Genetics and Developmental Biology, 5*, 259–266.

Goldman, R.M., & Fristoe, M. (1969). *Goldman–Fristoe Test of Articulation*. Circle Pines, MN: American Guidance Service.

Goodman, J.F. (1990). Technical note: Problems in etiological classifications of mental retardation. *Journal of Child Psychology and Psychiatry and Allied Disciplines, 31*, 465–469.

Goodman, L. (1998). The Human Genome Project aims for 2003. *Genome Research, 8*, 997–999.

Goodman, W.K., Price, L.H., Rasmussen, S.A., Mazure, C., Fleischmann, R.L.,

Hill, C.L., Heninger, G.R., & Charney, D.S. (1989). The Yale-Brown Obsessive-Compulsive Scale: Development, use and reliability. *Archives of General Psychiatry, 46,* 1006–1011.

Gosch, A., & Pankau, R. (1994). Social-emotional and behavioral adjustment in children with Williams syndrome. *American Journal of Medical Genetics, 53,* 335–339.

Gosch, A., & Pankau, R. (1996). Longitudinal study of the cognitive development in children with Williams-Beuren syndrome. *American Journal of Medical Genetics, 61,* 26–29.

Gosch, A., & Pankau, R. (1997). Personality characteristics and behavior problems in individuals of different ages with Williams syndrome. *Developmental Medicine and Child Neurology, 39,* 527–533.

Gould, S.J. (1980). Dr. Down's syndrome. In S.J. Gould, *The panda's thumb* (pp. 160–168). New York: W.W. Norton.

Greenberg, F., Guzzetta, V., de Oca-Luna, R.M., Magenis, R.E., Smith, A.C.M., Richter, S.F., Kondo, I., Dobyns, W.B., Patel, P.I., & Lupski, J.R. (1991). Molecular analysis of the Smith-Magenis syndrome: A possible continguous-gene syndrome associated with del(17) (p11.2). *American Journal of Human Genetics, 4,* 1207–1218.

Greenberg, F., Lewis, R.A., Potocki, L., Glaze, D., Parke, J., Killian, J., Murpha, M.A., Williamson, D., Brown, F., Dutton, R., McCluggage, C., Friedman, S., Sulek, M., & Lupski, J.R. (1996a). Multidisciplinary clinical study of Smith-Magenis syndrome: (deletion 17p11.2). *American Journal of Medical Genetics, 62,* 247–254.

Greenberg, F., Magenis, W., Finucane, B.M., Smith, A.C.M., Patel, L.I., & Lupski, J.R. (1996b). *Smith-Magenis and its clinical overlap with Prader-Willi syndrome.* Abstract presented to the American Society of Human Genetics Meeting.

Greenswag, L.R. (1987). Adults with Prader-Willi syndrome: A survey of 232 cases. *Developmental Medicine and Child Neurology, 29,* 145–152.

Greenswag, L.R. & Alexander, R.A. (Eds.). (1995). *Management of Prader-Willi syndrome* (2nd ed.) New York: Springer-Verlag.

Greer, M.K., Brown, F.R., Pai, G.S., Choudry, S.H., & Klein, A.J. (1997). Cognitive, adaptive, and behavioral characteristics of Williams syndrome. *American Journal of Medical Genetics, 74,* 521–525.

Gretjak, N. (1997). Educational tips. *Heart to Heart: Publication of the National Williams Syndrome Association, 14,* 6–7.

Gunay-Aygun, M., Heeger, S., Schwartz, S., & Cassidy, S.B. (1997). Delayed diagnosis in Prader-Willi syndrome due to uniparental disomy. *American Journal of Medical Genetics, 71,* 106–110.

Hagberg, B., & Kyllerman, M. (1983). Epidemiology of mental retardation—A Swedish survey. *Brain Devopment, 5,* 41–449.

Hagerman, R.J. (1996). Fragile X syndrome. *Child and Adolescent Psychiatric Clinics of North America, 5,* 895–911.

Hagerman, R.J., Hull, C.E., Safanda, J.F., Carpenter, I., Staley, L.W., O'Connor, R.A., Seydel, C., Mazzocco, M.M., Snow, K., Thibodeau, S.N., Kuhl, D., Nelson, D.L., Caskey, C.T., & Taylor, A.K. (1994). High functioning fragile X males: demonstration of an unmethylated fully expanded FMR-1 mutation associated with protein expression. *American Journal of Medical Genetics, 51,* 298–308.

Hagerman, R.J., Jackson, A.A., Levitas, A., Rimland, B., & Braden, M. (1986).

An analysis of autism in 50 males with fragile X syndrome. *American Journal of Medical Genetics, 23*, 359–374.

Hagerman, R.J., Murphy, M.A., & Wittenberger, M.D. (1988). A controlled trial of stimulant medication in children with the fragile X syndrome. *American Journal of Medical Genetics, 30*, 377–392.

Hagerman, R.J., Schreiner, R.A., Kemper, M., Wittenberger, M.D., Zahn, M., & Habicht, K. (1989). Longitudinal IQ changes in fragile X males. *American Journal of Medical Genetics, 33*, 513–518.

Hagerman, R.J., & Sobesky, W.E. (1989). Psychopathology in fragile X syndrome. *American Journal of Orthopsychiatry, 59*, 142–152.

Hall, J. (1991, July 16). *The New York Times.*

Hallahan, D.P., & Kauffman, J.M. (1997). *Exceptional children: Introduction to special education* (7th ed.). Needham Heights, MA: Allyn & Bacon.

Hanchett, J.M. (1998, July). *Treatment of self-abusive behavior in Prader-Willi syndrome.* Paper presented at the 20th Annual National Prader-Willi Syndrome Association Conference, Columbus, OH.

Hanson, D.M., Jackson, A., & Hagerman, R.J. (1986). Speech disturbances (cluttering) in mildly impaired males with the Martin-Bell/fragile X syndrome. *American Journal of Medical Genetics, 23*, 195–206.

Harris, N.G., Bellugi, U., Bates, E., Jones, W., & Rossen, M. (1997). Contrasting profiles of language development in children with Williams and Down syndromes. *Developmental Neuropsychology, 13*, 345–370.

Harris, S., Kasari, C., & Sigman, M. (1996). Shared attention and language gains in children with Down syndrome. *American Journal on Mental Retardation, 100*, 608–619.

Hathaway, S., & McKinley, J. (1989). Minnesota Multiphasic Personality Inventory-2. Minneapolis, MN: National Computer System.

Hauffa, B.P. (1997). One-year results of growth hormone treatment of short stature in Prader-Willi syndrome. *Acta Paediatrica* (Suppl.), *423*, 63–65.

Hauser-Cram, P., Warfield, M.E., Shonkoff, J.P., Krauss, M.W., Upshur, C., & Sayer, A. (1999). Family influences on adaptive development in young children with Down syndrome. *Child Development, 70*, 979–989.

Haxby, J.V. (1989). Neuropsychological evaluations of adults with Down's syndrome: Patterns of selective impairment in non-demented old adults. *Journal of Mental Deficiency Research, 88*, 193–210.

Hecht, F. (1991). Seizure disorders in the fragile X chromosome disorder. *American Journal of Medical Genetics, 28*, 509.

Hellings, J.A., & Warnock, J.K. (1994). Self-injurious behavior and serotonin in Prader-Willi syndrome. *Psychopharmacology Bulletin, 30*, 245–250.

Hennekam, R.C.M., Baselier, A.C.A., Beyaert, E., Bos, A., Blok, J.B., Jansma, H.B.M., Nilsen-Thorbecke, V.V., & Veerman, H. (1992). Psychological and speech studies in Rubinstein-Taybi syndrome. *American Journal on Mental Retardation, 96*, 645–660.

Hennekam, R.C.M., Boogaard, V.D., & Doorne, V. (1991). A cephalometric study in Rubinstein-Taybi syndrome. *Journal of Craniofacial Genetics and Developmental Biology, 20*, 33–40.

Hickok, G., Neville, H., Mills, D., Jones, W., Rossen, M., & Bellugi, U. (1995). Electrophysiological and quantitative analysis of the cortical auditory system in Williams syndrome. *Cognitive Neuroscience Society Abstracts, 2*, 66.

Ho, H.H., & Kalousek, D.K. (1989). Fragile X syndrome in autistic boys. *Journal of Autism and Developmental Disorders, 19*, 343–347.

Hodapp, R.M. (1994). Cultural-familial mental retardation. In R. Sternberg (Ed.), *Encyclopedia of intelligence* (pp. 711–717). New York: Macmillan.

Hodapp, R.M. (1995). Parenting children with Down syndrome and other types of mental retardation. In M. Bornstein (Ed.), *Handbook of parenting:* Vol. 1. *How children influence parents* (pp. 233–253). Mahwah, NJ: Lawrence Erlbaum Associates.

Hodapp, R.M. (1996a). Cross-domain relations in Down's syndrome. In J. Rondal, J. Perera, L. Nadel, & A. Comblain (Eds.), *Down's syndrome: Psychological, psychobiological, and socio-educational perspectives* (pp. 65–79). London: Whurr Publishers.

Hodapp, R.M. (1996b). Down syndrome: Developmental, psychiatric, and management issues. *Child and Adolescent Psychiatric Clinics of North America,* 5, 881–894.

Hodapp, R.M. (1997a). Cognitive functioning in adolescents with Down syndrome: Theoretical and practical issues. In S.M. Pueschel & M. Šuštrová (Eds.), *Adolescents with Down syndrome: Toward a more fulfilling life* (pp. 91–98). Baltimore: Paul H. Brookes Publishing Co.

Hodapp, R.M. (1997b). Direct and indirect behavioral effects of different genetic disorders of mental retardation. *American Journal on Mental Retardation,* 102, 67–79.

Hodapp, R.M. (1998). *Development and disabilities: Intellectual, sensory, and motor impairments.* New York: Cambridge University Press.

Hodapp, R.M. (1999). Indirect effects of genetic mental retardation disorders: Theoretical and methodological issues. *International Review of Research in Mental Retardation,* 22, 27–50.

Hodapp, R.M., & Burack, J.A. (1990). What mental retardation tells us about typical development: The examples of sequences, rates, and cross-domain relations. *Developmental Psychopathology,* 2, 213–225.

Hodapp, R.M., & Dykens, E.M. (1994). Mental retardation's two cultures of behavioral research. *American Journal on Mental Retardation,* 98, 675–687.

Hodapp, R.M., & Dykens, E.M. (1996). Mental retardation. In E.J. Mash & R.A. Barkley (Eds.), *Child psychopathology* (pp. 362–389). New York: Guilford Press.

Hodapp, R.M., & Dykens, E.M. (2000). The two cultures revisited: Behavioral research in genetic mental retardation syndromes. Manuscript submitted for publication.

Hodapp, R.M., Dykens, E.M., Fidler, D.J., & Rosner, B.A. (2000). *Social competence in children with Williams versus Down syndromes.* Submitted for publication.

Hodapp, R.M., Dykens, E.M., Hagerman, R.J., Schreiner, R., Lachiewicz, A.M., & Leckman, J.F. (1990). Developmental implications of changing trajectories of IQ in males with fragile X syndrome. *Journal of the American Academy of Child and Adolescent Psychiatry,* 29, 214–219.

Hodapp, R.M., Dykens, E.M., & Masino, L. (1997). Stress and support in families of persons with Prader-Willi syndrome. *Journal of Autism and Developmental Disorders,* 27, 11–24.

Hodapp, R.M., Dykens, E.M., Ort, S.I., Zelinsky, D., & Leckman, J.F. (1991). Changing patterns of intellectual strengths and weaknesses in males with fragile X syndrome. *Journal of Autism and Developmental Disorders,* 21, 503–516.

Hodapp, R.M., Evans, D., & Gray, F.L. (1999). Intellectual development in children with Down syndrome. In J.A. Rondal, J. Perera, & L. Nadel (Eds.),

Down's syndrome: A review of current knowledge (pp. 124–132). London: Whurr Publishers.

Hodapp, R.M., & Fidler, D.J. (1999). Special education and genetics: Connections for the 21st century. *Journal of Special Education, 33*(3) 130–137.

Hodapp, R.M., Fidler, D.J., & Smith, A.C.M. (1998). Stress and coping in families of children with Smith-Magenis syndrome. *Journal of Intellectual Disability Research, 42,* 331–340.

Hodapp, R.M., Freeman, S.F.N., Kasari, C. (1998). Parental educational preferences for students with mental retardation: Effects of etiology and current placement. *Education and Training in Mental Retardation and Developmental Disabilities, 33,* 342–349.

Hodapp, R.M., Leckman, J.F., Dykens, E.M., Sparrow, S.S., Zelinsky, D., & Ort, S.I. (1992). K-ABC profiles in children with fragile X syndrome, Down syndrome, and nonspecific mental retardation. *American Journal on Mental Retardation, 97,* 39–46.

Hodapp, R.M., & Ly, T.M. (in press). Visual processing strengths in Down Syndrome: A case for reading instruction? In S. Soraci & W.J. McIlvane (Eds.), *Perspectives on fundamental processes in intellectual functioning: Vol. 2. Visual information processing.* Stamford, CT: Ablex Publishing.

Hodapp, R.M., Wijma, C.A., & Masino, L.L. (1997). Families of children with 5p- (cri du chat) syndrome: familial stress and sibling reactions. *Developmental Medicine and Child Neurology, 39,* 757–761.

Hodapp, R.M., & Zigler, E. (1990). Applying the developmental perspective to children with Down syndrome. In D. Cicchetti & M. Beeghly (Eds.), *Children with Down syndrome: A developmental perspective* (pp. 1–28). New York: Cambridge University Press.

Hodapp, R.M., & Zigler, E. (1995). Past, present, and future issues in the developmental approach to mental retardation and developmental disabilities. In D. Cicchetti & D.J. Cohen (Eds.), *Manual of developmental psychopathology* (pp. 299–331). New York: John Wiley & Sons.

Hoffman, M. (1991). Unraveling the genetics of fragile X syndrome. *Science, 252,* 1070.

Holland, A.J., Treasure, J., Coskeran, P., & Dallow, J. (1995). Characteristics of the eating disorder in Prader-Willi syndrome: Implications for treatment. *Journal of Intellectual Disability Research, 39,* 373–381.

Holm, V.I. (1981). The diagnosis of Prader-Willi syndrome. In V.I. Holm, S. Sulzbacher, & P.L. Pipes (Eds.), *The Prader-Willi syndrome* (pp. 27–44). Baltimore: University Park Press.

Holm, V.A., Cassidy, S.B., Butler, M.G., Hanchett, J.M., Greenswag, L.R., Whitman, B.Y., & Greenberg, F. (1993). Prader-Willi syndrome: Consensus diagnostic criteria. *Pediatrics, 91,* 398–402.

Holroyd, J., & MacArthur, D. (1976). Mental retardation and stress on parents: A contrast between Down's syndrome and childhood autism. *American Journal of Mental Deficiency, 80,* 431–436.

Horn, J.L., & Hofer, S.M. (1992). Major abilities and development in the adult period. In R.J. Sternberg & C.A. Berg (Eds.), *Intellectual development* (pp. 44–99). New York: Cambridge University Press.

Hornby, G. (1995). Fathers' views of the effects on their families of children with Down syndrome. *Journal of Child and Family Studies, 4,* 103–117.

Hudgins, L.H., McKillop, J.A., & Cassidy, S.B. (1991). Hand and foot lengths in Prader-Willi syndrome. *American Journal of Medical Genetics, 41,* 5–9.

Jacobs, P.A., Mayer, M., Matsurura, J., Rhoads, F., & Yee, S.C. (1983). A cytogenetic study of a population of mentally retarded males with special reference to the marker (X) chromosome. *Human Genetics, 63,* 139–148.

Jacobsen, J., King, B.,H., Leventhal, B.L., Christian, S.L., Kedbetterm D.H., & Cook, E.H. (1998). Molecular screening for proximal 15q abnormalities in a mentally retarded population. *Journal of Medical Genetics, 35,* 534–538.

Jarrold, C., Baddeley, A.D., & Hewes, A.K. (1998). Verbal and nonverbal abilities in the Williams syndrome phenotype: Evidence for diverging developmental trajectories. *Journal of Child Psychology and Psychiatry and Allied Disciplines, 39,* 511–523.

Jernigan, T.L., & Bellugi, U. (1994). Neuroanatomical distinctions between Williams and Down syndromes. In S. Broman & J. Grafman (Eds.), *Atypical cognitive deficits in developmental disorders: Implications for brain function* (pp. 57–66). Mahwah, NJ: Lawrence Erlbaum Associates.

Jernigan, T.L., Bellugi, U., Sowell, E., Doherty, S.M., & Hesselink, J.R. (1993). Cerebral morphological distinctions between Williams and Down syndromes. *Archives of Neurology, 50,* 186–191.

Jones, O. (1980). Prelinguistic communication skills in Down's syndrome and normal infants. In T. Field, S. Goldberg, D. Stern, & A. Sostek (Eds.), *High-risk infants and children: Adult and peer interaction* (pp. 205–225). San Diego: Academic Press.

Jones, K.L., & Smith, D.W. (1975). The Williams elfin facies syndrome. *Journal of Pediatrics, 86,* 718–723.

Jones, W., Rossen, M., Hickok, G., Jernigan, T., & Bellugi, U. (1995). Links between behavior and brain: Brain morphological correlates of language, face, and auditory processing in Williams syndrome. *Society for Neuroscience Abstracts, 21*(3) 1926.

Jorgensen, J.W., Nielsen, K.B., Isager, T., & Mouridsen, S.E. (1984). Fragile X chromosome among child patients with disturbance of language and social relationships. *Acta Psychiatrica Scandinavica, 70,* 510–514.

Juyal, R.C., Finucane, B., Shaffer, L.G., Lupski, J.R., Greenberg, F., Scott, C.I. (1995). Apparent mosaicism for del(17)(p11.2) ruled out by FISH in a Smith-Magenis syndrome patient. *American Journal of Medical Genetics, 59,* 406–407.

Kahn, J.V. (1988). [Review of the book *Special education: A sourcebook*]. *American Journal on Mental Retardation, 92,* 550–551.

Kaplan, P., Kirschner, M., Watters, G., & Costa, T. (1989). Contractures in patients with Williams syndrome. *Pediatrics, 84,* 895–899.

Karmiloff-Smith, A., Grant, J., Berthoud, I., Davies, M., Howlin, P., & Udwin, O. (1997). Language and Williams syndrome: How intact is "intact"? *Child Development, 68,* 246–262.

Karmiloff-Smith, A., Klima, E., Bellugi, U., Grant, J., & Baron-Cohen, S. (1995). Is there a social processing module? Language, face processing and theory of mind in individuals with Williams syndrome. *Journal of Cognitive Neuroscience, 7,* 196–208.

Karmiloff-Smith, A., Tyler, L.K., Voice, K., Sims, K., Udwin, O., Howlin, P., & Davies, M. (1998). Linguistic dissociations in Williams syndrome: Evaluating receptive syntax in on-line and off-line tasks. *Neuropsychologia, 36,* 343–351.

Kasari, C., Freeman, S.F.N., & Hughes, M.A. (2000). *Emotion recognition of children with Down syndrome.* Manuscript submitted for publication.

Kasari, C., Freeman, S., Mundy, P., & Sigman, M. (1995). Attention regulation by children with Down syndrome: Coordinated joint attention and social referencing. *American Journal on Mental Retardation, 100,* 128–136.

Kasari, C., Mundy, P., Yirmiya, N., & Sigman, M. (1990). Affect and attention in children with Down syndrome. *American Journal on Mental Retardation, 95,* 55–67.

Kasari, C., & Sigman, M. (1997). Linking parental perceptions to interactions in young children with autism. *Journal of Autism and Developmental Disorders, 27,* 39–57.

Kasari, C., Sigman, M., Mundy, P., & Yirmiya, N. (1990). Affective sharing in the context of joint attention interactions. *Journal of Autism and Developmental Disabilities, 20,* 87–100.

Kataria, S., Goldstein, D., & Kushnick, T. (1984). Developmental delays in Williams syndrome. *Applied Research in Mental Retardation, 5,* 419–423.

Kaufman, A.S., & Kaufman, N.L. (1983). *Kaufman Assessment Battery for Children.* Circle Pines, MN: American Guidance Service.

Kaufman, A.S., & Kaufman, N.L. (1990). *Kaufman Brief Intelligence Test.* Circle Pines, MD: American Guidance Service.

Kaufman, A.S., Kaufman, N.L., & Goldsmith, B.Z. (1984). *K-SOS: Kaufman Sequential or Simultaneous?: A leaders guide.* Circle Pines, MN: American Guidance Service.

Kelley, G. (1991 June 9). New Hampshire Weekly: People and Places. Artist creates beauty from his period of grief. *Boston Sunday Globe.*

Kemper, M.B., Hagerman, R.J., & Altshul-Stark, D. (1988). Cognitive profiles of boys with fragile X syndrome. *American Journal of Medical Genetics, 30,* 191–200.

Kemper, S., Kynette, D., Rash, S., & O'Brien, K. (1989). Life span changes in adults' language. Effects of memory and genre. *Applied Psycholinguistics, 10,* 49–66.

Keogh, B., Bernheimer, L.R., & Gutherie, P. (1997). Stability and change over time in cognitive level of children with delays. *American Journal on Mental Retardation, 101,* 365–373.

Kerby, D.S., & Dawson, B. (1994). Autistic features, personality and adaptive behavior in males with the fragile X syndrome and no autism. *American Journal on Mental Retardation, 98,* 455–462.

Khan, N.L., & Wood, N.W. (1999). Prader-Willi and Angelman syndromes: Update on genetic mechanisms and diagnostic complexities. *Current Opinion in Neurology, 12,* 149–154.

Kingsley, J., & Levitz, M. (1994). *Count us in.* Orlando, FL: Harcourt Brace & Co., p. 44.

Kishino, T., Lalande, M., & Wagstaff, J. (1997). UBE3A/E6-AP mutations cause Angelman syndrome. *Nature Genetics, 15,* 70–73.

Klein, A.J., Armstrong, B.L., Greer, M.K., & Brown, F.R. (1990). Hyperacusis and otitis media in individuals with Williams syndrome. *Journal of Speech and Hearing Disorders, 55,* 339–344.

Klein, A.J., & Mervis, C.A. (in press). Cognitive strengths and weaknesses of 9- and 10-year-old children with Williams syndrome or Down syndrome. *Developmental Neuropsychology.*

Kleppe, S.A., Katayama, K.M., Shipley, K.G., & Foushee, D.R. (1990). The speech and language characteristics of children with Prader-Willi syndrome. *Journal of Speech and Hearing Disorders, 55,* 300–309.

Kok, L.L., & Solman, R.T. (1995). Velocardiofacial syndrome: learning difficulties and intervention. *Journal of Medical Genetics, 32,* 612–618.

Korenberg, J.R. (1995). Mental modeling. *Nature Genetics, 11,* 109–111.

Kumin, L. (1994). Intelligibility of speech in children with Down syndrome in natural settings: Parents' perspective. *Perceptual and Motor Skills, 78,* 307–313.

Kurtz, M.B., Finucane, B., Hyland, K., Bottiglieri, T., Sherwood, W.G., Bennett, M.J. (1994). Detection of metabolic disorders among selectively screened people with idiopathic mental retardation. *Mental Retardation, 32,* 328–333.

Kyllerman, M. (1995). On the prevalence of Angelman syndrome [Letter to the editor]. *American Journal of Medical Genetics, 59,* 405.

Laan, L.A.E.M., Boer, A.T.D., Hennekam, R.C.M., Reiner, W.O., & Brouwer, O.F. (1996). Angelman syndrome in adulthood. *American Journal of Medical Genetics, 66,* 356–360.

Lachiewicz, A.M. (1992). Abnormal behavior of young girls with fragile X syndrome. *American Journal of Medical Genetics, 43,* 72–77.

Lachiewicz, A.M., & Dawson, D.V. (1994). Behavior problems of young girls with fragile X syndrome: factor scores on the Conners parents questionnaire. *American Journal of Medical Genetics, 51,* 364–369.

Lachiewicz, A.M., Gullion, C., Spiridigliozzi, G., & Aylsworth, A. (1987). Declining IQs of young males with fragile X syndrome. *American Journal on Mental Retardation, 92,* 272–278.

Lacombe, D., Sabra, R., Taint, L., & Batten, J. (1992). Confirmation of an assignment of a locus for Rubinstein-Taybi syndrome gene to 16p13.3. *American Journal of Medical Genetics, 44,* 126–128.

Lamont, M.A., & Dennis, N.R. (1988). Aetiology of mild mental retardation. *Archives of Diseases in Children, 63,* 1032–1038.

Lane, D. (1985). After school: Work and employment for adults with Down's syndrome? In D. Lane & B. Stratford (Eds.), *Current approaches to Down's syndrome.* London: Holt, Rinehart, & Winston.

Lashkari, A., Smith, A.K., & Graham, J.M. (1999). Williams-Beuren syndrome: An update and review for the primary physician. *Clinical Pediatrics, 38,* 189–208.

Laws, G. (1998). The use of non-word repetition as a test of phonological memory in children with Down syndrome. *Journal of Child Psychology and Psychiatry and Allied Disciplines, 39,* 1119–1130.

Laws, G., Buckley, S., Bird, G., MacDonald, J., & Broadley, I. (1995). The influence of reading instruction on language and memory development in children with Down's syndrome. *Down's Syndrome: Research and Practice, 3,* 59–64.

Leckman, J.F., Goodman, W.K., North, W.J., Chappell, P.B., Price, L.H., Pauls, D.L. et al. (1994a). Elevated cerebrospinal fluid levels of oxytocin in obsessive-compulsive disorder: Comparison with Tourette's syndrome and healthy controls. *Archives of General Psychiatry, 51,* 782–792.

Leckman, J.F., Goodman, W.K., North, W.J., Chappell, P.B., Price, L.H., Pauls, D.L., Anderson, G.M., Riddle, M.A., McDougle, C.J., Barr, L.C., & Cohen, D.J. (1994b). The role of central oxytocin in obsessive compulsive disorder and related normal behavior. *Psychoneuroendocrinology, 19,* 723–749.

Ledbetter, D.H., Riccardi, V.M., Airhart, S.D., Strobel, R.J., Keenen, S.B., & Crawford, J.D. (1981). Deletion of chromosome 15 as a cause of Prader-Willi syndrome. *New England Journal of Medicine, 304,* 325–329.

Leddy, M. (1999). The biological bases of speech in people with Down syndrome. In J.F. Miller, M. Leddy, & L.A. Leavitt (Eds.), *Improving the communication of people with Down syndrome* (pp. 61–80). Baltimore: Paul H. Brookes Publishing Co.

Lejeune, J., Gautier, M., & Turpin, R. (1959). Etudes des chromosomes somatiques de neuf enfants mongoliens. [Somatic chromosome study of nine mongoloid children] *Comptes Rendus de l'Academie des Sciences, Série III, 248,* 1721.

Lejeune, J., Lafourcade, J., Berger, R., Vialatte, R., Boeswillwald, M., Seringe, P., & Turbin, R. (1963). Trois cas de deletion partielle du bras court d'un chromosome 5. [Three cases of partial deletion of the short arm of chromosome 3] *Comptes Rendus de l'Academie des Sciences, Série III, 257,* 3098–3102.

Lenhoff, H.M. (1998). Information sharing: Insights into the musical potential of cognitively impaired people diagnosed with Williams syndrome. *Music Therapy, 16,* 33–36.

Lenneberg, E.H. (1967). *Biological foundations of language.* New York: John Wiley & Sons.

Levine, K., & Wharton, R.K. (1993). *Children with Prader-Willi syndrome: Information for school staff.* Sarasota, FL Prader-Willi Syndrome Association.

Levitan, D.J., & Bellugi, U. (1998). Musical abilities in individuals with Williams syndrome. *Music Perception, 15,* 357–398.

Levitas, A., Hagerman, R.J., Braden, M., Rimland, B., McBogg, P., & Matus, I. (1983). Autism and the fragile X syndrome. *Developmental and Behavioral Pediatrics, 4,* 151–158.

Levitas, A.S., & Reid, C.S. (1998). Rubinstein-Taybi syndrome and psychiatric disorders. *Journal of Intellectual Disability Research, 42,* 284–292.

Lindgren, A.C., Hagenas, L., Muller, J., Blichfeldt, S., Rosenborg, M., Brismar, T., Rotzen, E. (1997). Effect of growth hormone treatment on growth and body composition in Prader-Willi syndrome: A preliminary study. *Acta Paediatrica* (Suppl.), *423,* 60–62.

Lindsay, E., Greenberg, F., Shaffer, L., Shapira, S., Scambler, P., & Baldini, A. (1995). Submicroscopic deletions at 22q11.2: Variability of the clinical picture and delineation of a commonly deleted region. *American Journal of Medical Genetics, 56,* 191–197.

Lipson, A., Yuille, D., Angel, M., Thompson, P., Vandervoord, J., Beckenham, E. (1991). Velocardiofacial syndrome: An important syndrome for the dysmorphologist to recognize. *Journal of Medical Genetics, 28,* 596–604.

Lopez-Rangel, A., Maurice, M., McGillivray, B., & Friedman, J.M. (1992). Williams syndrome in adults. *American Journal of Medical Genetics, 44,* 720–729.

Loveland, K.A., & Kelley, M.L. (1988). Development of adaptive behavior in adolescents and young adults with autism and Down syndrome. *American Journal on Mental Retardation, 93,* 84–92.

Loveland, K.A., & Kelley, M.L. (1991). Development of adaptive behavior in preschoolers with autism or Down syndrome. *American Journal on Mental Retardation, 96,* 13–20.

Lowery, M.C., Morris, C.A., Ewart, A., Brothman, L.J., Zhu, X.L., Leonard, C.O., Cary, J., Keating, M., & Brothman, A.R. (1995). Strong correlation of elastin deletions, detected by FISH, with Williams syndrome: Evaluation of 235 patients. *American Journal of Human Genetics, 57,* 49–53.

Lubs, H.A. (1969). A marker X chromosome. *American Journal of Human Genetics, 21,* 231–244.

Lupski, J.R., & Garcia, C.A. (1992). Molecular genetics and neuropathology of Charcot-Marie-tooth disease type 1A. *Brain Pathology, 2,* 337–349.

Lytton, H. (1990). Child and parent effects in boys' conduct disorder: A reinterpretation. *Developmental Psychology, 26,* 683–697.

MacDonald, G.W., & Roy, D.L. (1988). Williams syndrome: A neuropsychological profile. *Journal of Clinical and Experimental Neuropsychology, 10,* 125–131.

MacMillan, D. (1982). *Mental retardation in school and society* (2nd ed.). Boston: Little, Brown & Company.

Madison, L.S., George, C., & Moeschler, J.B. (1986). Cognitive functioning in the fragile X syndrome: A study of intellectual, memory and communication skills. *Journal of Mental Deficiency Research, 30,* 129–148.

Maes, B., Fryns, J.P., Van Walleghem, M., & Van den Berghe, H. (1994a). Cognitive functioning and information processing of adult mentally retarded men with fragile X syndrome. *American Journal of Medical Genetics, 50,* 190–200.

Maes, B., Fryns, J.P., Van Walleghem, M., & Van den Berghe, H. (1994b). Personal independence of adult mentally retarded men with fragile X syndrome. *Genetic Counseling, 5,* 129–139.

Mahoney, G. (1988). Enhancing the developmental competence of handicapped infants. In K. Marfo (Ed.), *Parent-child interaction and developmental disabilities* (pp. 203–219). New York: Praeger.

Marfo, K. (1990). Maternal directiveness in interactions with mentally handicapped children: An analytical commentary. *Journal of Child Psychology and Psychiatry and Allied Disciplines, 31,* 531–549.

Marfo, K. (1992). Correlates of maternal directiveness with children who are developmentally delayed. *American Journal of Orthopsychiatry, 62,* 219–233.

Marinescu, C.R., Johnson, E.I., Dykens, E.M., Hodapp, R.M., & Overhauser, J. (1999). No relationship between the size of the deletion and the level of developmental delay in cri-du-chat syndrome. *American Journal of Medical Genetics, 86,* 66–70.

Martin, A., State, M.W., North, W.G., Hanchette, J., & Leckman, J.F. (1998). Increased CSF oxytocin in patients with Prader-Willi syndrome. *Biological Psychiatry, 44,* 1349-1352.

Martin, J.P., & Bell, J. (1943). A pedigree of mental defect showing sex-linkage. *Journal of Neurological Psychiatry, 6,* 154–157.

Martin, N.D., Snodgrass, G., & Cohen, R.D. (1984). Idiopathic infantile hypercalcemia: A continuing enigma. *Archives of Diseases in Childhood, 59,* 605–613.

Mascari, M.J., Gottlieb, W., Rogan, P.K., Butler, M.G., Waller, D.A., Armour, J.A.L., Jeffreys, A.J., Ladda, R.L., & Nicholls, R.D. (1992). The frequency of uniparental disomy in Prader-Willi syndrome. *New England Journal of Medicine, 326,* 1599–1607.

Matalainen, R., Airaksinen, E., Mononen, T., Launiala, K., & Kaariainen, R. (1995). A population-based study on the causes of severe and profound mental retardation. *Acta Pediatrica, 84,* 261–266.

Matsuura, T., Sutcliffe, J.S., Fang, P., Galjaard, R. J., Jiang, Y., Benton, C.S., Rommens, J.M., & Beaudet, A.L. (1997). De novo truncation mutations in E6-AP ubinquitin-protein ligase gene (UBE3A) in Angelman syndrome. *Nature Genetics, 15,* 74–77.

Mazzocco, M.M., Baumgardner, T., Freund, L.S., & Reiss, A.L. (1998). Social functioning among girls with fragile X or Turner syndromes and their sisters. *Journal of Autism and Developmental Disorders, 28,* 509–517.

Mazzocco, M.M., Hagerman, R.J., & Pennington, B. (1992). Problem-solving limitations among cytogenetically expressing fragile X women. *American Journal of Medical genetics, 43,* 78–86.

Mazzocco, M.M., & Holden, J.A. (1996). Neuropsychological profiles of three sisters homozygious for the fragile X mutation. *American Journal of Medical Genetics, 64,* 323–328.

Mazzocco, M.M., Pennington, & Hagerman, R.J. (1993). The neurocognitive phenotype of female carriers of fragile X: Additional evidence of specificity. *Journal of Developmental and Behavioral Pediatrics, 14,* 328–335.

McCabe, E.R.B., de la Cruz, F., & Clapp, K. (1999) Workshop on fragile X: Future research directions. *American Journal of Medical Genetics, 85,* 317–322.

McConkie-Rosell, A., Spiridigliozzi, G.A., Iafolla, T., Tarleton, J., & Lachiewicz, A.M. (1997). Carrier testing in the fragile X syndrome: Attitudes and opinions of obligate carriers. *American Journal of Medical Genetics, 68,* 62–69.

McDonald-McGinn, D.M., Kirschner, R., Goldmuntz, E., Sullivan, K., Eicher, P., Gerdes, M., Moss, E., Solot, C., Wang, P., Jacobs, I., Handler, S., Knightly, C., Heher, K., Wilson, M., Ming, J.E., Grace, K., Driscoll, D., Pasquariello, P., Randall, P., Larossa, D., Emanuel, B.S., & Zackai, E.H. (1999). The Philadelphia story: The 22q11.2 deletion: Report on 250 patients. *Genetic Counseling, 10,* 11–24.

McGillivray, B.C., Herbst, D.S., Dill, F.J., Sandercock, H.J., & Tischler, B. (1986). Infantile autism: An occasional manifestation of fragile X mental retardation. *American Journal of Medical Genetics, 23,* 353–358.

McGuinness, D. (1997). Decoding strategies as predictors of reading skill: A follow-up study. *Annals of Dyslexia, 47,* 117–150.

Melyn, M., & White, D. (1973). Mental and developmental milestones of non-institutionalized Down's syndrome children. *Pediatrics, 52,* 542–545.

Merenstein, S.A., Sobesky, W.E., Taylor, A.K., Riddle, J.E., Tran, H.X., & Hagerman, R.J. (1996). Molecular-clinical correlations in males with an expanded FMR1 mutation. *American Journal of Medical Genetics, 64,* 388–394.

Mervis, C.B., & Bertrand, J. (1997). Developmenal relations between cognition and language: Evidence from Williams syndrome. In L.B. Adamson & M.A. Romski (Eds.), *Communication and language acquisition: Discoveries from atypical populations* (pp. 75–106). Baltimore: Paul H. Brookes Publishing Co.

Mervis, C.B., Morris, C.A., Bertrand, J.M. & Robinson, B.F. (1999). Williams syndrome: Findings from an integrated program of research. In H. Tager-Flusberg (Ed.), *Neurodevelopmental disorders: Contributions to a framework from the cognitive sciences* (pp. 65–110). Cambridge: MIT Press.

Mervis, C.B., & Robinson, B.F. (1999). Methodological issues in cross-syndrome comparisons: Matching procedures, sensitivity (Se), and specificity (Sp). Commentary on Sigman, M., & Ruskin, E. (1999). Continuity and change in the social competence of children with autism, Down syndrome, and developmental delays. *Monographs of the Society for Research in Child Development, 64*(No. 256), pp. 115–130.

Meryash, D.L. (1989). Perception of burden among at-risk women of raising a child with fragile X syndrome. *Clinical Genetics, 36,* 14–24.

Meryash, D.L., Szymanski, L.S., & Gerald, P. (1982). Infantile autism associated with the fragile X syndrome. *Journal of Autism and Developmental Disorders, 12,* 349–355.

Meyers, B.A. (1987). Psychiatric problems in adolescents with developmental disabilities. *Journal of the American Academy of Child and Adolescent Psychiatry, 26,* 74–79.

Meyers, B.A., & Pueschel, S.M. (1991). Psychiatric disorders in persons with Down syndrome. *The Journal of Nervous and Mental Disease, 179,* 609–613.

Miller, J. (1988). The developmental asynchrony of language development in children with Down syndrome. In L. Nadel (Ed.), *The psychobiology of Down syndrome* (pp. 167–198). Cambridge: MIT Press.

Miller, J. (1992). Lexical development in young children with Down syndrome. In R. Chapman (Ed.), *Processes in language acquisition and disorders* (pp. 202–216). St. Louis, MO: Mosby.

Miller, J., Leddy, M., Miolo, G., & Sedey, A. (1995). The development of early language skills in children with Down syndrome. In L. Nadel & D. Rosenthal (Eds.), *Down syndrome: Living and learning in the community* (pp. 115–120). New York: Wiley-Liss.

Milunsky, A., Jick, H., Jick, S.S., Bruell, C.L., MacLaughlin, D.S., Rothman, K.J., & Willett, W. (1989). Multivitamin/folic acid supplementation in early pregnancy reduces the prevalence of neural tube defects. *JAMA: Journal of the American Medical Association, 262,* 2847–2852.

Minassian, B.A., Delorey, T.M., Olsen, R.W., Philippart, M., Bronstein, Y., Zhang, Q., Guerrini, R., Ness, P.V., Livet, M.O., & Delgado-Escueta, A.V. (1998). Angelman syndrome: Correlations between epilepsy phenotypes and genotypes. *Annals of Neurology, 43,* 485–493.

Mink, I., Nihira, K., & Meyers, C. (1983). Taxonomy of family life styles: I. Homes with TMR children. *American Journal of Mental Deficiency, 87,* 484–497.

Mitchell, J., Schinzel, A., Langlois, S., Gillessen-Kaesbach, G., Schuffenhauer, S., Michaelis, R., Abeliovich, D., Lere, I., Christian, S., Guitart, M., McFadden, D.E., & Robinson, W.P. (1996). Comparison of phenotype in uniparental disomy and deletion Prader-Willi syndrome: Sex specific differences. *American Journal of Medical Genetics, 65,* 133–136.

Morgan, S.B. (1979). Development and distribution of intellectual and adaptive skills in Down Syndrome children: Implications for early intervention. *Mental Retardation, 17,* 247–249.

Morris, C.A., Demsey, S.A., Leonard, C.O., Dilts, C., & Blackburn, B.L. (1988). Natural history of Williams syndrome: Physical characteristics. *Journal of Pediatrics, 113,* 318–326.

Morris, C.A., Leonard, C.O., & Dilts, C. (1990). Adults with Williams syndrome. *American Journal of Medical Genetics* (Suppl. 6), *6,* 102–107.

Morris, C.A., Locker, J., Ensing, G., & Stock, A.D. (1993). Supravalvular aortic stenosis cosegregates with a familial 6;7 translocation which disrupts the elastin gene. *American Journal of Medical Genetics, 46,* 737–744.

Morris, C.A., Thomas, I.T., & Greenberg, F. (1993). Williams syndrome: Autosomal dominant inheritance. *American Journal of Medical Genetics, 47,* 478–481.

Morton, J., & Frith, U. (1993). What lesson for dyslexia from Down's syndrome? (Comments on Cossue, Rossini and Marshall, 1993). *Cognition, 48,* 289–296.

Moser, H.W. (1992). Prevention of mental retardation (genetics). In L. Rowitz (Ed.), *Mental retardation in the year 2000.* New York: Springer-Verlag.

Moser, H.W., & Naidu, S. (1996). The discovery and study of Rett Syndrome: Lessons for the understanding of developmental disabilities. In A.J. Capute and P.J. Accardo, (Eds.) Developmental disabilities in infancy and childhood: Vol. 1 (2nd. ed., pp. 379–386) Baltimore: Paul H. Brookes Publishing Co.

Moss, E.M., Batshaw, M.L., Solot, C.B., Gerdes, M., McDonald-McGinn, D.M., Driscoll, D.A., Emanuel, B.S., Zackai, E.H., & Wang, P.P. (1999). Psychoeducational profile of the 22q11.2 microdeletion: A complex pattern. *Journal of Pediatrics, 134,* 193–198.

Moss, S., Prosser, H., Ibbotson, B., & Goldberg, D. (1996). Respondent and informant accounts of psychiatric symptoms in a sample of patients with learning disability. *Journal of Intellectual Disability Research, 40,* 457–465.

Mostofsky, S.H., Mazzocco, M.M., Aakalu, G., Warsofsky, I.S., Denckla, M.D., & Reiss, A.L. (1998). Decreased cerebellar posterior vermis size in fragile X syndrome: Correlation with neurocognitive performance. *Neurology, 50,* 121–130.

Motzkin, B., Marion, R., Goldberg, R., Shpritzen, R., Saenger, P. (1993). Variable phenotypes in velocardiofacial syndrome with chromosomal deletion. *Journal of Pediatrics, 123,* 406–410.

Murphy, K.C., Jones, R.G., Griffiths, E., Thompson, P.W., & Owen, M.J. (1998). Chromosome 22q11 deletions: An under-recognized cause of idiopathic learning disability. *British Journal of Psychiatry, 172,* 180–183.

National Fragile X Foundation (1994). Denver, CO.

Naglieri, J.A., (1987). *Draw a Person: A Quantitative Scoring System.* San Antonio, TX: The Psychological Corporation.

Neibuhr, E. (1978). The cri du chat syndrome: Epidemiology, cytogenetics, and clinical features. *Human Genetics, 44,* 227–275.

Neville, H.J., Holcomb, P.J., & Mills, D.L. (1989). Auditory sensory and language processing in Williams syndrome: An ERP study. *Journal of Clinical and Experimental Neuropsychology, 11,* 52.

Neville, H.J., Mills, D.L., & Bellugi, U. (1994). Effects of altered auditory sensitivity and age of language acquisition on the development of language-relevant neural systems: Preliminary studies of Williams syndrome. In S. Broman & J. Grafman (Eds.), *Cognitive deficits in the developmental disorders: Implications for brain function* (pp. 67–83). Mahwah, NJ: Lawrence Erlbaum Associates.

Newborg, J., Stock, J.R., Wnek, L., Guidubaldi, J., & Svinicki, J. (1988). *Battelle Developmental Inventory (BDI).* Chicago: Riverside.

Newport, E. (1990). Maturational constraints on language learning. *Cognitive Science, 14,* 11–28.

Nicholls, R.D. (1993). Genomic imprinting and uniparental disomy in Angelman and Prader-Willi syndrome: A review. *American Journal of Medical Genetics, 46,* 16–25.

Nicholls, R.D., Knoll, J.H., Butler, M.G., Karam, S., & Lalande, M. (1989). Genetic imprinting suggested by maternal heterodisomy in nondeletion Prader-Willi syndrome. *Nature, 16,* 281–285.

Nicholson, W.R., & Hockey, K.A. (1993). Williams syndrome: A clinical study of children and adults. *Journal of Paediatric Child Health, 29,* 468–472.

Nielsen, K.B. (1983). Diagnosis of the fragile X syndrome (Martin Bell syndrome): Clinical findings in 27 males with the fragile site at Xq28. *Journal of Mental Deficiency Research, 27,* 211–226.

Nyhan, W.L. (1972). Behavioral phenotypes in organic genetic diseases: Presidential address to the Society for Pediatric Research (May 1, 1971). *Pediatric Research, 6,* 1–9.

Oberle, I., Rousseau, F., Heitz, D., Kretz, C., Devys, D., Hanauer, A., Boue, J., Bertheas, M.F., & Mandel, J.L. (1991). Instability of a 550 -base pair DNA segment and abnormal methylation in fragile X syndrome. *Science, 252,* 1097–1102.

O'Brien, G., & Yule, W. (Eds.). (1995). *Behavioural phenotypes.* London: MacKeith Press.

O'Callaghan, E., Larkin, C., Kinsella, A., & Waddington, J.L. (1991). Familial obstetric, and other clinical correlates of minor physical anomalies in schizophrenia. *American Journal of Psychiatry, 4,* 479–483.

Ollendick, T.H., King, N.J., & Frary, R.B. (1989). Fears in children and adolescents: Reliability and generalizability across age, gender, and nationality. *Behaviour Research and Therapy, 27*, 19–26.

Olsen, R.W., & Avoli, M. (1997). GABA and epileptogenesis. *Epilepsia, 38*, 399–407.

Opitz, J.M. (1996, March). *Historiography of the causal analysis of mental retardation.* Speech to the 29th annual Gatlinburg Conference on Reseach and Theory in Mental Retardation and Developmental Disabilities, Gatlinburg, TN.

Overhauser, J., Huang, X., Gersh, M., Wilson, W., McMahon, J., Bengtsson, U., Rojas, K., Meyer, M., & Wasmuth, J.J. (1994). Molecular and phenotypic mapping of the short arm of chromosome 5: Sublocalization of the critical region for the cri-du-chat syndrome. *Human Molecular Genetics, 3*, 247–252.

Owens, R.E., Jr., & MacDonald, J.D. (1982). Communicative uses of the early speech of non-delayed and Down syndrome children. *American Journal of Mental Deficiency, 86*, 503–510.

Padfield, C.J., Partington, M.W., & Simpson, N.E. (1968). The Rubinstein-Taybi syndrome. *Archives of Diseases in Children, 43*, 94–101.

Pankau, R., Partsch, C.J., Winter, M., Gosch, A., & Wessel, A. (1996). Incidence and spectrum of renal abnormalities in Williams-Beuren syndrome. *American Journal of Medical Genetics, 63*, 301–304.

Papolos, D.F., Faedda, G.L., Veit, S., Goldberg, R., Morrow, B., Kucherlapati, R., & Shpritzen, R.J. (1996). Bipolar spectrum disorders in patients diagnosed with vel-cardio-facial syndrome: Does a hemizygous deletion on chromosome 22q11 result in bipolar affective disorder? *American Journal of Psychiatry, 153*, 1541–1547.

Park, V., Howard-Peebles, P., Sherman, S., Taylor, A., & Wulfsberg, E. (1994). American College of Medical Genetics Policy Statement: Fragile X syndrome: Diagnostic and carrier testing. *American Journal of Medical Genetics, 53*, 380–381.

Partington, M.W. (1984). The fragile X syndrome: II. Preliminary data on growth and development in males. *American Journal of Medical Genetics, 17*, 175–194.

Partsch, C.J., Dreyer, G., Gosch, A., Winter, M., Schneppenheim, R., Wessel, A., & Pankau, R. (1999). Longitudinal evaluation of growth, puberty, and bone maturation in children with Williams syndrome. *Journal of Pediatrics, 134*, 82–89.

Partsch, C.J., Pankau, R., Blum, W.F., Gosch, A., & Wessel, A. (1994). Hormonal regulation in children and adults with Williams syndrome. *American Journal of Medical Genetics, 51*, 251–257.

Pary, R. (1992). Differentail diagnosis of functional decline in Down syndrome. *The Habilitative Medical Healthcare Newsletter, 11*, 37–41.

Paul, R., Cohen, D.J., Breg, R., Watson, M., & Herman, S. (1984). Fragile X syndrome: Its relations to speech and language disorders. *Journal of Speech and Hearing Disorders, 49*, 326–336.

Paul, R., Dykens, E.M., Leckman, J.F., Watson, M., Breg, R., & Cohen, D.J. (1987). A comparison of language characteristics of mentally retarded adults with fragile X syndrome and those with nonspecific mental retardation and autism. *Journal of Autism and Developmental Disorders, 17*, 457–468.

Payton, J.B., Steele, M.W., Wenger, S.L., & Minshew, N. J. (1989). The fragile X marker and autism in persepctive. *Journal of the American Academy of Child and Adolescent Psychiatry, 28*, 417–468.

Penner, K.A., Johnston, J., Faircloth, B.H., Irish, P., & Williams, C.A. (1993).

Communication, cognition, and social interaction in the Angelman syndrome. *American Journal of Medical Genetics, 46,* 34–39.

Pennington, B., O'Connor, R., & Sudhalter, V. (1991). Toward a neuropsychology of fragile X syndrome. In R.J. Hagerman & A.C. Silverman (Eds.), *Fragile X syndrome: Diagnosis, treatment, and research* (pp. 173–201). Baltimore: The Johns Hopkins University Press.

Penrose, L.S. (1933). *Mental defect.* London: Sidgwick & Jackson.

Pezzini, G., Vicari, S., Volterra, V., Milani, L., & Ossella, M.T. (1999). Children with Williams syndrome: Is there a single neuropsychological profile? *Developmental Neuropsychology, 15,* 141–155.4

Piaget, J. (1954). *The construction of reality in the child.* New York: Ballantine.

Piaget, J., & Inhelder, B. (1947). Diagnosis of mental operations and theory of intelligence. *American Journal of Mental Deficiency, 51,* 401–406.

Pike, A.C., & Super, M. (1997). Velocardiofacial syndrome. *Postgraduate Medical Journal, 73,* 771–775.

Pitcairn, T.K., & Wishart, J.G. (1994). Reactions of young children with Down syndrome to an impossible task. *British Journal of Developmental Psychology, 12,* 485–489.

Plissart, L., Borghgraef, M., Volcke, P., Van den Berghe, H., & Fryns, J.P. (1994). Adults with Williams syndrome: Evaluation of the medical, psychological, and behavioral aspects. *Clinical Genetics, 46,* 161–167.

Pober, B.R., & Dykens, E.M. (1996). Williams syndrome: An overview of medical, cognitive, and behavioral features. *Child and Adolescent Psychiatric Clinics of North America, 5,* 929–943.

Pober, B.R., Lacro, R.V., Rice, C., Mandell, V., & Teele, R.L. (1993). Renal findings in 40 individuals with Williams syndrome. *American Journal of Medical Genetics, 46,* 271–274.

Powell, L., Houghton, S., & Douglas, G. (1997). Comparison of etiology-specific cognitive functioning profiles for individuals with Fragile X and individuals with Down syndrome. *Journal of Special Education, 31,* 362–376.

Power, T.J., Blum, N.J., Jones, S.M., & Kaplan, P.E. (1997). Brief report: Response to methylphenidate in two children with Williams syndrome. *Journal of Autism and Developmental Disorders, 27,* 79–87.

Prader, A., Labhart, A. & Willi, A. (1956). Ein syndrom von aidositas, kleinwuchs, kryptorchismus und oligophrenie nach myotonieartigem zustand im neugeborenenalter [A syndrome of obesity, hypogonadism, and learning disability, with hypotonia during the neonatal period]. *Schweizerische Medizinische Wochenschrift, 86,* 1260–1261.

Prasher, V.P. (1995). Overweight and obesity amongst Down syndrome adults. *Journal of Intellectual Disability Research, 39,* 437–441.

Proops, R., and Webb, T. (1981). The 'fragile' X chromosome in the Martin-Bell-Renpenning syndrome and in males with other forms of familial mental retardation. *Journals of Medical Geneticies, 18,* 366–373.

Pueschel, S.M. (1990). Clinical aspects of Down syndrome from infancy to adulthood. *American Journal of Medical Genetics,* [Suppl. 7], 52–56.

Pueschel, S.M., Bernier, J.C., & Pezzullo, J.C. (1991). Behavioral observations in children with Down's syndrome. *Journal of Mental Deficiency Research, 35,* 502–511.

Pueschel, S.M., Gallagher, P., Zartler, A., & Pezzullo, J. (1987). Cognitive and learning processes in children with Down syndrome. *Research in Developmental Disabilities, 8,* 21–37.

Pueschel, S.M., Herman, R., & Groden, G. (1985). Screening children with autism for fragile X syndrome and phenylketonuria. *Journal of Autism and Developmental Disorders, 15,* 335–338.

Pueschel, S.M., & Hopmann, M.R. (1993). Speech and language abilities of children with Down syndrome: A parent's perspective. In A.P. Kaiser & D.B. Gray (Ed.), *Enhancing children's communication: Vol. 2. Research foundations for intervention* (pp. 335–362). Baltimore: Paul H. Brookes Publishing Co.

Pulver, A.E., Nestadt, G., Shpritzen, R.J., Lamacz, M., Wolyniec, P.S., Morrow, B., Karayiorgou, M., Antonarakis, S.E., Housman, D., & Kucherlapati, R. (1994). Psychotic illness in patients diagnosed with velo-cardio-facial syndrome and their relatives. *Journal of Nervous and Mental Disease 182,* 476–478.

Punnett, H.H., & Zakai, E.H. (1990). Old syndromes and new cytogenetics. *Developmental Medicine and Child Neurology, 32,* 820–831.

Rasore-Quartino, A., & Cominetti, M. (1995). Clinical follow-up of adolescents and adults with Down syndrome. In L. Nadel & D. Rosenthal (Eds.), *Down syndrome: Living and learning in the community* (pp. 238–245). New York: Wiley-Liss.

Reilly, J.S., Klima, E.S., & Bellugi, U. (1991). Once more with feeling: Affect and language in atypical populations. *Developmental Psychopathology, 2,* 367–391.

Reiss, S. (1988). Reiss Screen for Maladaptive Behavior. Chicago: International Diagnostic Systems, Inc.

Reiss, A.L., Abrams, M.T., Greenlaw, R., Freund, L., & Denckla, M.B. (1995). Neurodevelopmental effects of the FMR-1 full mutation in humans. *Nature Medicine, 1,* 159–167.

Reiss, A.L., Aylward, E., Freund, L.S., Joshi, P.K., & Bryan, R.N. (1991). Neuroanatomy of Fragile X syndrome: the posterior fossa. *Annals of Neurology, 29,* 26–32.

Reiss, A.L., Feinstein, C., Rosenbaum, K.N., Borengasser-Caruso, & Goldsmith, B.M. (1985). Autism associated with Williams syndrome. *The Journal of Pediatrics, 106,* 247–249.

Reiss, A.L., & Freund, L. (1990). Fragile X syndrome, DSM-III-R and autism. *Journal of the American Academy of Child and Adolescent Psychiatry, 29,* 855–891.

Reiss, A.L., & Freund, L. (1992). Behavioral phenotype of fragile X syndrome: DSM-III-R autistic behavior in male children. *American Journal of Medical Genetics, 43,* 35–46.

Reiss, A.L., Freund, L., Abrams, M.T., Boehm, C., & Kazazian, H. (1993). Neurobehavioral effects of the fragile X premutation in adult women: A controlled study. *American Journal of Human Genetics, 52,* 884–894.

Reiss, A.L., Freund, L.S., Baumgardner, T.L., Abrams, M.T., & Denckla, M.B. (1995). Contribution of the FMR-1 gene mutation to human intellectual dysfunction. *Nature Genetics, 11,* 331–334.

Reiss, A.L., Freund, L., Vinogradov, S., Hagerman, R.J., & Cronister, A. (1989). Parental inheritance and psychological disability in fragile X females. *American Journal of Human Genetics, 45,* 697–705.

Reiss, A.L., Hagerman, R.J., Vinogradov, A., Abrams, M., & King, R.J. (1988). psychiatric disability in female carriers of the fragile X chromosome. *Archives of General Psychiatry, 45,* 25–30.

Reiss, A.L., Lee, J., & Freund, L. (1994). Neuroanatomy of fragile X syndrome: The temporal lobe. *Neurology, 44,* 1317–1324.

Reiss, S., & Havercamp, S.M. (1998). Toward a comprehensive assessment of fundamental motivation: The factor structure of the Reiss profiles. *Psychological Assessment, 10,* 97–106.

Rhoads, F.A. (1984). Fragile X syndrome in Hawaii: A summary of clinical experience. *American Journal of Medical Genetics, 17,* 209–214.

Riccardi, V.M. (1977). Trisomy 8: An international study of 70 patients. In D.

Bergsma (Ed.), *Birth defects: Original article series, Vol. XIII, No. 3C* (pp. 171–184). White Plains, NY: National Foundation.

Riddle, J.E., Cheema, A., Sobesky, W.E., Gardner, S.C., Taylor, A.K., Pennington, B.F., & Hagerman, R.J. (1998). Phenotypic involvement in females with the FMR1 gene mutation. *American Journal on Mental Retardation, 102,* 590–601.

Robinson, W.P., Bottani, A., Yagang, X., Balakrishman, J., Binkert, F., Machler, M., Prader, A., & Schinzel, A. (1991). Molecular, cytogenetic and clinical investigations of Prader-Willi syndrome patients. *American Journal of Human Genetics, 49,* 1219–1234.

Robinson, W.P., Bernasconi, F., Mutiranguara, A., Ledbetter, D.H., Langlois, S., Malcom, S., Morris, M., & Schinzel, A.A. (1993). Non-disjunction of chromosome 15: Origin and recombination. *American Journal of Human Genetics, 53,* 740–751.

Robinson, H., Wake, S., Wright, F., Laing, S., & Turner, G. (1996). Informed choice in fragile X syndrome and its effects on prevalence. *American Journal of Medical Genetics, 64,* 198–202.

Rodrigue, J.R., Morgan, S.B., & Geffken, G.R. (1991). A comparative evaluation of adaptive behavior in children and adolescents with autism, Down syndrome, and normal development. *Journal of Autism and Developmental Disorders, 21,* 187–196.

Rohr, A., & Burr, D.B. (1978). Etiological differences in patterns of psycholinguistic development of children of IQ 30 to 60. *American Journal of Mental Deficiency, 87,* 549–553.

Roizen, N.J. (1996). Down syndrome and associated medical disorders. *Mental Retardation and Developmental Disability Research Reviews, 2,* 85–89.

Roizen, N.J., Luke, A., Sutton, M., & Schoeller, D.A. (1995). Obesity and nutrition in children with Down syndrome. In L. Nadel & D. Rosenthal (Eds.), *Down syndrome: Living and learning in the community* (pp. 213–215). New York: Wiley-Liss.

Roizen, N.J., Walters, C., Nicol, T., & Blondes, T.A. (1993). Hearing loss in children with Down syndrome. *Journal of Pediatrics, 123,* S9–S12.

Rondal, J. (1977). Maternal speech in normal and Down's Syndrome children. In P. Mittler (Ed.), *Research to practice in mental retardation: Education and training* (Vol. 3, pp. 239–243). Baltimore: University Park Press.

Rondal, J. (1995). *Exceptional language development in Down syndrome.* New York: Cambridge University Press.

Rondal, J. (1996). Oral language in Down's syndrome. In J. Rondal, J. Perera, L. Nadel, & A. Comblain (Eds.), *Down's syndrome: Psychological, psychobiological, and socio-educational perspectives* (pp. 99–117). London: Whurr Publishers.

Rondal, J., Ghiotto, M., Bredart, S., & Bachelet, J.F. (1988). Mean length of utterance of children with Down syndrome. *American Journal on Mental Retardation, 93,* 64–66.

Rosenberg, & Abbeduto, L. (1993). *Language and communication in mental retardation: Development, processes, and intervention.* Mahwah, NJ: Lawrence Erlbaum Associates.

Rosin, M. M., Swift, E., Bless, D., & Vetter, D. K. (1988). Communication profiles of adolescents with Down syndrome. *Journal of Childhood Communication Disorders, 12,* 49–64.

Rourke, B.P. (1995). (Ed.). *Syndrome of nonverbal learning disabilities: Neurodevelopmental manifestations.* New York: Guilford Press.

Rousseau, F., Rouillard, P., Morel, M.L., Khandjian, E.W., & Morgan, K. (1995).

Prevalence of carriers of premutation-size alleles of the FMR-1 gene- and implications for the population genetics of fragile X syndrome. *American Journal of Human Genetics, 57,* 1006–1018.

Rubinstein, J.H. (1990). Broad thumb-hallux (Rubinstein-Taybi) syndrome. *American Journal of Medical Genetics Supplement, 6,* 3–16.

Rubinstein, J.H., & Taybi, H. (1963). Broad thumbs and toes and facial abnormalities: A possible mental retardation syndrome. *American Journal of Diseases in Children, 105,* 88–108.

Rumsey, J.M. (1996). Neuroimaging studies of autism. In G.Rein Lyon & J.M. Rumsey (Eds.), *Neuroimaging: A window to the neurological foundations of learning and behavior in children* (pp. 119–146). Baltimore: Paul H. Brookes Publishing Co.

Ruskin, E., Kasari, C., Mundy, P., & Sigman, M. (1994). Attention to people and toys during social and object mastery in children with Down syndrome. *American Journal of Mental Retardation, 99,* 103–111.

Rutter, M., Bailey, A., Bolton, P., & Le Couteur, A. (1994). Autism and known medical conditions: Myth and substance. *Journal of Child Psychology and Psychiaty, 35,* 311–322.

Rutter, M., Simonoff, E., & Plomin, R. (1996). Genetic influences on mild mental retardation: Concepts, findings, and research implications. *Journal of Biosocial Science, 28,* 509–526.

Saitoh, S., Buiting, K., Cassidy, S.B., Conroy, J.M., Driscoll, D.J., Gabriel, J.M., Gillessen-Kaesbach, G., Clenn, C.C., Greenswag, L.R., Horsthemke, B., Kondo, I., Kuwajima, K., Niikawa, N., Rogan, P.K., Schwartz, S., Seip, J., Williams, C.A., Wiznitzer, M., & Nicholas, R.D. (1997). Clinical spectrum and molecular diagnosis of Angelman and Prader-Willi syndrome imprinting mutation patients. *American Journal of Medical Genetics, 68,* 195–206.6,

Salthouse, T.A. (1984). Effects of age and skill in typing. *Journal of Experimental Psychology: General, 113,* 345–371.

Sarimski, K. (1997). Behavioural phenotypes and family stress in three mental retardation syndroems. *European Child and Adolescent Psychiatry, 6,* 26–31.6

Scarr, S. (1993). Developmental theories for the 1990s: Development and individual differences. *Child Development, 63,* 1–19.

Scharfenaker, S., Hickman, L., & Braden, M. (1991). An integrated approach to intervention. In R.J. Hagerman & A.C. Silverman (Eds.), *Fragile X syndrome: Diagnosis, treatment, and research* (pp. 327–372). Baltimore: The Johns Hopkins University Press.

Scheerenberger, R. (1983). *A history of mental retardation.* Baltimore: Paul H. Brookes Publishing Co.

Schreinmachers, D.M., Cross, P.K., & Hook, E.B. (1982). Rates of trisomies 21, 18, 13 and other chromosome abnormalities in about 20,000 prenatal studies compared with estimated rates in live births. *Human Genetics, 61,* 318.

Scott, P., Mervis, C.B., Bertrand, J., Klein, B.P., Armstrong, S.C., & Ford, A.J. (1995). Semantic organization and word fluency in 9- and 10-year-old children with Williams syndrome. *Genetic Couseling, 6,* 172–173.

Seguin, J.A., & Hodapp, R.M. (1998). *Transition from school to adult services in Prader-Willi syndrome: What parents need to know.* Roslyn Heights, NY: Prader-Willi Perspectives. (Available from the PWSA-USA, 1-800-926-4797).

Seguin, J.A., & Hodapp, R.M. (1999). *Transition issues of individuals with Prader-Willi syndrome versus with Down syndrome.* Manuscript submitted for publication.

Seltzer, M., Krauss, M.W., & Tsunematsu, N. (1993). Adults with Down syndrome and their aging mothers: Diagnostic group differences. *American Journal on Mental Retardation, 97,* 496–508.

Seltzer, M., & Ryff, C. (1994). Parenting across the lifespan: The normative and nonnormative cases. *Life-Span Development and Behavior, 12,* 1–40.

Shepperdson, B. (1995). Two longitudinal studies of the abilities of people with Down's syndrome. *Journal of Intellectual Disability Research, 39,* 419–431.

Silverstein, A.B., Legutki, G., Friedman, S.L., & Takayama, D.L. (1982). Performance of Down syndrome individuals on the Stanford-Binet Intelligence Scale. *American Journal of Mental Deficiency, 86,* 548–551.

Simon, E.W., & Finucane, B.M. (1996). Facial emotion identification in males with fragile X syndrome. *American Journal of Medical Genetics, 67,* 77–80.

Simon, E.W., Rappaport, D.A., Papka, M., & Woodruff-Pak, D.S. (1995). Fragile-X and Down's syndrome: Are there syndrome-specific cognitive profiles at low IQ levels? *Journal of Intellectual Disability Research, 39,* 326–330.

Skuse, D.H., James, R.S., Bishop, D.V.M., Coppins, B., Dalton, P., Aamodt-Leeper, G., Bacarese-Hamilton, M., Creswell, C., McGurk, R., & Jacobs, P.A. (1997). Evidence from Turner's syndrome of an imprinted X-linked locus affecting cognitive function. *Nature, 387,* 705–708.

Sloper, P., Cunningham, P., Turner, S., & Knussen, C. (1990). Factors related to the academic attainment of children with Down's syndrome. *British Journal of Educational Psychology, 60,* 284–298.

Sloper, P., & Turner, S. (1996). Progress in social-independent functioning of young people with Down's syndrome. *Journal of Intellectual Disability Research, 40,* 39–48.

Smith, A., Field, B., Murray, R., Nelson, J. (1990). Two cases of cri-du-chat syndrome with mild phenotypic effect but with different size of 5p deletion. *Journal of Paediatrics and Child Health, 26,* 152–154.

Smith, A., Marks, R., Haan, E., Dixon, J., & Trent, R.J. (1997). Clinical features in four patients with Angelman syndrome resulting from paternal uinparental disomy. *Journal of Medical Genetics, 34,* 426–429.

Smith, A., Robson, L., & Buchholz, B. (1998). Normal growth in Angelman syndrome due to paternal UPD. *Clinical Genetics, 53,* 223–225.

Smith, A., Wiles, C., Haan, E., McGill, J., Wallace, G., Dixon, J., Selby, R., Cooley, A., Marks, R., & Trent, R.J. (1996). Clinical features in 27 patients with Angelman syndrome reulting from DNA deletion. *Journal of Medical Genetics, 22,* 107–112.

Smith, A.C.M., Dykens, E.M., & Greenberg, F. (1998a). The behavioral phenotype of Smith-Magenis syndrome. *American Journal of Medical Genetics, 81,* 179–185.

Smith, A.C.M., Dykens, E.M., & Greenberg, F. (1998b). Sleep disturbance in Smith-Magenis syndrome. *American Journal of Medical Genetics, 81,* 186–191.

Smith, A.C.M., McGavran, L., Robinson, J., Waldstein, G., Macfarlane, J., Zonona, J., Reiss, J., Lahr, M., Allen, L., & Magenis, E. (1986). Interstitial deletion of (17)(p11.2 p11.2) in nine patients. *American Journal of Medical Genetics, 24,* 393–414.

Smith, A.C.M., McGavran, L., Waldstein, G., & Robinson, J. (1982). Deletion of the 17 short arm in two patients with facial clefts and congenital heart disease. *American Journal of Human Genetics, 34,* A410.

Snow, C.P. (1993). *The two cultures.* New York: Cambridge University Press (Original work published 1959)

Sobesky, W.E., Hull, C.E., & Hagerman, R.J. (1994). Symptoms of schizotypal personality disorder in fragile X women. *Journal of American Academy of Child and Adolescent Psychiatry, 33,* 247–255.

Sobesky, W.E., Pennington, B.F., Porter, D., Hull, C.E., & Hagerman, R.J. (1994). Emotional and neurocognitive deficits in Fragile X. *American Journal of Medical Genetics, 51,* 378–385.

Sobesky, W.E., Porter, D., Pennington, B.F., & Hagerman, R.J. (1995). Dimensions of shyness in fragile X females. *Developmental Brain Dysfunction, 8,* 280–292.

Sobesky, W.E., Taylor, A.K., Pennington, B.F., Bennetto, L., Porter, D., Riddle, J., & Hagerman, R.J. (1996). Molecular/clinical correlations in females with fragile X. *American Journal of Medical Genetics, 64,* 340–345.

Sohner, L., & Mitchell, P. (1991). Phonatory and phonetic characteristics of prelinguistic vocal development in cri du chat syndrome. *Journal of Communication Disorders, 24,* 13–20.

Solnit, A., & Stark, M. (1961). Mourning and the birth of a defective child. *The Psychoanalytic Study of the Child, 16,* 523–537.

Songster, T.B., Smith, G., Evans, M., Munson, D., & Behen, D. (1997). Special Olympics and athletes with Down syndrome. In S.M. Pueschel & M. Šustrová (Eds.), *Adolescents with Down syndrome: Toward a more fulfilling life* (pp. 341–357). Baltimore: Paul H. Brookes Publishing Co.

Sovner, R., Hurley, A.D., & Labrie, R. (1985). Is mania compatible with Down's syndrome? *British Journal of Psychiatry, 146,* 319–320.

Sparrow, S., Balla, D., & Cicchetti, D. (1984). *Vineland Adaptive Behavior Scales–Interview Edition.* Circle Pines, MN: American Guidance Service.

Stalker, H.J., & Williams, C.A. (1998). Genetic counseling in Angelman syndrome: The challenge of multiple causes. *American Journal of Medical Genetics, 77,* 54–59.

State, M., Dykens, E.M., Rosner, B., Martin, A., & King, B.H. (1999). Obsessive-compulsive symptoms in Prader-Willi and "Prader-Willi-like" patients. *Journal of the American Academy of Child and Adolescent Psychiatry, 38,* 329–334.

Stavrou, E. (1990). The long-term stability of WISC-R scores in mildly retarded and learning disabled children. *Psychology in the Schools, 27,* 101–110.

Stein, D.J., Keating, K., Zar, H.J & Hollander, E. (1994). A survey of the phenomenology and pharmacotherapy of compulsive and impulsive-aggressive symptoms in Prader-Willi syndrome. *The Journal of Neuropsychiatry and Clinical Neuroscience, 6,* 23–29.

Stevens, C.A., Carey, J.C., & Blackburn, B.L. (1990). Rubinstein-Taybi syndrome: A natural history study. *American Journal of Medical Genetics Supplement, 6,* 30–37.

Steyaert, J., Decruyevaere, M., Bohrgraef, M., & Fryns, J. P. (1994). Personality profile in adult female fragile X carriers: Assessed with the Minnesota Multiphasic Personality Profile (MMPI). *American Journal of Medical Genetics, 51,* 370–373.

Stoneman, Z. (1998). Research on siblings of children with mental retardation: Contributions of developmental theory and etiology. In J.A. Burack, R.M. Hodapp, & E. Zigler (Eds.), *Handbook on mental retardation and development.* New York: Cambridge University Press.

Stratton, R.F., Dobyns, W.B., Greenberg, F., DeSana, J.B., Moore, C., Fidone, G., Runge, G.H., Feldman, P., Sekhon, G.S., Pauli, R.M., & Ledbetter, D.H. (1986). Interstitial deletion of (17)(p11.2 p11.2): Report of six additional patients with a new chromosome deletion syndrome. *American Journal of Medical Genetics, 24,* 421–432.

Sudhalter, V., Cohen, I., Silverman, W., & Wolf-Schein, E. (1990). Conversational analyses of males with fragile X syndrome, Down syndrome, and autism: Comparison of the emergence of deviant language. *American Journal on Mental Retardation, 94,* 431–441.

Sulzbacher, S., Crnic, K., & Snow, J. (1981). Behavioral and cognitive disabilities in Prader-Willi syndrome. In V.A. Holm, S. Sulzbacher, & P. Pipes (Eds.), *Prader-Willi syndrome* (pp. 147–169). Baltimore: University Park Press.

Summers, J.A., Allison, D.B., Lynch, P.S., & Sandler, L. (1995). Behaviour problems in Angelman syndrome. *Journal of Intellectual Disability Research, 39,* 97–106.

Summers, J.A., & Feldman, M.A. (1999). Distinctive pattern of behavioral functioning in Angelman syndrome. *American Journal on Mental Retardation, 104,* 376–384.

Sutherland, G.R. (1977). Fragile cites on human chromosomes, demonstration of their dependence on the type of tissue culture medium. *Science, 197,* 265–266.

Swaab, D.F. (1997). Prader-Willi syndrome and the hypothalamus, *Acta Paediatrica* (Suppl.) *423,* 50–54.

Swaab, D.F., Purba, J.S., & Hofman, M.A. (1995). Alterations in the hypothalamic paraventricular nucleus and its oxytocin neurons (putative satiety cells) in Prader-Willi syndrome: A study of 5 cases. *Journal of Clinical Endocrinology and metabolism, 80,* 573–579.

Swillen, A., Devriendt, K., Legius, E., Eyskens, B., Dumoulin, M., Gewillig, M., & Fryns, J.P. (1997). Intelligence and psychosocial adjustment in velocardiofacial syndrome: A study of 37 children and adolescents. *Journal of Medical Genetics, 34,* 453–458.

Symons, F.J., Butler, M.G., Sanders, M.D., Feurer, I.D., & Thompson, T. (1999). Self-injurious behavior and Prader-Willi syndrome: Behavioral forms and body locations. *American Journal on Mental Retardation, 104,* 260–269.

Szymanski, L.S. & Biederman, J. (1984). Depression and anorexia nervosa of persons with Down syndrome. *American Journal of Mental Deficiency, 89,* 246–251.

Tager-Flusberg, H., Boshart, J., & Baron-Cohen, S. (1998). Reading the windows to the soul: Evidence of domain-specific sparing in Williams syndrome. *Journal of Cognitive Neuroscience, 10,* 631–639.

Tannock, R. (1988). Mothers' directiveness in their interactions with children with and without Down syndrome. *American Journal on Mental Retardation, 93,* 154–165.

Tassabehji, M., Metcalfe, K., Karmiloff-Smith, A., Carette, M.J., Grant, J., Dennis, N., Reardon, W., Splitt, M., Read, A.P., & Donnai, D. (1999). Williams syndrome: Use of chromosomal microdeletions as a tool to dissect cognitive and physical characteristics. *American Journal of Human Genetics, 64,* 118–125.

Tassone, F.L., Hagerman, R.J., Ikle, D., Dyer, P.N., Lampe, M., Willemsen, R., Oostra, B.A., & Taylor, A.K. (1999). FMRP expression as a potential prognostic indicator in fragile X syndrome. *American Journal of Medical Genetics, 84,* 250–261.

Taylor, R.L. (1988). Cognitive and behavioral features. In M.L. Caldwell & R.L. Taylor (Eds.), *Prader-Willi syndrome: Selected research and management issues* (pp. 29–42). New York: Springer-Verlag.

Taylor, R.L., & Caldwell, M.L. (1985). Type and strength of food preferences of individuls with Prader-Willi syndrome. *American Journal of Mental Deficiency, 29,* 109–112.

Terman, L.M., & Merrill, M.A. (1960). *Stanford-Binet Intelligence Scale.* Boston: Houghton Mifflin.

Thapar, A., Gottesman, I.I., Owen, M.J., O'Donovan, M.C., & McGuffin, P. (1994). The genetics of mental retardation. *British Journal of Psychiatry, 164:,* 747–758.

Thase, M.E., Liss, L., Smeltzer, D.J., & Maloon, J. (1982). Clinical evaluation of dementia in Down's syndrome: A preliminary report. *Journal of Mental Deficiency Research, 26,* 239–244.

Thase, M.E., Tigner, R., Smeltzer, D.J., & Liss, L. (1984). Age-related neuropsychological deficits in Down's syndrome. *Biological Psychiatry, 19,* 571–585.

Thomas, V., & Olsen, D.H. (1993). Problem families and the circumplex model: Observational assessment using the clinical rating scale (CRS). *Journal of Marital and Family Therapy, 19,* 159–175.

Thompson, N.M., Gulley, M.L., Rogeness, G.A., Clayton, R.J., Johnson, C., Hazelot, B., Cho, C.G., & Zellmer, V.T. (1994). Neurobehavioral characteristics of CGG amplification status in fragile X females. *American Journal of Medical Genetics, 54,* 378–383.

Thompson, M.M., Rogeness, G.A., McClure, E., Clayton, R., & Johnson, C. (1996). Influence of depression on cognitive functioning in fragile X females. *Psychiatry Research, 64,* 97–104.

Thompson, T., Roof, E., Dimitropoulos, A., Feurer, I., Stone, W., & Butler, M.G. (1999, July). *Obsessive-compulsive and maladaptive features of Prader-Willi syndrome.* Presentation to the 13th annual meeting of the Prader-Willi Syndrome Association Scientific Conference, Columbus, OH.

Thorndike, R.L., Hagen, E.P., & Sattler, J.M. (1986). *Technical manual: Stanford-Binet Intelligence Scale* (4th ed.). Chicago: Riverside Publishing.

Tint, G.S., Irons, M., Elias, E.R., Batta, A.K., Frieden, R., Chen, T.S., & Salen, G. (1994). Defective cholesterol biosynthesis associated with the Smith-Lemli-Opitz syndrome. *New England Journal of Medicine, 330,* 107–113.

Tomc, S.A., Williamson, N.K., & Pauli, R.M. (1990). Temperament in Williams syndrome. *American Journal of Medical Genetics, 36,* 345–352.

Torff, B., & Gardner, H. (1999). The vertical mind—the case for multiple intelligences. In M. Anderson (Ed.), *The development of intelligence* (pp. 139–159). East Sussex, England: Psychology Press, Ltd.

Tranebjaerg, L., & Kure, P. (1991). Prevalence of fra(X) and other specific diagnoses in autistic individuals in a Danish county. *American Journal of Meidcal Genetics, 38,* 212–214.

Turk, J., & Cornish, K. (1998). Face recognition and emotion perception in boys with fragile X syndrome. *Journal of Intellectual Disability Research, 42,* 490–499.

Turner, G., Webb, T., Wake, S., & Robinson, H. (1996). Prevalence of fragile X syndrome. *American Journal of Medical Genetics, 64,* 197–197.

Tyler, L.K., Karmiloff-Smith, A., Voice, K., Stevens, T., Grant, J., Udwin, O., Davies, M., & Howlin, P. (1997). Do individuals with Williams syndrome have bizarre semantics? Evidence for lexical organization using an on-line task. *Cortex, 33,* 515–527.

Udwin, O. (1990). A survey of adults with Williams syndrome and idiopathic infantile hypercalcemia. *Developmental Medicine and Child Neurology, 32,* 129–141.

Udwin, O., Davies, M., & Howlin, P. (1996). A longitudinal study of cognitive abilities and educational attainment in Williams syndrome. *Developmental Medicine and Child Neurology, 38,* 1020–1029.

Udwin, O., & Dennis, J. (1995). Psychological and behavioural phenotypes in genetically determined syndromes: A review of research findings. In G. O'Brien & W. Yule (Eds.), *Behavioural phenotypes* (pp. 90–208). London: MacKeith Press.

Udwin, O., Howlin, P., Davies, M., & Mannion, E. (1998). Community care for adults with Williams syndrome: How families cope and the availability of support networks. *Journal of Intellectual Disability Research, 42,* 238–245.

Udwin, O., & Yule, W. (1988). *Children with Williams syndrome: Guidelines for teachers.* Essex, UK: Infantile Hypercalcaemia Foundation Limited.

Udwin, O., & Yule, W. (1990). Expressive language of children with Williams syndrome. *American Journal of Medical Genetics Supplement, 6,* 108–114.

Udwin, O., & Yule, W. (1991). A cognitive and behavioral phenotype in Williams syndrome. *Journal of Clinical and Experimental Neuropsychology, 13,* 232–244.

Udwin, O., Yule, W., & Martin, N. (1987). Cognitive abilities and behavioral characteristics of children with idiopathic infantile hypercalcemia. *Journal of Child Psychology and Psychiatry, 13,* 232–244.

Van Borsel, J., Curfs, L.M.G., & Fryns, J.P. (1997). Hyperacusis in Williams syndrome: A sample survey. *Genetic Counseling, 8,* 121–126.

van Lieshout, C.F.M., de Meyer, R.E., Curfs, L.M.G., & Fryns, J.P. (1998). Family contexts, parental behaviour, and personality profiles of children and adolescents with Prader-Willi, fragile X, or Williams syndrome. *Journal of Child Psychology and Psychiatry, 39,* 699–710.

Venter, P.A., Op'lHof, J., Coezee, D.S., Van de Wa, H.C., & Retie, F. (1984). No marker X chromosome in autistic children. *Human Genetics, 67,* 107.

Verhoeven, W.M.A., Curfs, L.M.G., & Tuinier, S. (1998). Prader-Willi syndrome and cycloid psychoses. *Journal of Intellectual Disability Research, 42,* 455–462.

Verkerk, A.J., Pieretti, M., Sutcliffe, J.S., Fu, Y.-H, Kuhi, D.P., Pizzuti, A., Reiner, O., Richards, S., Victoria, M.F., Zhang, F., Eussen, B.E., Van Ommen, G.J., Blonden, L.A., Riggens, G.J., Chastain, J.L., Kunst, C.B., Galjaard, H., Caskey, C.T., Nelson, D.L., Oostra, B.A., & Warren, S.T. (1991). Identification of a gene (FMR-1) containing a CHGG repeat coincident with a breakpoint cluster region exhibiting length variation in fragile X syndrome. *Cell, 65,* 905–914.

Vicari, S., Brizzolara, D., Carlesimo, G.A., Pezzini, G., & Volterra, V. (1996). Memory abilities in children with Williams syndrome. *Cortex, 32,* 503–514.

Vicari, S., Carlesimo, G., Brizzolara, D., & Pezzi, G. (1996). Short-term memory in Williams syndrome: A reduced contribution of lexical-semantic knowledge to word span. *Neuropsychologia, 34,* 919–925.

Vietze, P., Abernathy, S., Ashe, M., & Faulstich, G. (1978). Contingency interaction between mothers and their developmentally delayed infants. In G.P. Sackett (Ed.), *Observing behavior.* (Vol. 1, pp. 115–132). Baltimore: University Park Press.

Vitiello, B., Spreat, S., & Behar, D. (1989). Obsessive-compulsive disorder in mentally retarded patients. *Journal of Nervous and Mental Disease, 177,* 232–236.

Volterra, V., Capirci, O., Pezzini, G., Sabbadini, L., & Vicari, S. (1996). Linguistic abilities in Italian children with Williams syndrome. *Cortex, 32,* 663–677.

von Armin, G., & Engel, P. (1964). Mental retardation related to hypercalcemia. *Developmental Medicine and Child Neurology, 6,* 366–377.

Vygotsky, L. (1993). Defect and compensation. In R.W. Rieber & A.S. Carton

(Eds.), *The collected works of L.S. Vygotsky: Vol. 2. The fundamentals of defectology* (pp. 52–64). New York: Plenum. (Original work published 1927)

Wahlstrom, J., Gillberg, C., Gustavson, K.H., & Holgren, G. (1986). Infantile autism and the fragile X: A Swedish multicenter study. *American Journal of Medical Genetics, 23,* 403–408.

Wahlstrom, J., Steffenberg, S., Helgren, L., & Gillberg, C. (1989). Chromosome findings in twins with early-onset autistic disorder. *American Journal of Medical Genetics, 32,* 19–21.

Waisbren, S.E., Brown, M.J., de Sonneville, L.M.J., & Levy, H.L. (1994). Review of neuropsychological functioning in treated phenylketonuria. *Acta Paediatrica* (Suppl. 407), 98–103.

Wallerstein, R., Anderson, C.E., Hay, B., Gupta, P., Gibas, L., Ansari, K., Cowchock, F.S., Weinblatt, V., Reid, C., Levitas, A., & Jackson, L. (1997). Submicroscopic deletions at 16p13.1 in Rubinstein-Taybi syndrome: Frequency and clinical manifestations in a North American population. *Journal of Medical Genetics, 34,* 203–206.

Wang, P.P. (1996). A neuropsychological profile of Down syndrome: Cognitive and brain morphology. *Mental Retardation and Developmental Disability Research Reviews, 2,* 102–108.

Wang, P.P., & Bellugi, U. (1994). Evidence from two genetic syndromes for a dissociation between verbal and visual-spatial short-term memory. *Journal of Clincal and Experimental Neuropsychology, 16,* 317–322.

Wang, P.P., Doherty, S., Hesselink, J.R., & Bellugi, U. (1992). Callosal morphology concurs with neurobehavioral and neuropathological findings in two neurodevelopmental disorders. *Archives of Neurology, 49,* 407–411.

Wang, P.P., Doherty, S., Rourke, S.B., & Bellugi, U. (1995). Unique profile of visuo-perceptual skills in a genetic syndrome. *Brain and Cognition, 29,* 54–65.

Warnock, J.K., & Kestenbaum, T. (1992). Pharmacologic treatment of severe skin-picking behaviors in Prader-Willi syndrome. *Archives of Dermatology, 128,* 1623–1625.

Warren, A.C., Holroyd, S., & Folstein, M.F. (1989). Major depression in Down's syndrome. *British Journal of Psychiatry, 155,* 202–205.

Warren, J., & Hunt, E. (1981). Cognitive processing in children with Prader-Willi syndrome. In V.A. Holm, S. Sulzbacher, & P. Pipes (Eds.), *Prader-Willi syndrome* (pp. 161–177). Baltimore: University Park Press.

Waters, J., Clarke, D.J., & Corbett, J.A. (1990). Educational and occupational outcome in Prader-Willi syndrome. *Child: Care, Health, and Development, 16,* 271–282.

Watson, J.D., & Crick, F.H.C. (1953). Molecular structure of nucleic acids: A structure for deoxyribose nucleic acid. *Nature, 171,* 737–738.

Watson, M.S., Leckman, J.F., Annex, B., Breg, R.W., Boles, D., Volkmar, R.R., Cohen, D.J., & Carter, C. (1984). Fragile X syndrome in a survey of 75 autistic males. *New England Journal of Medicine, 301,* 1462.

Wechsler, D. (1974). *Manual for the Wechsler Intelligence Scale for Children–Revised.* San Antonio, TX: The Psychological Corporation.

Wechsler, D. (1981). *Manual for the Wechsler Adult Intelligence Scale–Revised.* San Antonio, TX: The Psychological Corporation.

Wechsler, D. (1991). *Manual for the Wechsler Intelligence Scale for Children* (3rd ed.). San Antonio, TX: The Psychological Corporation.

Weller, E.L., & Mahoney, G. (1983). A comparison of oral and total communication modalities on the language training of young mentally handicapped children. *Education and Training in Mental Retardation, 18,* 103–110.

Werner, E. (1993). Risk, resilience, and recovery: Perspectives from the Kauai longitudinal study. *Development and Psychopathology, 5,* 503–515.

Werner, H., & Strauss, A. (1939). Problems and methods of functional analysis in mentally deficient children. *Journal of Abnormal and Social Psychology, 34,* 37–62.

Wessel, A., Pankau, R., Berdau, W., & Leons, P. (1997). Aortic stiffness with the Williams-Beuren syndrome. *Pediatric Cardiology, 18,* 244.

Wessel, A., Pankau, R., Kececioglu, D., Rushewski, W., & Beursch, J.H. (1994). Three decades of follow-up of aortic and pulmonary vascular lesions in the Williams-Beuren syndrome. *American Journal of Medical Genetics, 52,* 297–301.

Whitman, B.Y., & Accardo, P. (1987). Emotional problems in Prader-Willi adolescents. *American Journal of Medical Genetics, 28,* 897–905.

Wiegers, A.M., Curfs, L.M.G., Vermeer, E.L. M.H., & Fryns, J.P. (1993). Adaptive behavior in the fragile X syndrome: profile and development. *American Journal of Medical Genetics, 47,* 216–220.

Wiig, E.H., Secord, W., & Semel, E. (1992). *Clinical Evaluation of Language Fundamentals Manual.* San Antonio, TX: The Psychological Corporation.

Wilkins, L.E., Brown, J.A., & Nance, W.E., Wolf, B. (1983). Clinical heterogeneity in 80 home-reared children with cri du chat syndrome. *The Journal of Pediatrics, 102,* 528–533.

Willems, P.J., Reyniers, E., & Oostra, B.A. (1995). An animal model for fragile X syndrome. *Mental retardation and Developmental Disability Research Reviews, 1,* 298–302.

Williams, C.A., Zori, R.T., Hendrickson, J., Stalker, H., Marum, T., Whidden, E., & Driscoll, D.J. (1995). Angelman syndrome. *Current Problems in Pediatrics, 25,* 216–231.

Williams, J.C., Barrett-Boyes, B.G., & Lowe, J.B. (1961). Supravalvular aortic stenosis. *Circulation, 24,* 1311–1318.

Winter, M., Pankau, R., Amm, M., Gosch, A., & Wessel, A. (1996). The spectrum of ocular features in the Williams-Beuren syndrome. *Clinical Genetics, 49,* 28–31.

Wishart, J.G. (1995). Cognitive abilities in children with Down syndrome: Developmental instability and motivational deficits. In C.J. Epstein, T. Hassold, I.T. Lott, L. Nadel, & D. Patterson (Eds.), *Etiology and pathogenesis of Down syndrome* (pp. 57–91). New York: Wiley-Liss.

Wishart, J.G., & Johnston, F.H. (1990). The effects of experience on attribution of a stereotyped personality to children with Down's syndrome. *Journal of Mental Deficiency Research, 34,* 409–420.

Wisniewski, K.E., Wisniewski, H.M., & Wen, G.Y. (1985). Occurrence of Alzheimer's neuropathology and dementia in Down syndrome. *Annals of Neurology, 17,* 278–282.

Wolf-Schein, E.G., Sudhalter, V., Cohen, I., Fisch, G.S., Hanson, D., Pfadt, A.G., Hagerman, R.J., Jenkins, E., & Brown, W.T. (1987). Speech-language and the fragile X syndrome: Initial findings. *Journal of the American Speech-Language-Hearing Association, 29,* 35–38.

Wolff, P.H., Gardner, J., Paccia, J., & Lappen, J. (1989). The greeting behavior of fragile X males. *American Journal on Mental retardation, 93,* 406–411.

Woodcock, R. (1987). *Woodcock Reading Mastery Tests–Revised.* Circle Pines, MN: American Guidance Service.

Wright, H.H., Young, S.R., Edwards, J.G., Abramson, R.K., & Duncan, J. (1986). Fragile X syndrome in a population of autistic children. *Journal of the American Academy of child and Adolescent Psychiatry, 25*, 641–644.

Wright-Talamante, C., Cheema, A., Riddle, J.E., Luckey, D.W., Taylor, A.K., & Hagerman, R.J. (1996). A controlled study of longitudinal IQ changes in females and males with fragile X syndrome. *American Journal of Medical Genetics, 64*, 350–355.

Zebrowitz, L.A. (1997). *Reading faces: Window to the soul?* Boulder, CO: Westview Press

Zebrowitz, L.A., Kendall-Tackett, K.A., & Fafel, J. (1991). The influence of children's facial maturity on parental expectations and punishments. *Journal of Experimental Child Psychology, 52*, 221-238.

Zebrowitz, L.A., & Montepare, J.M. (1992). Impressions of babyfaced males and females across the lifespan. *Developmental Psychology, 28*, 1143–1152.

Zellweger, H. (1977). Down syndrome. In P.J. Vinker & G.W. Bruyn (Eds.), *Handbook of clinical neurology* (Vol. 31, pp. 367–469). Amsterdam: North Holland Publishing Co.

Zigler, E. (1967). Familial mental retardation: A continuing dilemma. *Science, 155*, 292–298.

Zigler, E. (1969). Developmental versus difference theories of retardation and the problem of motivation. *American Journal of Mental Deficiency, 73*, 536–556.

Zigler, E., & Hodapp, R.M. (1986). *Understanding mental retardation.* New York: Cambridge University Press.

Zigman, W.B., Schupf, N., Lubin, R.A., & Silverman, W. (1987). Premature regression of adults with Down syndrome. *American Journal of Mental Deficiency, 92*, 161–168.

Zigman, W.B., Schupf, N., Zigman, A., & Silverman, W. (1993). Aging and Alzheimer Disease in people with mental retardation. *International Review of Research in Mental Retardation, 19*, 41–70.

Zigman, W., Silverman, W., & Wisniewski, H.M. (1996). Aging and Alzheimer's disease in Down syndrome: Clinical and pathological changes. *Mental Retardation and Developmental Disability Research Reviews, 2*, 73–79.

Ziler, H. (1971): Der Mann-Zeichen-Test in Detailstatisticischer Auswertun, Münster: Aschondorffsche Verlagsbuchhandlung.

Zori, R.T., Hendrickson, J., Woolven, S., Whidden, E.M., Gray, B., & Williams, C.A. (1992). Angelman syndrome: A clinical profile. *Journal of Child Neurology, 7*, 270–280.

Resources

SYNDROME-SPECIFIC ORGANIZATIONS

Angelman Syndrome Foundation
Post Office Box 12437
Gainsville, FL 32604
800-432-6435

CHARGE Syndrome Foundation
(for information on
velocardiofacial syndrome)
2004 Parkade Blvd
Columbia, MO 65202-3121
800-442-7604

Cri du Chat Syndrome
5p- Society
7108 Katella #502
Stanton, CA 90680
888-970-0777
http://www.fivepminus.org

National Down Syndrome
Society
666 Broadway, 8th Floor
New York, NY 10012-2317
800-221-4602
http://www.ndss.org

National Down Syndrome
Congress
1605 Chantilly Drive, Suite 250
Atlanta, GA 30324
800-232-6372
http://www.members.carol.net/
ndsc

National Fragile X Foundation
1441 York Street, Suite 303
Denver, CO 80206
800-688-8765
http://www.nfxf.org

Prader-Willi Syndrome
Association (USA)
5700 Midnight Pass Road, Suite 6
Sarasota, FL 34242
800-926-4797
http://www.pwsausa.org

PRISMS: Parents and
Researchers Interested in
Smith-Magenis Syndrome
11875 Fawn Ridge Lane
Reston, VA 22094
703-709-0568
acmsmith@nchgr.nih.gov

Rubinstein-Taybi Parent Group
Post Office Box 146
Smith Center, KS 66967
785-697-2984
http://www.tucson.com/crier.rts
.htm

Velo-Cardio-Facial Syndrome
Parent Support Group
110-45 Queens Blvd
Forest Hills, NY 11375-5501
718-261-8049
http://www.kumc.edu/GEC/prof/
vcfhome.html

Williams Syndrome Association
Post Office Box 297
Clawson, MI 48017-0297
248-541-3630
http://www.williams-
   syndrome.org

OTHER SUPPORT AND INFORMATIONAL ORGANIZATIONS

Alliance of Genetic Support
   Groups
35 Wisconsin Circle, Suite 440
Chevy Chase, MD 20815-7015
200-336-GENE
http://medhlp.netusa.net/www/
   agsg.htm

The Arc of the United States
1010 Wayne Avenue
Suite 650
Silver Spring, MD 20910
301-565-3842
http://www.thearc.org

Exceptional Parent Magazine:
555 Kinderkamack Road
Oradell, NJ 07649
http://www.eparent.com

genetwork: Bridging the Gap
   between Genetic Diagnosis
   and Special Education
Genetic Services at Elwyn
Elwyn, Training and Research
   Institute
111 Elwyn Road
Elwyn, PA 19063

Mothers United for Moral
   Support (MUMS)
150 Custer Court
Green Bay, WI 54301-1243
414-336-5333

National Information Center for
   Children & Youth with
   Disabilities
Post Office Box 1492
Washington, DC 20013
800-695-0285

National Organization for Rare
   Disorders (NORD)
Post Office Box 8923
New Fairfield, CT 06812-8923
800-999-NORD
http://www.NORD-
   rbd.com/~orphan

Sibling Information Network
1775 Ellington Road
South Windsor, CT 06074
203-648-1205

Special Olympics International
1325 G Street, NW, Suite 500
Washington, DC 20005-3104
202-628-3630
www.specialolympics.org

Index

Page numbers followed by *f* indicate figures; those followed by *t* indicate tables.